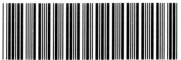

This book is due for return on or before the last date

Radiation Oncology in Palliative Cancer Care

Radiation Oncology in Palliative Cancer Care

Edited by

Stephen Lutz, MD MS

Radiation Oncologist
Department of Radiation Oncology
Blanchard Valley Regional Cancer Center
Findlay, OH, USA

Edward Chow, MBBS MSc PhD FRCPC

Professor, Department of Radiation Oncology
University of Toronto;
Senior Scientist, Sunnybrook Research Institute
Chair, Rapid Response Radiotherapy Program and Bone Metastases Site Group
Sunnybrook Health Sciences Centre
Toronto, ON, Canada

Peter Hoskin, MD FRCP FRCR

Professor in Clinical Oncology, University College London;
Clinical Oncologist
Mount Vernon Hospital
Northwood, London, UK

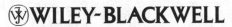

WILEY-BLACKWELL

A John Wiley & Sons, Ltd., Publication

This edition first published 2013 © 2013 by John Wiley & Sons, Ltd.

Registered office: John Wiley & Sons, Ltd., The Atrium, Southern Gate, Chichester, West Sussex, PO19 8SQ, UK

Editorial offices: 9600 Garsington Road, Oxford, OX4 2DQ, UK
The Atrium, Southern Gate, Chichester, West Sussex, PO19 8SQ, UK
350 Main Street, Malden, MA 02148-5020, USA
111 River Street, Hoboken, NJ 07030-5774, USA

For details of our global editorial offices, for customer services and for information about how to apply for permission to reuse the copyright material in this book please see our website at www.wiley.com/wiley-blackwell

Library of Congress Cataloging-in-Publication Data
Radiation oncology in palliative cancer care / edited by Stephen Lutz, Edward Chow, Peter Hoskin.
    p. ; cm.
  Includes bibliographical references and index.
  ISBN 978-1-118-48415-9 (hardback : alk. paper)
  I. Lutz, Stephen. II. Chow, Edward. III. Hoskin, Peter J.
  [DNLM: 1. Neoplasms–radiotherapy. 2. Palliative Care–methods. 3. Radiation Oncology–methods. 4. Radiotherapy–methods. QZ 269]
  616.99'407572–dc23

                              2012044508

ISBN: 9781118484159

A catalogue record for this book is available from the British Library.

Wiley also publishes its books in a variety of electronic formats. Some content that appears in print may not be available in electronic books.

Cover image: (Top) iStockphoto.com Courtesy of Simon Lo
Cover design by Modern Alchemy LLC

Set in 9.5/12pt Palatino by Toppan Best-set Premedia Limited, Hong Kong
Printed and bound in Singapore by Markono Print Media Pte Ltd

1   2013

Contents

Contributor list

Shaun Baggarley, MSc
Chief Radiation Physicist
Department of Radiation Oncology
National University Cancer Institute
National University Health System
Republic of Singapore

Elizabeth A. Barnes, MD FRCP(C)
Assistant Professor
Department of Radiation Oncology
University of Toronto
Odette Cancer Centre
Toronto, ON, Canada

Susannah Batko-Yovino, MD
Assistant Professor
Department of Radiation Oncology, and Program
of Palliative Medicine
John Hopkins University
Baltimore, MD, USA

Lawrence B. Berk, MD PhD
Chair, Radiation Oncology
Director, Radiation Oncology at Tampa General
Hospital
University of South Florida
Tampa, FL, USA

Sean Bydder, BHB MBChB MBA
FRANZCR
Consultant Radiation Oncologist
Department of Radiation Oncology
Sir Charles Gairdner Hospital;
Professor
School of Surgery
The University of Western Australia
Perth, Australia

Eric L. Chang, MD
Professor and Chair
Department of Radiation Oncology
Keck School of Medicine at
University of Southern California
Los Angeles, CA, USA

Samuel T. Chao, MD
Assistant Professor
Cleveland Clinic Lerner College of Medicine
Cleveland, OH, USA

Haris Charalambous, BM MRCP
FRCR
Consultant in Clinical Oncology
Department of Radiation Oncology
Bank of Cyprus Oncology Centre
Nicosia, Cyprus

Caroline Chung, MD MSc FRCPC CIP
Radiation Oncologist and Clinician-Scientist
University Health Network-Princess Margaret
Assistant Professor
Department of Radiation Oncology
University of Toronto
Toronto, ON, Canada

June Corry, FRANZCR FRACP MD
Consultant Radiation Oncologist
Chair Head and Neck Service
Peter MacCallum Cancer Centre
Melbourne, Victoria, Australia

Henry Ddungu, MD
UCI Hutchinson Center Cancer Alliance
Upper Mulago Hill Road
P O Box 3935 Kampala
Kampala, Uganda

Gillian M. Duchesne, MB MD FRCR
FRANZCR Gr Ct Health Econ
Professor of Radiation Oncology
Peter MacCallum Cancer Centre
University of Melbourne and Monash University
Melbourne, Victoria, Australia

Alysa Fairchild, BSc MD FRCPC
Associate Professor
Department of Radiation Oncology
Cross Cancer Institute
University of Alberta
Edmonton, AB, Canada

Frank D. Ferris, MD FAAHPM
Executive Director
Palliative Medicine Research and Education
OhioHealth
Columbus, OH, USA

Robert Glynne-Jones, MB BS FRCP FRCR
Macmillan Lead Clinician in Gastrointestinal Cancer
Mount Vernon Cancer Centre
Northwood, London, UK

Charles F. von Gunten, MD PhD FAAHPM
Vice President
Medical Affairs
Hospice and Palliative Medicine
OhioHealth
Columbus, OH, USA

Mark Harrison, MB.BC PhD
Consultant Oncologist
Mount Vernon Cancer Centre
Northwood, London, UK

James A. Hayman, MD MBA
Professor
Department of Radiation Oncology
University of Michigan
Ann Arbor, MI, USA

David D. Howell, MD FACR FAAHPM
Assistant Professor
Department of Radiation Oncology
University of Toledo College of Medicine
Toledo, OH, USA

Candice A. Johnstone, MD MPH
Assistant Professor
Medical Director of the Froedtert and Medical College of Wisconsin Cancer Network
Department of Radiation Oncology
Medical College of Wisconsin
Milwaukee, WI, USA

Joshua Jones, MD MA
Fellow
Palliative Care Service
Massachusetts General Hospital
Boston, MA, USA

Andre Konski, MD MBA MA FACR
Professor and Chair
Department of Radiation Oncology
Wayne State University School of Medicine
Barbara Ann Karmanos Cancer Center
Detroit, MI, USA

Ian H. Kunkler, MA MB BCHIR FRCPE CRCR
Honorary Professor of Clinical Oncology
University of Edinburgh
Edinburgh Cancer Centre
Edinburgh, Scotland, UK

Yvette van der Linden, MD PhD
Radiation oncologist
Department of Clinical Oncology
University Medical Centre
Leiden, The Netherlands

Simon S. Lo, MD
Director
Radiosurgery Services and Neurologic Radiation Oncology;
Associate Professor
University Hospitals Seidman Cancer Center
Case Comprehensive Cancer Center
Case Western Reserve University
Cleveland, OH, USA

Jiade J. Lu, MD MBA
Head and Associate Professor
Department of Radiation Oncology
National University Cancer Institute
National University Health System
Republic of Singapore

Ernesto Maranzano, MD
Director
Radiation Oncology Centre
Santa Maria Hospital
Terni, Italy

Nina A. Mayr, MD
Professor
Radiation Oncology
Arthur G. James Cancer Hospital
The Ohio State University
Columbus, OH, USA

Erin McMenamin, MSN CRNP AOCN ACHPN
Oncology Nurse Practitioner
Department of Radiation Oncology
Hospital of the University of Pennsylvania
Philadelphia, PA, USA

Marcia Meldrum, PhD
Associate Researcher
Center for Health Services and Society
Semel Institute for Neuroscience and Human Behavior
University of California, Los Angeles
Los Angeles, CA, USA

Benjamin Movsas, MD
Chairman
Department of Radiation Oncology
Henry Ford Health System
Detroit, MI, USA

Arno J. Mundt, MD
Professor and Chair
Center for Advanced Radiotherapy Technologies
(CART)
Department of Radiation Medicine and Applied
Sciences
University of California, San Diego
San Diego, CA, USA

Firuza Patel, MD
Professor
Department of Radiotherapy and Oncology
Post Graduate Institute of Medical Education and
Research
Chandigarh, India

Rinaa S. Punglia, MD MPH
Assistant Professor
Department of Radiation Oncology
Dana-Farber Cancer Institute and the Brigham
and Women's Hospital
Harvard Medical School
Boston, MA, USA

Dirk Rades, MD PhD
Professor
Head of Department
Department of Radiotherapy
University Hospital Lübeck
Lübeck, Germany

George Rodrigues, MD MSc FRCPC
Clinician Scientist and Radiation Oncologist
Departments of Radiation Oncology and
Epidemiology/Biostatistics
London Health Sciences Centre and University of
Western Ontario
London, ON, Canada

Daniel E. Roos, BSc(Hons) DipEd
MBBS MD FRANZCR
Senior Radiation Oncologist
Department of Radiation Oncology
Royal Adelaide Hospital;
Professor
University of Adelaide School of Medicine
Adelaide, South Australia, Australia

Arjun Sahgal, MD
Associate Professor
Radiation Oncology
Princess Margaret Hospital and the Sunnybrook
Health Sciences Center
University of Toronto,
Toronto, ON, Canada

Thomas Smith, MD FACP
Harry J. Duffey Family Professor of Palliative
Medicine;
Professor of Oncology
Department of Oncology and Program of
Palliative Medicine
John Hopkins University
Baltimore, MD, USA

Bin S. Teh, MD
Professor, Vice Chair and Senior Member
The Methodist Hospital, Cancer Center and
Research Institute
Weill Cornell Medical College
Houston, TX, USA

Albert Tiong, MB BS M.App.Epi.
FRANZCR
Consultant Radiation Oncologist
Peter MacCallum Cancer Centre
Melbourne, Victoria, Australia

Fabio Trippa, MD
Vice Chair
Radiation Oncology Centre
Santa Maria Hospital
Terni, Italy

May Tsao, MD FRCPC
Assistant Professor
Department of Radiation Oncology, University of
Toronto;
Sunnybrook Odette Cancer Centre
Toronto, ON, Canada

Vassilios Vassiliou, MD PhD
Consultant in Radiation Oncology
Department of Radiation Oncology
Bank of Cyprus Oncology Centre
Nicosia, Cyprus

Tamara Vern-Gross, DO FAAP
Department of Radiation Oncology
Wake Forest Baptist Health
Comprehensive Cancer Center
Winston-Salem, NC, USA

Anushree M. Vichare, MBBS MPH
Measures Development Manager
American Society for Radiation Oncology
Fairfax, VA, USA

Deborah Watkins Bruner, RN PhD
FAAN
Robert W. Woodruff Professor of Nursing
Nell Hodgson Woodruff School of Nursing
Professor of Radiation Oncology
Associate Director for Outcomes Research
Winship Cancer Institute
Emory University
Atlanta, GA, USA

Michelle Winslow, BA PhD
Research Fellow
Academic Unit of Supportive Care
University of Sheffield
Sheffield, South Yorkshire, UK

Aaron H. Wolfson, MD
Professor and Vice Chair
Department of Radiation Oncology
University of Miami Miller School of Medicine
Miami, FL, USA

Foreword

"The final causes, then, of compassion are to prevent and to relieve misery."
Joseph Butler [1692–1752]

This textbook, *Radiation Oncology in Palliative Cancer Care*, represents the full evolution of radiation therapy, and of oncology in general. This evolution in radiation oncology is in response to the changing priorities of cancer care.

More than a century ago, radiotherapy was the only treatment available for cancer, palliating the suffering from large masses and open wounds from the disease. The priority was to relieve the suffering from the disease, as the cure of cancer was rare. As medical science evolved, especially in anesthesia and surgery, the principles of cancer resection were developed. Cure of cancer became the priority, often at the accepted price of disfigurement. In the latter half of the 20th century, the development of chemotherapeutic agents dominated. Cure of cancer remained the priority, but now at the price of toxicity. Acute toxicity often limited the patient's ability to receive chemotherapy on schedule or complete the prescribed number of courses of chemotherapy. Late chemotherapeutic toxicity risked significant end-organ damage. Despite the "War on Cancer," the sacrifice of cure at any human cost was beginning to be questioned.

Quality of life, during and after cancer therapy, became a priority commensurate with cancer cure. Although often not fully recognized as such, palliative care principles were applied to improve the cancer patient's quality of life. In its broadest definition, palliative care relieves the symptoms of cancer and its treatment at any stage of disease, and maintains or restores the dignity of function. For every patient, spanning all age groups from young children to elderly adults, the palliative principles of comfort in positioning, reassurance, and beneficence, and the avoidance of treatment-related symptoms are paramount.

These principles of palliative care invoked the priority of delivering effective cancer treatment with the fewest side effects. Most notably, acute chemotherapy toxicity was significantly reduced with the development of more effective anti-emetic agents. The development of sophisticated linear accelerators, including electron beam and intensity modulated radiation, allowed improved outcomes due to the targeted delivery of higher radiation doses with fewer side effects. Previously unthinkable, advancements in radiation therapy technology also allowed multi-modality therapy, the combination of chemotherapy and radiation with function-sparing surgery for virtually every anatomic region. This exciting period both expanded the potential for cancer cure and improved the cancer patient's quality of life because side effects of cancer therapy were more effectively controlled.

While most of the focus in cancer treatment over the latter half of the 20th century was, very understandably, on these multi-modality developments, a smaller, but concerted, effort was formally launched for patients with incurable disease. Hospice care was exported from the groundbreaking work of Dame Cicely Saunders in Great Britain. Meanwhile, the contributing role and significant impact of radiotherapy in palliative care was often relegated to "service work" within academic centers. Palliative radiotherapy was neither the topic of scientific research, nor acknowledged as a valuable sub-specialty within the field.

Palliative radiotherapy finally began to be recognized as an integral aspect of radiation oncology through the convergence of multiple factors. First and foremost were advocacy efforts to improve cancer patients' quality of life. The expanding role of medical ethics within health-care systems also reinforced the responsibility to relieve suffering. Meanwhile, clinical research documented improved rates of survival among incurable cancer patients with effective symptom control.

The second factor was the continued development of systemic agents used for palliation. Expanding beyond supportive care that reduced the side effects of cancer treatment, drug development then prioritized the treatment of metastatic disease. This was exemplified most prominently by the clinical trials of bisphosphonates for bone metastases. Radiation oncology recognized the scope of palliative care within its practices as the number of patients who received bisphosphonates, instead of palliative radiation, increased. It was then determined that palliative care, even at tertiary care cancer centers, accounted for more than one-third of the requests for radiotherapeutic consultation, and represented an untapped research potential.

The third factor involved both the economics of health care, and the limited health-care resources faced in all nations. In the United States, last-year-of-life expenditures constituted 26% of the entire Medicare budget [1]. Many governments have dealt with spiraling health-care costs by developing guidelines for care that incorporate comparative effectiveness research. The potential impact and main priority for comparative effectiveness research is based on prevalence, disease burden, variability in outcomes, and costs of care. The most efficient means of delivering effective cancer treatment is an economic priority for all nations. Additionally, access to care with limited health-care resources is especially prevalent in middle and low-income nations. These economic and resource issues in health care prompted international clinical trials that evaluated the most efficient radiotherapeutic fractionation for the treatment of bone metastases. Clinical trials that address economics as well as outcomes, like that of the international palliative bone metastases trial, will not only influence palliative treatment approaches, but every aspect of cancer therapy in the future.

This textbook is an acknowledgment that palliative radiotherapy is now a sub-specialty of radiation oncology. This formally makes palliative radio-therapy a priority within patient care, academic research, quality assurance, and medical education. However, the principles of palliation were the first precepts of cancer treatment, and were first applied by radiation oncologists. The priorities of the past have now evolved to the priorities of the future.

Nora Janjan, MD MPSA MBA
National Center for Policy Analysis, Dallas, TX, USA

Reference

1. Hoover DR, Crystal S, Kumar R, *et al*. Medical expenditures during the last year of life: findings from the 1992-1996 Medicare current beneficiary survey. *Health Serv Res* 2002; **37**: 1625–1642.

PART 1

General principles of radiation oncology

CHAPTER 1

A brief history of palliative radiation oncology

Joshua Jones
Palliative Care Service, Massachusetts General Hospital, Boston, MA, USA

Introduction

A simple chronology of scientific and technologic developments belies the complexity of the history of palliative radiotherapy. The diversity of palliative radiation treatments utilized today reflects a dichotomy evident in the earliest days of therapeutic radiation, namely that radiation can be utilized to extend survival or to address anticipated or current symptoms. However, the line between "curative" and "palliative" treatments is not always obvious. Furthermore, even "palliative" radiotherapy has an impact on local tumor control, potentially improving survival and complicating the balance between effective and durable palliation with possible short- or long-term side effects of therapy. This introduction provides a basic overview of developments in the history of radiation therapy that continue to inform the complex thinking on how best to palliate symptoms of advanced cancer with radiation therapy.

The early years

Within a few short months of Wilhelm Roentgen's publication of his monumental discovery in January 1896, several early pioneers around the world began treating patients with the newly discovered X-rays [1]. Early reports detailed treatments of various conditions of the hair, skin (lupus and "rodent ulcers") and "epitheliomata," primarily cancers of the skin, breast, and head and neck [2] (Figure 1.1). Other early reports, as championed by Emile Grubbe in a 1902 review, touted both the cure of malignancy as well as "remarkable results" in "incurable cases" including relief of pain, cessation of hemorrhage or discharge and prolongation of life without suffering [3]. Optimism was high that X-rays would soon be able to transform many of the "incurable cases" to curable.

Radiation Oncology in Palliative Cancer Care, First Edition. Edited by Stephen Lutz, Edward Chow, and Peter Hoskin.
© 2013 John Wiley & Sons, Ltd. Published 2013 by John Wiley & Sons, Ltd.

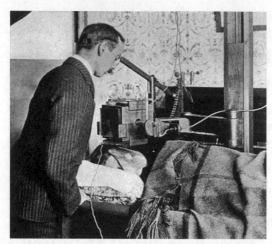

Figure 1.1 An early radiotherapy machine delivering low energy X-rays with shielding of the face by a thin layer of lead. Reproduced from Williams [4].

In his 1902 textbook, Francis Williams, one of the early pioneers from Boston, described his optimism that radiation therapy would eliminate growths on the skin: "The best way of avoiding the larger forms of external growths is by prevention; that is, by submitting all early new growths, whether they seem of a dangerous nature or not, to the X-rays. No harm can follow their use in proper hands and much good will result from this course [4]." He went on to state that, while "internal new growths" could not yet be treated with X-ray therapy, he was optimistic that such treatments would be possible in the future. In this setting, he put forward an early treatment algorithm for cancer that divided tumors into those treatable with X-ray therapy, those treatable with surgery and X-ray therapy post-operatively, and those amenable to palliation with X-ray therapy. He further described that the specific treatment varied from patient to patient but could be standardized between patients based on exposure time and skin erythema.

Other early radiology textbooks took a more measured approach to X-ray therapy. Leopold Freund's 1904 textbook described in great detail the physics of X-rays and again summarized the early clinical outcomes. In his description of X-ray therapy, he highlighted the risks of side effects, including ulceration, with prolonged exposures to X-rays without sufficient breaks. He noted that the mechanism of action of radiation was still not understood, with theories at the time focusing on the electrical effects of radiation, the production of ozone, or perhaps direct effects of the X-rays themselves. Freund highlighted early attempts at measuring the dose of radiation delivered, emphasizing the necessity of future standardization of dosing and research into the physiologic effects of X-ray therapy [2]. As foreshadowed in the textbooks of Williams and Freund, early research in radiation therapy focused on clinical descriptions of the effectiveness of X-rays contrasted with side effects of X-rays, the determination of what disease could be effectively treated with radiotherapy, the standardization of equipment and measurement of dose, and attempts to understand the physiologic effects of X-ray therapy.

The history of radium therapy in many ways parallels developments in the history of Roentgen ray therapy. After the discovery of radium by the Curies in 1898, the effects of radium on the skin were described by Walkoff and Giesel in early 1901. This description was offered prior to the famed "Becquerel burn" in which Henri Becquerel noticed a skin burn after leaving a piece of radium in a pocket of his waistcoat [5]. Radium quickly found many formulations of use: as a poultice on the skin, as an "emanation" that could be inhaled, consumed in water, or absorbed via a bath, or in needles that could be implanted deep into the body [6]. The reports of the effectiveness of radium therapy appeared more slowly than those of X-ray therapy, however, owing to its cost and rarity.

The future of radium mining in the United States for use in medical treatments was pushed forward by the incorporation of the National Radium Institute in 1913, a joint venture by a Johns Hopkins physician, Howard Kelly, a philanthropist and mine executive, James Douglas, and the US Bureau of Mines. However, the notion of protecting lands for radium mining was vigorously debated in Congress in 1914 and 1915. The debate focused on therapeutic uses of radium, risks to radium workers, and the nuances of the economics, given that radium had previously been exported for processing and re-imported at much higher cost. The debate over the use of radium treatments escaped from the medical literature into the public consciousness [7]. Kelly championed the curative effects of radium therapy, but there was significant opposition to the use of radium in medicine due to a reported lack of efficacy. In 1915, Senator John Works from California made a speech before the United States Senate urging no further use of radium in the treatment of cancer:

> The claim that radium is a cure for cancer has been effectually exploded by actual experience and declared by numerous competent authorities on the subject to be ineffectual for that purpose . . . If radium is not a specific [cure] for cancer, the passage of the radium bill would be an act of inhuman cruelty. It would be taken as an indorsement [sic] by the Government of that remedy and would bring additional suffering, disappointment, and sorrow to sufferers from the disease, their relatives and friends, and bring no compensating results [8].

In spite of these concerns and the growth and subsequent decline of popular radium treatments including radium spas and radium baths in the 1920s and 1930s, radium therapy continued to grow and develop an evidence base for both the curative treatment of cancer and the relief of symptoms from advanced cancer.

With publicity surrounding the development of cancer and later death among radium dial workers (the first death coming in 1921), radium therapy was again under attack in the early 1920s. In 1922, in an address to the Medical Society of New York, Kelly sought to "emphasize the *palliative results*." As reported in the Medical Record, Kelly believed "If he could do nothing more than improve and relieve his patients, as he had been able to do, never curing one, it would still be worth his while to continue this work [9]." Palliative radiotherapy, with the explicit goal of palliation and not cure, had been recognized as a legitimate area of study.

Fractionation

A challenge that has persisted through the history of the treatment of cancer is how best to improve the therapeutic ratio: specifically, how best to target cancer cells while minimizing damage to surrounding normal tissue. In the earliest years of radiation therapy, minimizing toxicity to the skin was a significant challenge as the kilovoltage X-rays delivered maximum dose to the skin, creating brisk erythema, desquamation, and even ulceration (Figure 1.2). In the 1920s, Regaud conducted a series of experiments demonstrating that dividing a total dose of radiation into smaller fractions could obtain the same target effect (sterilization of a ram) while minimizing skin damage [10]. These observations were later applied by Coutard in the radiotherapy clinic to the treatment of cancer, both superficial and deep tumors. By the mid-1930s, the

Treatment plans and isodose curves: 1919–1925 and 1980

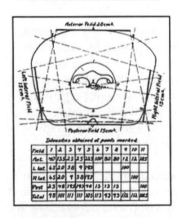

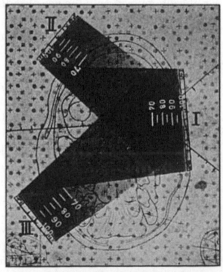

Figure 1.2 Isodose curves from 1919 and 1925. Reproduced from Mould [32], with permission from Taylor and Francis Publishing.

concept of fractionating radiotherapy to give three to five doses per week over a period of 5 to 6 weeks had become a standard method for the protection of normal tissues [11].

After Coutard's publication, studies demonstrating the efficacy of fractionated radiotherapy also suggested palliation from radiotherapy could be achieved with lower delivered doses. One specific article, published by Lenz and Freid in *Annals of Surgery* in 1931, highlighted challenges with fractionation and set forth suggestions for palliation of symptomatic metastases from breast cancer. The study explored the natural history of breast cancer metastases to the brain, spine, and bones and the effect of radiotherapy in the treatment of these metastases [12]. The study retrospectively analyzed two time periods in the course of illness: the pre-terminal period (up to one year prior to death or two-thirds of the time of illness if the patient lived less than one year) and the terminal period (the final one-third of time of illness if the patient lived less than one year). Lenz correlated the impact of grade of cancer as visualized under the microscope with the length of time of survival, finding that higher grade tumors led to shorter survival and a shorter terminal period. He also described the increased recognition of bone metastases with the use of diagnostic X-rays and indicated that diagnosis of metastases to the brain or spinal cord was still difficult to evaluate.

It was unclear to practitioners at that time if neurologic symptoms were from bone metastases causing mass effect on the central nervous system or if the metastases resided within the nervous system itself. The author subsequently evaluated the effect of radiotherapy on relief of symptoms in both the terminal and pre-terminal patients. Ten of 19 patients in the terminal stage had improvement of symptoms (primarily pain) with radiotherapy and 12 of 12 in the pre-terminal stage had improvement of symptoms, lasting a few weeks to 3 years. The dose of radiotherapy, however, did not correlate with symptomatic relief, and relief was often obtained within 24 to 48 hours after starting treatment. As Lenz described it, a treatment "series" consisted of the total amount of radiation delivered over about two months. Dose was measured according to skin erythema: less than one erythema dose was a "small" dose, one to two erythema doses was a "moderate" dose, and more than two erythema doses was a "large" dose. Treatment was certainly fractionated over the course of two months, but Lenz's work provided an early suggestion that moderate doses of radiotherapy could produce effective palliation of metastatic disease.

Advances in radiotherapy technique: the 1950s and 1960s

While the field of radiotherapy experienced many advances in technology such as increases in the understanding of dose distribution and in the biologic effects of radiation through the 1930s and 1940s, the next significant clinical breakthrough in radiotherapy came in the 1950s. The first supervoltage machines capable of producing X-rays greater than 1 MeV were put into

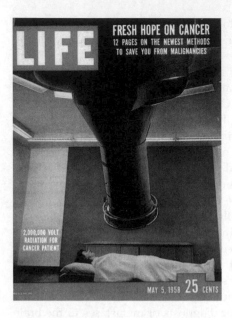

Figure 1.3 Supervoltage radiotherapy machine at Hospital for Joint Disease in NY, aiming at patient with bladder cancer. Reproduced from [13], with permission from Time & Life Pictures/Getty Images.

clinical use in the early 1950s with cobalt teletherapy machines, betatrons, van de Graaf generators, and linear accelerators (Figure 1.3). These "supervoltage" machines allowed deeper penetration of the radiation beam, sparing the skin and allowing easier treatment of internal tumors. The excitement at the prospect of a cure was exemplified by the May 1958 cover of *Life* magazine which featured a new supervoltage X-ray machine. The article inside highlighted surgery and radiation as the only two possible cures for cancer and boasted "These standard approaches have now been perfected almost to their limit [13]." While expectations for curative radiotherapy had certainly increased, palliative outcomes were also being explored with the new technology.

A review of palliative radiotherapy for lung and breast cancer in the *British Medical Journal* in 1957 reported that radiotherapy was most commonly employed in palliation of symptoms of advanced cancer, but that "the question has been asked whether patients later suffer more while dying if they have had such treatment than if they had not." [14] According to the review, the indications for palliative treatment of lung cancer symptoms, including vena cava obstruction, hemoptysis, dyspnea and cough, required a standard dose of 3000 rad as sufficient for palliation (though the fractionation was not described). The effect on life span is "difficult to assess" but prolongation is not the goal of therapy. In answering their posed question about the effectiveness of therapy, the authors responded that when radiotherapy caused more symptoms than it helped, "this suggests a failure of judgment by the radiotherapist." The review also indicated that complication rates from palliation of breast cancer bone metastases, including fibrosis of muscle and necrosis of

TABLE 3
OVER-ALL RESULTS OF RADIATION THERAPY
FOR BRAIN METASTASES

Prim. tum.	Tot. pt.	No. avail. evaluat.			No. pt. lost fol.-up	No. pt. incomplete treat.
		Treat.	Respond.	Fail.		
Breast	85	64	55	9	5	16
Lung	74	54	45	9	1	19
Lymphoma	11	6	5	1	2	3
Melanoma	10	5	2	3	3	2
Bone & soft tis. sarcoma	10	10	7	3	0	0
Other	28	19	9	10	1	8
TOTAL	218	158	123	35	12	48

Figure 1.4 Early results of palliative whole brain radiotherapy. Reproduced from [16], with permission from Wiley.

bone, were diminishing. Balancing benefit with harm from palliative radiotherapy was now the task of the radiotherapist.

Early reports of the palliative treatment of brain metastases, confirmed with lumbar puncture, encephalogram, and angiography, revealed symptomatic relief in many patients, even though the earliest report (1954) still used orthovoltage X-rays (Figure 1.4) [15]. In 1961, Chu provided an update on the first study to evaluate whole brain radiotherapy. Patients presented with headache, dizziness, nausea, vomiting, incontinence, visual changes, and changes in mentation; many suffered from hemiparesis or hemiplegia at the start of radiotherapy. The report detailed treatment of 218 patients with opposed orthovoltage X-ray fields to a median dose of 3000 rad over 3 weeks, starting with low daily doses and increasing to higher daily doses to avoid acute side effects of treatment. Therapy was well-tolerated with improvement in symptoms in 77.8% (123 of 158) of evaluable patients who received the prescribed dose [16].

One final episode from the early years of supervoltage therapy deserves mention. In preparation for experiments to understand the role of oxygenation on high dose irradiation, the radiotherapy group at Columbia treated 63 patients with advanced metastatic cancer with once weekly radiation treatments using a 22.5 MeV betatron with doses ranging from 800 rad to 1250 rad to total doses of 1250 to 4000 rad over 4 weeks [17]. Degree of response was complicated by short survival and many symptoms, but the authors described subjective responses in 37 of 63 patients and objective responses in 29 of 63 patients. Treatment was generally well-tolerated with mild nausea being the most common. Serious complications included edema in head and neck cancer in patients who had previously had radical surgery; radiation fibrosis of the lung in two patients previously irradiated to the lung; myelitis in one patient; and esophageal perforation in one patient who received 4000 rad in

4 weeks and who exhibited no evidence of cancer at autopsy. The authors concluded that massive dose irradiation in one week interval doses is both feasible and justified in order to provide rapid relief with minimal inconvenience to the patient. The risk of severe radiation injury, the authors reported, limits total dose (they suggested 3000 rad as the maximum permissible dose) and selection of patients who might be candidates for high dose palliative radiotherapy.

In 1964, Robert Parker, of the University of Washington, published a clinical management guideline in *JAMA* describing the role of palliative radiotherapy in the management of patients with advanced cancer. He described the importance of determining whether radiation is palliative up front:

> When the initial objective of radiation therapy is palliation, new ground rules must be applied. Possible serious complications or even slowly self-limiting side effects are no longer acceptable. Overall treatment time must be short. Cost must be minimized. Convenience of treatment must be considered [18].

While the "ground rules" for palliative radiotherapy could be accepted by most, the line between purely palliative and definitively curative has continued to be an evolving target.

Fractionation revisited: explicit palliation

In 1969, the newly formed Radiation Therapy Oncology Group organized its first clinical trials in the use of radiotherapy in the treatment of cancer. The combined publication of two early studies (RTOG 6901 and RTOG 7361) evaluated patients with brain metastases treated with either short (one or two fractions) or long (1 to 4 weeks) courses of radiotherapy [19]. The studies demonstrated similar outcomes among the short- and long-course treatment arms with comparable rates of improvement in neurologic function, treatment morbidities, and overall survival rates, but with decreased durability of palliation in the short course arms. The authors recommended more fractionated courses with higher radiation doses for palliation of patients with brain metastases due to the durability of palliation. Subsequent trials on brain metastases sought to improve the therapeutic ratio through the addition of radiation sensitizers.

Several studies by the RTOG and other groups similarly evaluated different dose-fractionation schemes for painful bone metastases. Early studies including RTOG 7402 evaluated various dose/fractionation schemes ranging from five to fifteen fractions for solitary or multiple bony metastases. Overall improvement in pain and complete pain relief were not statistically different between regimens [20]. Further studies have evaluated single- versus multi-fraction regimens with the overall response rates being similar with a single fraction of 8 Gy (800 rad) in comparison with more protracted dose-fractionation schedules with slightly higher retreatment rates in the single treatment groups, but without significant increase in late toxicity [21,22].

Stereotactic radiotherapy

Beginning in the 1950s, Leksell and his neurosurgical team developed a "stereotactic" approach to the treatment of deep brain lesions including arteriovenous malformations, craniopharyngiomas and acoustic neuromas [23]. Simultaneously, advances in anatomic and functional imaging from the 1970s to the present day have contributed to earlier detection of metastatic disease with computed tomography (CT), magnetic resonance imaging (MRI), and positron emission tomography (PET). When the advanced imaging was combined with computer treatment planning and the stereotactic approach of Leksell, high doses of radiation could be delivered in a conformal manner to small areas in the brain with either multiple cobalt sources (i.e. Gammaknife) or a linear accelerator. Early experience with stereotactic treatment of brain metastases that had previously been irradiated revealed minimal toxicity with significant improvement in neurologic symptoms and ability to have patients discontinue corticosteroids [24].

These stereotactic techniques were applied in the RTOG 9005 dose escalation study of stereotactic radiosurgery for the treatment of previously irradiated brain metastases or primary brain tumors [25]. Subsequently, the RTOG 9508 study combining whole brain radiotherapy with or without stereotactic radiotherapy boost demonstrated that combined stereotactic radiosurgery and whole brain radiotherapy led to an improvement in performance status at 6 months and a survival advantage for patients with a single brain metastasis [26]. Such studies that demonstrate improvement in length of life have complicated the previously purely palliative nature of radiation for brain metastases. The safety, efficacy, and possible enhancement of survival with stereotactic radiotherapy to the brain have led to questions seen earlier in history: when is highly conformal radiotherapy appropriate in the treatment of brain metastases? When is surgical resection appropriate in the treatment of brain metastases? When is whole brain radiotherapy appropriate in the treatment of brain metastases? And when is palliative care, without radiotherapy or surgical intervention, appropriate in the management of brain metastases?

Prognostication and tailoring palliative radiotherapy to anticipated survival

In an attempt to further characterize the results of the early trials of stereotactic radiosurgery for brain metastases, the RTOG conducted a recursive partitioning analysis (RPA) to evaluate factors predictive of survival in patients with brain metastases [27]. The RPA analyzed patients from three RTOG studies of different dose fractionation schemes with and without sensitizers. The RPA revealed three categories of patients from 1200 eligible patients, divided into classes based on Karnofsky performance status, age, and presence or absence of extracranial metastases (see Chapter 22 for full study details). This RPA was validated [28], and new models for survival prediction (namely the diagnosis-specific Graded Prognostic Assessment or GPA) have been developed to further refine estimates of prognosis. The RPA, GPA, and other models of prognosis (for other sites of metastatic disease) may assist in developing treatment algorithms, but challenges remain in tailoring treatment to survival estimate.

As an example of the challenge with tailoring treatment to survival, Gripp and colleagues analyzed a group of 216 patients with advanced cancer admitted to the hospital for palliative radiotherapy. All patients had survival estimates completed by physicians and data were collected to help inform prognosis. Thirty-three patients died within 30 days of hospital admission and were analyzed in a pre-planned subgroup analysis to determine adequacy of treatment [29]. Physician survival estimates (characterized as less than one month, 1 to 6 months, or more than 6 months) were more likely to be greater than 6 months (21%) than less than 1 month (16%), although all patients died within 30 days of admission. Half of the patients were on treatment more than 60% of their remaining lives. In this setting, Gripp retrospectively asks the question: can we tailor treatment to anticipated survival? In an accompanying editorial, Hartsell responds by applauding the conclusion (that patients are often over-treated toward the end of life), but reaffirms previously described principles of palliative radiotherapy, namely that the treatment should be delivered in the shortest time possible with the fewest side effects possible. Incorporating the goals of providing evidence-based, convenient, palliative radiotherapy with the fewest possible side effects while being aware of long-term side effects in possible long-term survivors is a challenge; determining the role of stereotactic radiotherapy in this mix is one of the pressing tasks within the palliative radiotherapy community.

Conclusion

The prevalence of abstracts presented at the American Society for Radiation Oncology (ASTRO) Annual Meetings from 1993 to 2000 that focused on symptom control and palliative care remained steady and low, ranging from 0.9% to 2.2% of all abstracts presented during those years. In 2004, ASTRO made "palliative care" a discrete topic for submission of abstracts [30]. While the total number of abstracts on symptom control and palliative care has increased from 2001 to 2010, the majority of the increase is related to the use of stereotactic radiotherapy in the treatment of metastatic disease. Even with this increase, the proportion of abstracts related to symptom control and palliative care remains low at about 5% of all abstracts [31]. Upwards of 40% of all radiotherapy treatments have palliative intent; with the increasing complexity of palliative radiotherapy treatment options and treatments, it is incumbent upon the fields of palliative care and radiotherapy to continue to work to implement best practices in the treatment of patients with palliative radiotherapy.

References

1. Leszczynski K, Boyko S. On the controversies surrounding the origins of radiation therapy. Radiotherapy and oncology? *J Eur Soc Ther Radiol Oncol* [Internet] 1997; **42**: 213–217. Available at: http://www.ncbi.nlm.nih.gov/pubmed/9155069 (accessed November 16, 2012).
2. Freund L. *Elements of general radio-therapy for practitioners.* [Internet] New York: Rebman, 1904; Available at: http://books.google.com/books?id=goCGUdSHOPwC (accessed November 16, 2012).
3. Grubbe E. X-rays in the treatment of cancer and other malignant diseases. *Med Rec* [Internet] 1902; **62**: 692–695. Available at: http://onlinelibrary.wiley.com/doi/10.1002/cbdv.200490137/abstract (accessed March 31, 2012).
4. Williams FH. The Roentgen rays in medicine and surgery [Internet]. Macmillan; 1902. Available at: http://books.google.com/books?id=lSKI4azQxkoC (accessed November 16, 2012).
5. Mould R. The discovery of radium in 1898 by Maria Sklodowska-Curie (1867-1934) and Pierre Curie (1859-1906) with commentary on their life and times. *Br J Radiol* [Internet] 1998; **71**: 1229–1254. Available at: http://bjr.birjournals.org/content/71/852/1229.short (accessed April 1, 2012).
6. Simpson F. *Radium Therapy*. St. Louis: CV Moseby Company, 1922.
7. Viol C. The radium situation in America. *Radium* [Internet] 1915; **4**: 105–112. Available at: http://www.archive.org/details/n06radium04came (accessed November 16, 2012).
8. Works JD. The Public Health Service: Speech in the Senate of the United States. 1915.
9. Wightman O. Is radium worthwhile? *Med Rec* 1922; **101**: 516–522.
10. Hall EJ, Giaccia AJ. *Radiobiology for the Radiologist*, 6th edn. Philadelphia: Lippincott Williams and Wilkins, 2006.
11. Coutard H. The results and methods of treatment of cancer by radiation. *Ann Surg* [Internet] 1937; **106**: 584–598. Available at: http://www.ncbi.nlm.nih.gov/pmc/articles/PMC1390613/ (accessed March 31, 2012).
12. Lenz M, Freid J. Metastases to the skeleton, brain and spinal cord from cancer of the breast and the effect of radiotherapy. *Ann Surg* [Internet] 1931; **93**: 278–293. Available at: http://www.ncbi.nlm.nih.gov/pubmed/17866472 (accessed November 16, 2012).
13. Cancer – On Brink of Breakthroughs. Life. 1958; 102–113.
14. Palliative radiotherapy. *BMJ* 1957; **2**: 455–456.
15. Chao JH, Phillips R, Nickson JJ Roentgen-ray therapy of cerebral metastases. *Cancer* 1954; **7**: 682–689.
16. Chu FCH, Hilaris B, Chu FC, et al. Value of radiation therapy in the management of intracranial metastases. *Cancer* [Internet] 1961; **14**: 577–581. Available at: http://www.ncbi.nlm.nih.gov/pubmed/13693470 (accessed March 31, 2012).
17. Horrigan WD, Alto P, Brunswick N. Massive-dose rapid palliative radiotherapy. 1961; 439–444.
18. Parker RG. Palliative radiation therapy. *JAMA* 1964; **190**: 1000–1002.

19. Borgelt B, Gelber R, Larson M, *et al*. Ultra-rapid high dose irradiation schedules for the palliation of brain metastases: final results of the first two studies by the Radiation Therapy Oncology Group. *Int J Radiat Oncol Biol Phys* [Internet] 1981; 7: 1633–1638. Available at: http://www.ncbi.nlm.nih.gov/pubmed/6174490 (accessed November 16, 2012).

20. Tong D, Gillick L, Hendrickson FR. The palliation of symptomatic osseous metastases: final results of the Study by the Radiation Therapy Oncology Group. *Cancer* [Internet] 1982; 50:893–899. Available at: http://www.ncbi.nlm.nih.gov/pubmed/6178497 (accessed November 16, 2012).

21. Lutz S, Berk L, Chang E, *et al*. Palliative radiotherapy for bone metastases: an ASTRO evidence-based guideline. *Int J Radiat Oncol Biol Phys* [Internet] 2011; 79: 965–976. Available at: http://www.ncbi.nlm.nih.gov/pubmed/21277118 (accessed November 16, 2012).

22. Hartsell WF, Scott CB, Bruner DW, *et al*. Randomized trial of short- versus long-course radiotherapy for palliation of painful bone metastases. *J Natl Canc Inst* 2005; 97: 798–804. Available at: http://www.ncbi.nlm.nih.gov/pubmed/15928300 (accessed November 16, 2012).

23. Leksell L. Occasional review Stereotactic radiosurgery. *J Neurol Neurosurg Psychiatry* 1983; 46: 797–803.

24. Loeffler JS, Kooy HM, Wen PY, *et al*. The treatment of recurrent brain metastases with stereotactic radiosurgery. *J Clin Oncol* [Internet] 1990; 8: 576–582. Available at: http://www.ncbi.nlm.nih.gov/pubmed/2179476 (accessed November 16, 2012).

25. Shaw E, Scott C, Souhami L, *et al*. Single dose radiosurgical treatment of recurrent previously irradiated primary brain tumors and brain metastases: final report of RTOG protocol 90-05. *Int J Radiat Oncol Phys* [Internet] 2000; 47: 291–298. Available at: http://www.ncbi.nlm.nih.gov/pubmed/10802351 (accessed November 16, 2012).

26. Andrews DW, Scott CB, Sperduto PW, *et al*. Whole brain radiation therapy with or without stereotactic radiosurgery boost for patients with one to three brain metastases: phase III results of the RTOG 9508 randomised trial. *Lancet* [Internet] 2004; 363: 1665. Available at: http://linkinghub.elsevier.com/retrieve/pii/S0140673604162508 (accessed November 16, 2012).

27. Gaspar L, Scott C, Rotman M, *et al*. Recursive partitioning analysis (RPA) of prognostic factors in three Ratiation Therapy Ongolocy Group (RTOG) brain metastases trials. *Int J Radiat Oncol Biol Phys* 1997; 37: 745–751.

28. Gaspar LE, Scott C, Murray K, *et al*. Validation of the RTOG recursive partitioning analysis (RPA) classification for brain metastases. *Int J Radiat Oncol Biol Phys* [Internet] 2000; 47: 1001–1006. Available at: http://www.ncbi.nlm.nih.gov/pubmed/17056192 (accessed November 16, 2012).

29. Gripp S, Mjartan S, Boelke E, *et al*. Palliative radiotherapy tailored to life expectancy in end-stage cancer patients: reality or myth? *Cancer* [Internet] 2010; 116: 3251–3256. Available at: http://www.ncbi.nlm.nih.gov/pubmed/20564632 (accessed March 31, 2012).

30. Barnes E, Palmer JL, Bruera E. Prevalence of symptom control and palliative care abstracts presented at the Annual Meeting of the American Society for Therapeutic Radiology and Oncology. *Int J Radiat Oncol Biol Phys* [Internet] 2002; 54: 211–214. Available at: http://www.ncbi.nlm.nih.gov/pubmed/12182994 (accessed November 16, 2012).

31. Jones J, Lutz S. Abstract 2907: trends in symptom control and palliative care abstracts at ASTRO 2001 to 2010. *Int J Radiat Oncol Biol Phys* 2011; 81(2S): 645.

32. Mould R. *A Century of X-Rays and Radioactivity in Medicine with Emphasis on Photographic Records of the Early Years*. Bristol, UK: Institute of Physics Publishing, 1993.

CHAPTER 2

The radiobiology of palliative radiation oncology

Candice A. Johnstone
Department of Radiation Oncology, Medical College of Wisconsin, Milwaukee, WI, USA

Introduction

The biologic basis for the effects of radiation on living cells dictates the potential benefits and limitations of radiotherapy for the palliation of end-of-life cancer symptoms. The goals of curative intent therapy are to eradicate all tumor cells, with treatment directed both toward macroscopically evident disease as well as anatomic areas that may be harboring microscopically occult disease. Alternatively, radiotherapy may successfully provide palliative relief of symptomatic tumors by fractionally decreasing the size of macroscopic tumor masses while ignoring areas of microscopic involvement [1]. The radiobiologic basis of radiotherapy is relevant to the discussion of either of these treatment approaches. The understanding of radiobiology involves the definition of several terms (Table 2.1). For those seeking a more detailed discussion of radiation biology, please refer to Hall's classic text [2].

Radiation effect on cells

Direct and indirect effect of radiation

Therapeutic radiation uses ionizing radiation to treat cancer. Radiation either affects DNA *directly* by creating double- and single-strand DNA breaks or *indirectly* by interacting with water and other small molecules to create reactive oxygen species which cause DNA damage [3]. Photons may interact with tumor cells in a number of different ways, depending upon the energy of the incident photon. The absorption of photons used for therapeutic radiation is dominated by the Compton effect, which depends upon the electron density of the irradiated tissue [4].

Radiation Oncology in Palliative Cancer Care, First Edition. Edited by Stephen Lutz, Edward Chow, and Peter Hoskin.

Table 2.1 Glossary of terms commonly used in radiobiology.

Term	Definition
Direct effect	Formation of single- and double-stranded DNA breaks due to interactions of photons with cellular DNA.
Indirect effect	Interactions of photons with water or other small molecules which then create reactive oxygen molecules that cause DNA strand breaks.
Compton effect	The most prevalent means by which photons of therapeutic energies interact with matter.
Cell survival curve	The ratio of cells that survive a radiation dose versus the size of that dose.
Linear quadratic equation	A mathematical model that predicts the biologic effectiveness of radiotherapy, taking into account both direct and indirect effects of photon interactions with DNA.
Linear energy transfer (LET)	An estimate of energy deposition as a charged particle travels through matter.
Alpha-beta ratio	The relative contributions of radiotherapy-induced DNA effects caused by non-repairable (alpha) and repairable (beta) damage, respectively.
Cell cycle	Characterization of a sequence of events that lead individual cells to progress through replication.
Fractionation	The division of a single radiotherapy dose into smaller doses, or fractions, that allow for cellular repair between treatments.
Standard fractionation	By convention, standard fractionation for curative radiation therapy involves delivery of 1.8–2.0 Gy per fraction to a total dose of 30–80 Gy, depending upon the diagnosis.
Hyperfractionation	A means of delivering more than one fraction per day in an attempt to control rapidly growing tumors.
Hypofractionation	Delivery of a smaller number of larger sized fractions commonly employed in palliative care situations to minimize time investment to patients and caretakers.
Four "R's" of radiobiology	The most basic radiobiology principles, including cellular repair, tissue reoxygenation, cell cycle reassortment, and cellular repopulation.
Biologically equivalent dose (BED)	An equation that estimates comparable biologic effectiveness from different radiotherapy fractionation schemes.

Shape of the cell survival curves

The effects of radiation on cells in tissue cultures may be described by plotting the percent of cells that survive radiation exposure versus the amount of dose delivered. These *cell survival curves* differ from one cell type to another, with the characteristics exhibited by cell cultures thought to correlate in some ways with the behavior of those cells in humans. The shape of the cell survival curves seen after radiation dose delivery is best described by a shape that has both linear and quadratic components [5,6]. The linear component of cell kill relates directly to the radiation dose, and it is thought to be caused by double-stranded DNA breaks that are not repaired (Figure 2.1). This aspect of cell kill is more prevalent in radiation beams that have a higher linear energy transfer (LET), such as alpha particles. The quadratic component of cell kill relates to repair of single strand breaks, a capability that differs between cell types.

The alpha/beta ratio describes the dose at which the linear and quadratic components of cell death are equal. Cell types with a low alpha/beta ratio are late reacting normal cell types and tumors that are more radiation resistant [7]. Those with a high alpha/beta ratio are early reacting normal tissues and most tumors. There are also differences in the radiosensitivity of tissue types based upon the structural organization of the organ. For example, the esophagus and spinal cord are organized in series, where damage to any part along the length of the organ can interfere with function. Thus, these types of organs are limited by the maximum dose and generally have a higher total organ

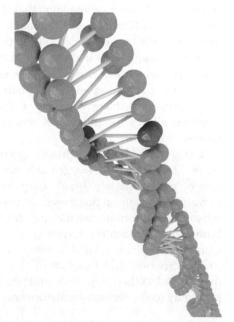

Figure 2.1 A stylized representation of a length of double-stranded DNA with breaks in both strands due to radiotherapy damage. Reproduced with permission from Dreamstime.

tolerance to radiation. Organs that are arranged in parallel, such as the lungs or the liver, can tolerate very high doses of radiation to small portions of the organ, but have a low total organ tolerance to radiation.

Cell cycle characteristics

Human cells follow a well-choreographed cell cycle that includes the following phases: quiescent or "G0 phase," active growth or "G1 phase," DNA replication or "synthesis phase," mitotic preparation or "G2" phase, and active mitosis or "M phase" [2]. *In vivo*, cells move throughout the cell cycle at a pace that relates to the tissue type and cell type. The pace of the cell cycle correlates mostly with the amount of time a cell spends in the first gap (G1) phase. Thus, the proportion of cells in a particular phase of the cell cycle varies over time. From *in vitro* experiments, cells have been found to be most sensitive to ionizing radiation in the late G2 or mitosis phases. This cell cycle-specific sensitivity to radiation led to the concept of fractionation.

Interaction of cell cycle and radiotherapy fractionation

The "four R's" of radiobiology define the ways that radiation therapy fractionation combines with the realities of the cell cycle to influence cell survival curves [8].

Repair of DNA damage is generally more efficient in normal cells than tumor cells, thereby allowing for a therapeutic ratio. Ionizing radiation causes lethal, sublethal, and potentially lethal DNA damage. Lethal damage always results in cell death, while sublethal damage can usually be repaired in the absence of additional insult or injury. Sublethal repair explains the relative increase in the surviving cell population if a radiation dose is split into two fractions. Potentially lethal damage is thought to represent DNA damage that can be repaired if the post-irradiation environment is not optimal for growth. This concept is incompletely understood at the cellular level. *In vitro* and *in vivo* experiments have demonstrated that a minimum of 6 hours between fractions allows for maximum repair of sublethal damage to the normal tissues.

Reoxygenation is thought to work to the tumor's disadvantage in two major ways. The presence of oxygen enhances the DNA damage of ionizing radiation by approximately 3-fold compared to anaerobic conditions. Most solid tumors stimulate angiogenesis; however, the tumor vasculature is not as robust as the normal vasculature and there are often hypoxic areas that are both transient (acutely hypoxic) and more permanent (chronic hypoxia). Chronic hypoxia is related to temporary blockage of tumor vasculature due to the structure and function of the vessels. *Reoxygenation* works through oxygenated cells dying first, and thus the hypoxic cells become closer in proximity to the tumor vasculature and chronic hypoxic elements are reversed as chronically hypoxic cells become more exposed to oxygen. Secondly, because of the nature of tumor vasculature, different parts of the tumor may be oxygenated or hypoxic depending on the collapse or blockage of different branches of these abnormal vessels. Cells which are acutely hypoxic at the time of one fraction of radiation may not be the same as those that are hypoxic the next day.

Reassortment of cells throughout the cell cycle over time allows for a different proportion of tumor cells to be in a more radiation-sensitive phase of the cell cycle, thus distributing potentially lethal effects over a wider population of tumor cells. Obviously, reassortment is more common in cells which have a relatively short cell cycle time. Radiotherapy induced death is therefore less common for cells that reside in the relatively radiation-insensitive gap phases for lengthy periods of time.

Repopulation describes the proliferation of cells in response to an injury, such as radiation. It is more pronounced in the reaction of early responding tissues, such as skin and fast growing tumors, than it is in late responding tissues. By virtue of the fact that repopulation leads to a larger number of tumor cells that must be killed to totally eradicate a cancer or to diminish the size of a macroscopic tumor, it is an instance where the effects of fractionation may be deleterious to treatment goals. During the course of a fractionated course of radiation, accelerated repopulation may be seen as a response to the first few weeks of radiation damage. Accelerated radiotherapy describes an approach in which the overall treatment time is minimized to overcome any effects of repopulation. It is also the reason why gaps in treatment may have a negative impact on outcome.

Radiotherapy fractionation characteristics

Curative standard fractionation schemes have developed over several decades into daily fractions of 1.8–2.0 Gy given to a total dose of between 40 Gy and 80 Gy, depending upon the tumor type. There are few palliative care scenarios where the time intensiveness of protracted treatment would be justified. More appropriately, hypofractionated regimens of 3–10 Gy delivered in 1–10 fractions has been found to provide excellent symptom relief for a variety of palliative care situations.

Fractionation has different effects on acute and late responding tissues. Late effects are more pronounced with larger fraction sizes than with smaller fractions. In other words, increasing the fraction size does not necessarily increase the acute side effects, but it can increase the risk of late side effects. Conversely, the larger fraction but lower total dose regimens have been shown to be associated with less acute toxicity. Late toxicity occurs several months to years after the radiation dose is delivered. In palliative radiation, the time course of the patient's expected survival may influence whether they will live long enough to experience late toxicity. Concerns about severe side effects in those who live longer than expected may serve to limit the use of hypofractionated treatment but are rarely well-founded.

Various methods have been used to compare different fractionation regimens. The first model of the isoeffect of fractionation regimens was the Strandquist plot. This was later replaced by the nominal standard dose (NSD) system by Ellis. The current, most widely used model, is the biologic equivalent dose (BED) which enables doses using different fraction sizes to be converted to a common schedule, typically the equivalent dose in 2 Gy fractions (EQDI). The formula is based on: BED = nd $(1 + (n$ / alpha-beta ratio)), where d is the dose per fraction and n is the number of fractions. More complex derivations will add components to account for repair and treatment time. While helpful in defining a common metric for radiation dose, it is important to realize that they can only provide a guide and are based upon a number of assumptions related to the biologic characteristics of a particular tumor. The situation is even more complex in palliation where the target may be normal (e.g. pain mediating or osteoclasts) rather than tumor cells. They should therefore be interpreted against the background of clinical data and experience.

Conclusion

A basic understanding of radiobiology is needed to assess the most appropriate palliative radiotherapy fractionation schemes. Radiotherapy either directly or indirectly causes DNA strand breaks that can lead to cell death. Radiobiology principles that influence cell kill include DNA repair, tissue reoxygenation, cell cycle reassortment, and repopulation. The principles of radiobiology explain that the acute effects of treatment depend upon total dose while late effects depend upon both total dose and dose per fraction. Therefore, the choice of palliative radiotherapy fractionation scheme requires a rigorous review of the available data as well as an educated estimate of patient prognosis.

References

1. Kirkbride P, Barton R. Palliative radiation therapy. *J Palliat Med* 1999; **2**: 87–97.
2. Hall E, Giaccia A. *Radiobiology for the Radiobiologist*, 6th edn. Philadelphia: Lippincott Williams and Wilkins, 2012.
3. Ward J. *DNA Damage Produced by Ionizing Radiation in Mammalian Cells: Identities, Mechanisms of Formation, and Repairability*. San Diego: Academic Press, 1988, pp. 104–106.
4. Jayaraman S, Lanzl L. *Clinical Radiotherapy Physics*. Berlin: Springer, 2004, p. 81.
5. Brenner D. The linear-quadratic model is an appropriate methodology for determining isoeffective doses at large doses per fraction. *Semin Radiat Oncol* 2008; **18**: 234–239.
6. Kirkpatrick J, Meyer J, Marks L. The linear-quadratic model is inappropriate to model high dose per fraction effects in radiosurgery. *Semin Radiat Oncol* 2008; **18**: 240–243.

7. Williams M, Denekamp J, Fowler J. A review of alpha/beta ratios for experimental tumors: implications for clinical studies of altered fractionation. *Int J Radiat Oncol Biol Phys* 1985; **11**: 87–96.
8. Pajonk F, Vlashi E, McBride H. Radiation resistance of cancer stem cells. The 4 R's of radiobiology revisited. *Stem Cells* 2008; **28**: 639–648.

CHAPTER 3

The physics of radiation oncology

Shaun Baggarley, Jiade J. Lu

Department of Radiation Oncology, National University Cancer Institute, National University Health System, Republic of Singapore

Introduction

Radiation therapy is the medical use of ionizing radiation for curative or palliative treatment of cancer. Ionizing radiation refers to different types of energy in the form of high frequency electromagnetic (EM) waves (X-rays, gamma rays) or highly accelerated particles (electrons, protons) [1]. These high-energy EM waves and particles interact with matter by transferring some or all of their energy to atomic electrons and nuclei in a material. This deposition of energy results in the production of ions and the breaking of molecular bonds. In the case of living tissue, ionizing radiation can directly damage DNA molecules or create ions from other molecules such as water that will chemically interact with DNA molecules, resulting in cell damage [2].

The description of medical physics requires the understanding of several terms (Table 3.1). The quantity used to describe the amount of ionizing radiation delivered to a material is called *absorbed dose*, and its *Système international d'unités* (SI) unit is the gray (Gy). Within living tissue or organs, there is a relationship between the absorbed dose delivered and the resultant biologic effect, such as cell damage. This relationship is dependent on a number of factors, including the amount of dose delivered, the type of radiation, the tissue type, the rate at which radiation is delivered, and the frequency of delivery. The primary goal of radiation therapy is to preferentially destroy cancerous cells without affecting normal cells. However, the anatomic location of tumor adjacent to unaffected normal tissue structures usually makes it impossible to limit dose solely to the cancer. The probability of a successful therapeutic or palliative outcome relative to the incidence of side effects in normal tissue is called the *therapeutic ratio*.

Radiation Oncology in Palliative Cancer Care, First Edition. Edited by Stephen Lutz, Edward Chow, and Peter Hoskin.

Table 3.1 Glossary of terms commonly used in medical physics for the delivery of radiation therapy.

Term	Definition
X-ray therapy	A form of electromagnetic radiation with a shorter wavelength than light and with the capability of penetrating solid materials.
Electron therapy	An electron is a negatively charged subatomic particle normally bound to the nucleus of an atom but which may be ejected and used as one category of "particle treatment" in radiotherapy.
Absorbed dose	The amount of energy actually absorbed in some material, most commonly referring to treatment of human tissue.
Gray (Gy)	One measure of absorbed dose, equal to one joule of energy deposited in one kg of a material. Alternative measures of absorbed dose include the Roentgen (R), radiation absorbed dose (rad), Roentgen equivalent man (REM), and Curie (Ci).
Therapeutic ratio	The ratio of lethal dose divided by the therapeutic dose of radiation in a living system.
Teletherapy	Radiation oncology treatment in which a radioactive source is placed at some defined distance from the body. Cobalt-60 and cesium-137 machines are two examples of teletherapy.
Linear accelerator	A device that produces high energy photons (i.e. X-rays) or charged particles (i.e. electrons) for use in radiation therapy.
Intensity modulated radiation therapy	A type of three-dimensional radiation therapy that uses thousands of small radiation beamlets which enter the body from different angles and overlap within target regions.
Volumetric modulated arc therapy	A specific type of IMRT in which three-dimensional therapy is delivered as multi-leaf collimators move concurrently with a single gantry rotation about the patient.
Image guided radiation therapy	A method of delivering radiation treatments using radiographic equipment to better define the target volume in the patient. The implantation of radiopaque devices, or "fiducial markers," may aid these efforts.
Proton therapy	A specialized type of linear accelerator treatment that uses a cyclotron to deliver charged particles in the form of protons to a cancer patient. Protons have a specialized deposition of dose in tissue that can improve sparing of adjacent, normal tissues.
Brachytherapy	Placement of a sealed radiotherapy source into a body cavity or tissue to dose a tumor target while limiting exposure to adjacent tissues because of decreasing dose with distance.
Simulation	The process of setting up a patient in a comfortable and reproducible position that will be recreated with each subsequent treatment.
Dosimetry	Accurately measuring the dose to be delivered to specific anatomic sites in a patient treated with radiotherapy. It is usually computer-aided, and it most commonly evaluates dose in reference to diagnostic studies such as a CT simulation.

The development of radiation therapy technology

The early understanding of radiation therapy

The drive behind the development of technology for radiation therapy has been largely based on the need to improve the therapeutic ratio. Historically, radiation therapy began shortly after the discovery of X-rays by Wilhelm Röntgen in 1895 and radioactivity by Henri Becquerel in 1896 [3]. Early radiation therapy was based on simple treatments using a single low energy X-ray beam or radioactive radium-226 placed adjacent to or placed interstitially in the tumor [4]. From early observations it was realized that a relationship existed between the amount of radiation delivered and the efficacy of treatment and the generation of side effects. However, the exact nature of the relationship and the factors associated with tumor cell kill and normal tissue side effects were not known, and the technology did not exist at that time to significantly improve the therapeutic ratio.

The development of teletherapy machines

During the 1950s, dedicated radiation treatment machines containing cesium-137 or cobalt-60 sources, also known as *Teletherapy Machines*, were used to direct and shape beams of gamma rays at tumors [5]. The concept of directing multiple beams to intersect at the target and shaping the beam to match the tumor shape meant the dose was more concentrated at the cancerous tissue relative to normal tissue. Thus, technologic advances translated into an improvement in the therapeutic ratio. However, further improvements were still required, particularly with regards to the penetrating power of the beams, the conformality of the beams, and the ability to accurately locate the tumor position and extent.

The proliferation of linear accelerators

Further development in the delivery of ionizing radiation occurred in the 1980s and 1990s with the introduction of linear accelerators, or *linacs*, that produced more highly penetrating X-ray beams and electron beams compared to the earlier teletherapy machines. Linear accelerators are manufactured in a number of configurations and sizes, but all are similar in that they produce ionizing radiation "artificially" by accelerating electrons to very high energies [6]. These high-energy electrons are either used directly or they are used to create X-rays that are aimed as beams at the tumor (Figure 3.1).

Linacs came to have specialized beam-shaping devices in the form of customized blocks placed in the path of the beams to enhance conformality. The use of multiple, static, conformed X-ray beams is often referred to as three-dimensional (3D) conformal radiation therapy, or 3D-CRT, and is also known in more modern times as "conventional therapy" [7]. The 3D aspect of 3D-CRT refers to the type of imaging technology (3D reconstructed axial CT images)

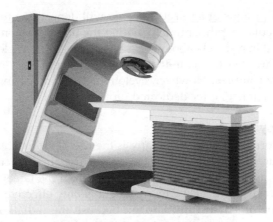

Figure 3.1 A common linear accelerator has a movable table and a gantry that rotates around the patient. The beam is produced in the neck of the gantry, and it is shaped as it leaves the head of the gantry toward the patient. Reproduced with permission from Dreamstime.

used to plan and calculate the radiation dose to the patient. While 3D-CRT can often provide excellent beam conformity, the static nature of the beam does not offer much scope for optimizing the dose within the tumor or to normal tissues adjacent to the tumor. Thus the therapeutic ratio can only be enhanced to a certain extent with 3D-CRT.

The advent of intensity modulated radiation therapy

Dose shaping capabilities were enhanced with the invention of multiple movable leaves in the delivery pathway of the linac beam. These *multi-leaf collimators* (MLCs) can deliver *intensity modulated radiation therapy* (IMRT) by either forming a static shape when the machine is delivering dose or by moving during the treatment to produce a dynamic change in the shape of the dose delivered over time [8]. To improve dose optimization, IMRT was developed. IMRT uses MLCs to modify the intensity of the beam by dividing each beam into smaller components called *beamlets*. So, instead of several intersecting static beams as in 3D-CRT, IMRT has literally hundreds of smaller intersecting beams, each made up of multiple and variable intensity beamlets. Through the use of computerized optimization algorithms, it possible to plan IMRT beams to deliver the dose to the tumor and the surrounding tissue with enhanced precision. A further development of IMRT is stereotactic radiation therapy where the machine will rotate in one or more arcs, dynamically delivering the radiation beamlets as it rotates [9].

Finally, the past two decades have also ushered in the use of proton therapy machines that utilize cyclotron technology to produce ionizing radiation with special spatial properties. Protons have a unique dosing characteristic in that they deliver most of their energy at the end of their travel path. This means that a beam of protons of a selected energy will deposit the majority of their dose at a particular depth, optimally within the tumor. Proton therapy originally developed in research laboratories, inasmuch as the accelerators (known as cyclotrons) needed to create the proton beams are large, expensive, and technologically complex. However, cyclotrons have increasingly been introduced into the clinic to offer dedicated proton therapy [10].

Brachytherapy radiation

The simplest form of radiation therapy is the use of radioactive sources that are placed adjacent to, or inside, the tumor. The use of radioactive sources for radiation therapy is known as brachytherapy (from the Greek word *brachys*, meaning "short-distance") [1]. The treatment is only effective within a small radius from the brachytherapy implant because the radiation dose from a single radioactive source will decrease rapidly with distance. The radioactive sources used typically emit gamma rays or beta particles (electrons). Brachytherapy is most easily utilized where a tumor is readily accessible and is not too large in size, though sources may be placed into internal sites with needles directed through the skin or by applicators placed during a surgical procedure. Brachytherapy may be achieved through the placement of either permanent or temporary sources. In most modern facilities, temporary sources are commonly placed with an afterloading machine containing a single source that emits gamma rays, with the source positioned within specialized interstitial or intracavitary catheters inside the patient. The source position and duration of delivery can be programmed to optimize the dose to the tumor.

The impact of diagnostic improvements on radiotherapy delivery

Mirroring the technologic advances of radiotherapy, modern diagnostic imaging capabilities began in the 1970s when Godfrey Hounsfield invented the first Computed Tomography (CT) scanner [11]. For the first time, this diagnostic capability enabled radiation oncologists to visualize anatomy in two-dimensional (2D) axial planes and to improve the accuracy of locating the tumor relative to adjacent tissues. The CT information was also used to more accurately calculate radiation dose distributions in the patient with the aid of computers.

Later, as computing technology improved, 2D axial CT planes were reconstructed into 3D representations of the anatomy, and 3D radiation dose calculations were also performed. The ability to place radiopaque fiducial markers in the body to account for movement of target structures, known as *image guided radiation therapy* (IGRT), has also aided the therapeutic ratio for the treatment of some cancer types [12]. The precision of radiotherapy has also been improved by further improvements in CT scanners and magnetic resonance imaging scanners, as well as by the introduction of positron emission tomography (PET) scanners that help to define functional imaging in addition to anatomic imaging [13] (Figure 3.2).

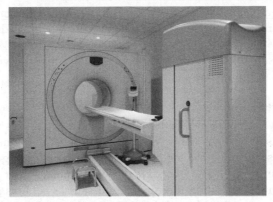

Figure 3.2 A positron emission tomography/computerized tomography (PET/CT) scanner provides diagnostic information about the anatomic and functional characteristics of cancers. The information from a PET/CT can provide significant information to the radiation oncologist, medical physicist, and medical dosimetrist in their efforts to plan appropriate treatment for the patient. Reproduced with permission from Dreamstime.

Process of radiation therapy

Simulation

Just as is true in any other processes of cancer management, palliative radiation therapy requires careful planning and quality assurance. Once the diagnosis is confirmed and treatment strategy is determined, radiation oncologists and their colleagues will plan for the courses of radiotherapy. This planning usually includes two steps: simulation and dosimetry planning. Simulation can be completed with a "simulator" in the form of a simple X-ray device, though nowadays simulation is most commonly performed using a planning CT machine, with which the localization of tumor is more precise and accurate. Newer technologies allow simulations with magnetic resonance imaging (MRI) or PET scanners, but those capabilities have not yet become commonplace in radiotherapy clinics. Patients with a very poor prognosis who are suffering a great deal of pain may sometimes undergo a "clinical set up" using anatomic landmarks, avoiding time that would be spent completing a more complex simulation.

Dosimetry

Computerized dose planning takes place after simulation, and it may require anywhere from several minutes to several days of time depending upon the complexity of the calculations, the quality of the dose planning software, and the availability of qualified dosimetrists. During planning, radiation dosimetrists work closely with the attending physician to determine the dose arrangement of radiation to the targets of treatment. The purpose of this process is to ensure sufficient doses to be delivered to the targets and to minimize unwanted treatment to the surrounding normal organs and tissues. Once the planning is completed, the patient can start the radiation therapy. In some palliative care situations where patients are consulted, simulated, and treated in the same visit, treatment planning may consist of very simple calculations with limited computer aid [14].

Initiation of therapy

Although early start of radiation therapy is preferred in most scenarios, radiation therapy usually starts within a few days in most non-emergency palliation to allow sufficient time for planning. In medical emergencies such as spinal cord compression and excessive bleeding from a tumor uncontrollable by other measures, radiation therapy should start as soon as possible, often the same day as consultation and simulation. Delaying the initiation of radiation in such situations may cause unrecoverable functional loss or even jeopardize the patient's life.

Patient immobilization

One of the critical factors in any external beam treatment is the immobilization of the patient during the delivery [15]. In order to reduce patient movement and improve setup accuracy between and during treatments, immobilization devices are commonly fashioned to maximize the chances that the dose is delivered to the treatment volume as had been planned during simulation and dose planning. In cases where sub-millimeter accuracy is required, specialized stereotactic frames are combined with radiation therapy. This approach to treatment is referred to as stereotactic radiosurgery (SRS) or stereotactic radiation therapy (SRT) for cranial treatment and stereotactic body radiation therapy (SBRT) for all other anatomic sites, but their use is limited to a specific subset of palliative cases.

Management of patients during treatment

During the course of radiation therapy, the radiation oncologist sees the patient at least once per week in "on-treatment visits" to complete an interval history and a focused physical examination to assess treatment response and to manage toxicities. In addition, radiation oncologists are required to verify the treatment field defined during simulation and planning with an X-ray taken at least weekly during treatment to ensure the consistency of the patient set-up and beam accuracy. In cases where palliative patients suffer a marked decline after treatment, follow-up can be offered by telephone to limit travel requirements.

Special considerations in developing countries

Resource limitations in developing countries can create circumstances where the cost of linacs may be prohibitive. Teletherapy machines have the advantage of being technically simple, reliable, and cheaper to purchase and operate.

Conversely, they have the disadvantages of a relatively low beam energy, low beam output, and poor dose conformity compared to a linear accelerator. Furthermore, the radiation-producing sources diminish in strength as their energy decays, thereby requiring lengthier treatment times to produce equivalent doses. This slower throughput may cause scheduling difficulties in countries where the ratio of treatment machines to population is low. Also, the cost for subsequent source changes may be prohibitive in some locales. Still, because of the advantages that teletherapy machines offer, they are still commonly used in developing countries.

Conclusion

Radiation therapy has provided successful palliative therapy since its original discovery in the late 1800s. The main goal of technologic advances in radiation therapy is to improve the ratio of tumor cell kill to normal tissue toxicity, otherwise known as the therapeutic ratio. Palliative radiation therapy may be delivered with machinery ranging from cobalt-60 teletherapy machines to highly sophisticated linacs that provide stereotactic body radiation therapy. Still, regardless of the method of radiotherapy delivery, optimization of palliative care requires treatment that is effective, time-efficient, and well-coordinated with other palliative interventions.

References

1. Khan F. *The Physics of Radiation Therapy*, 4th edn. Philadelpia, PA: Lippincott Williams and Wilkins, 2009.
2. Hall EJ, Giaccia AJ. *Radiobiology for the Radiologist*, 6th edn. Philadelphia: Lippincott Williams and Wilkins, 2006.
3. Freund L. *Elements of general radio-therapy for practitioners.* [Internet] New York: Rebman, 1904; Available at: http://books.google.com/books?id=goCGUdSHOPwC (accessed November 16, 2012).
4. Simpson F. *Radium Therapy.* St. Louis: CV Moseby Company, 1922.
5. Comas F, Brucer M. First impressions of therapy with Cesium 137. *Radiology* 1957; **69**: 231–235.
6. Baker M. Medical linear accelerator celebrates 50 years of treating cancer. 2007 (April 18), Stanford News. Available at: http://news.stanford.edu/news/2007/april18/med-accelerator-041807.html (accessed June 25, 2012).
7. Palo Alto Medical Foundation. Three-Dimensional Conformal Radiotherapy. 2012. Available at: http://www.pamf.org/radonc/tech/3d.html (accessed June 25, 2012).
8. Memorial Sloan-Kettering Cancer Center. *Intensity Modulated Radiation Therapy.* Madison, WI: Medical Physics Publishing, 2003.
9. Otto K. Volumetric modulated arc therapy: IMRT in a single gantry arc. *Med Phys* 2008; **35**: 310–317.
10. Paganetti H. *Proton Therapy Physics.* Boca Raton, FL: CRC Press, Taylor & Francis Group, LLC, 2012.

11. Philips CT Marketing, Philips Healthcare. Development of CT imaging. 2006. Available at: http://clinical.netforum.healthcare.philips.com/us_en/Explore/White-Papers/CT/Development-of-CT-imaging (accessed June 25, 2012).

12. Jaffray D, Siewerdsen J, Wong J, *et al.* Flat-panel cone-beam computed tomography for image guided radiation therapy. *Int J Radiat Oncol Biol Phys* 2002; **53**: 1337–1349.

13. Society for Nuclear Medicine. Fact Sheet: What is PET? 2012. Available at: http://interactive.snm.org/index.cfm?PageID=11123 (accessed June 25, 2012).

14. Bentel G. *Radiation Therapy Planning*, 2nd edn. New York, NY: McGraw Hill, 1996.

15. Bentel G. *Patient Positioning and Immobilization in Radiation Oncology*. New York, NY: McGraw Hill, 1999.

CHAPTER 4

Curative intent versus palliative intent radiation oncology

Vassilios Vassiliou, Haris Charalambous
Department of Radiation Oncology, Bank of Cyprus Oncology Centre, Nicosia, Cyprus

Introduction

Radiotherapy (RT) plays an important role in the management of cancer patients, given that about half of all cancer patients undergo RT at some point during their illness [1]. The treatment of malignant neoplasms with RT has historically been separated by goals of care, dividing those who are treated with "curative intent" from those who are treated with "palliative intent." The basis of this separation has been based mainly on anatomic staging, with patients who have metastatic disease receiving short courses of palliative RT, while patients with localized or locally advanced disease receiving more protracted courses of radiation therapy, often combined with chemotherapy. In fact, many radiotherapy prescription sheets are pre-printed with boxes for the practitioner to designate the goal of therapy.

The rationale behind these two approaches ignores the clinical reality that patients with localized or locally advanced disease have symptoms in need of palliation and the true definition of palliative care, namely that it is the practice of attending disease symptoms and treatment toxicities in any patient with a life-threatening illness. The World Health Organization's (WHO) definition of palliative care (PC) in 1990 still projects the most meaningful framework to evaluate this patient group [2]. PC is "the active, holistic care of patients with advanced, progressive illness, including management of pain and other symptoms whilst provision of psychological, social, and spiritual support is paramount. The goal of PC is achievement of the best quality of life for patients and their families." Furthermore, it is recognized that "many aspects of PC are also applicable earlier in the course of the illness in conjunction with other treatments," which particularly applies to patients receiving curative RT or chemoradiation (CRT) [2].

Radiation Oncology in Palliative Cancer Care, First Edition. Edited by Stephen Lutz, Edward Chow, and Peter Hoskin.
© 2013 John Wiley & Sons, Ltd. Published 2013 by John Wiley & Sons, Ltd.

This definition has been accepted by most oncology societies worldwide. The National Cancer Policy Board of the United States adopted the WHO definition of PC in 2001, and in its *"Improving Palliative Care for Cancer"* report stated "the importance of PC beginning at the time of cancer diagnosis and increasing in amount and intensity throughout the course of the patient's illness, until death" [3]. A recent provisional clinical opinion (PCO) from the American Society of Clinical Oncology (ASCO) in 2012 advocated integration of palliative care early in the management of any patient with progressive or advanced cancer [4]. The ASCO statement recognizes the importance of PC in terms of improvement of patients' symptoms, quality of life, and satisfaction, while reducing the caregiver's burden. Finally, the American Society for Radiation Oncology (ASTRO) has gone a step further, recognizing the need for expertise in PC amongst its members so that they can deliver both radiation and PC to their patients [5].

This chapter will highlight those circumstances where patients may receive radiation therapy that provides palliative relief while also aiming for cure. Table 4.1 delineates the difference in approaches of RT for those treated for cure plus still aiming for palliation of their symptoms versus those treated solely with palliative intent [6]. Those who are solely treated for palliation

Table 4.1 Differences between curative plus palliative RT and palliative RT, alone.

	Curative plus palliative RT	Palliative RT, alone
Aim	Tumor eradication Symptom management	Solely for symptom management
Total dose	45–50 Gy for microscopic disease 60–70 Gy for macroscopic disease	8–30 Gy
Fractionation	1.8–2.0 Gy fractions	3.0–8.0 Gy fractions
Duration	5–8 weeks	1–2 weeks
Acute toxicity	Increased incidence and severity due to higher total dose and lengthier treatment duration	Reduced incidence and severity due to smaller overall dose and shorter treatment duration
Late toxicity	Decreased incidence due to smaller fraction size	Increased incidence due to larger fraction size
Chemotherapy	Given sequentially or concurrently in an effort to increase cure rates	May be given sometimes sequentially, but almost never concurrently (to minimize toxicity)

appropriately receive courses that have a lower total dose, a larger fraction size, and a smaller number of fractions, termed "hypofractionation." This approach diminishes the chances of acute toxicity, while creating a higher risk for late toxicity, an acceptable trade-off when one considers that most patients treated solely with palliative intent will not survive long enough to face the delayed risks caused by hypofractionation. In contrast, patients treated for cure plus palliation receive a larger total dose of radiation given in a larger number of small dose fractions in an effort to maximize tumor cell kill while minimizing the risks of late side effects.

While survival rates are well-known for most primary tumor types and stages, the outcome of any individual patient is not pre-destined. The minimization of symptoms is of immediate importance to patients whether they die from their cancer, or not. Furthermore, some patients with limitations such as poor performance status (PS) or concurrent comorbid illnesses may begin curative intent radiotherapy but be unable to complete their course as it was intended. Alternatively, patients with poor performance status who are treated solely with palliative intent may respond so well to treatment as to survive a great deal longer than their clinical circumstance would have first predicted. Sadly, for some locally advanced tumors there is often little difference in survival outcome whether RT is given with curative doses versus those more commonly treated solely with palliative intent. Table 4.2 outlines these common, poor prognosis tumor types and compares their symptoms and survival rates.

The determination of cure plus palliation intent versus pure palliative intent

Several factors may help determine which patients are to be treated with any curative goals and which are to be treated solely with palliative goals. Those factors may relate to the patient, the disease, the treatment, or resource availability (Figure 4.1).

In general, the variables which correlate with palliative only treatments include:
• patient – poor performance status, limited functional capabilities, elderly age, significant weight loss, presence of severe comorbid disease, overall poor quality of life
• disease – diagnosis known to have a poor prognosis, disease too extensive to be safely encompassed in a radical RT treatment volume, presence of metastatic disease
• treatment – poor response to previous treatment, anticipated high toxicity risks with RT dosed to cure the disease, previous RT
• resource availability – lack of access to necessary treatment types, decreased RT capacity, large distance to nearest RT center.

Table 4.2 Cancers that may be treated with curative intent radiotherapy but which should also receive palliative care intervention from the time of initial diagnosis.

Diagnosis	Symptoms	Expected Survival
High grade glioma	Seizures	Grade III: Surgery + CRT = 3 years
	Neurologic impairment	Grade IV: good prognosis (young, good PS, methylated MGMT) Surgery + CRT = 2 years
	Headaches	
		Grade IV: intermediate prognosis (young, good PS, no methylated MGMT) surgery + RT = 1 year
		Grade IV poor prognosis (old, poor PS) suboptimal surgery + RT = 6 months
Pancreatic and hepatobiliary cancer	Anorexia/nausea	Pancreatic cancer: 5 year <5%
	Pain	Inoperable cholangiocarcinoma: median survival 9–14 months
	Obstructive jaundice	
Advanced lung cancer	Cough/Hemoptysis	Non-small cell lung cancer (NSCLC) locally advanced disease: 12–18 months.
	Dyspnea	
	Pain	Small cell Lung Cancer (SCLC) limited stage: 12–18 months
	SVC syndrome	
	Airway obstruction	
Esophageal tumor	Dysphagia	5 year <20%
	Hemoptysis	
	Pain	
Locally advanced or recurrent gynecologic, gastrointenstinal, genitourinary	Pain	Stage IVA cervical cancer: 5 year 16–25%
	Relief hydronephrosis	Advanced bladder cancer: 7.5–14.4 months
	Urinary retention	Unresectable gastric cancer: 5 year 10%
	Intestinal obstruction	Pelvic mass from recurrent or metastatic colorectal ca: 6–14 months
	Bleeding/hematuria	
Locally advanced head-neck cancer	Pain	Early stage (T1/T2, N-ve) 5-year local control 80–90%, 5-year survival 60–80%
	Bleeding	
	Dysphagia	Locally advanced disease (T3/T4, N+ve) 5-year local control 50–60%, 5-year survival 40%

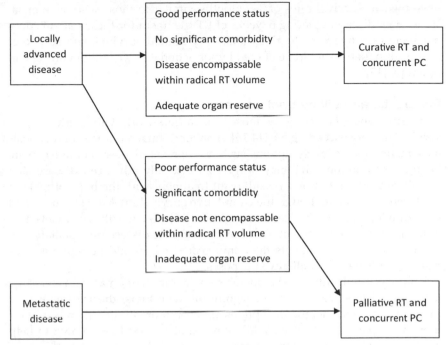

Figure 4.1 Clinical decision tree for curative RT plus PC palliative versus purely palliative RT plus PC radiotherapy.

Clinical diagnoses

High grade glioma

High grade gliomas, WHO grade III or IV, are the most common primary brain tumors in adults. World Health Organization grade IV tumors are predominantly (up to 90%) glioblastoma multiforme (GBM), the most aggressive primary malignant brain tumor histology [7,8]. Patients with high grade tumors present with non-specific symptoms like headaches relating to raised intracranial pressure, specific symptoms relating to the specific location of the tumor for example hemiparesis, aphasia, or hemianopia, in about 50% of tumors, and finally seizures in about 25% of patients [9]. Prognosis in patients with high grade gliomas is related to pathologic grade, patient age, and clinical/neurologic state at diagnosis [10]. On average, patients with grade III tumors (anaplastic astrocytomas) after conventional aggressive treatment with surgery, RT, and chemotherapy have a median survival close to 3 years, compared to 1 year for grade IV tumors, i.e. GBM [11]. Even the most favorable subgroup of GBM patients (i.e. those with young age, good PS, hypermethylation of O-6-methylguanine-DNA methyltransferase, and tolerance of concurrent and adjuvant temozolamide) have only a 2-year median survival [12]. Conversely, elderly patients with poor PS and fixed neurologic deficit have median survival rates of 3–9 months, similar to those who have metastatic brain disease. Offering 6 weeks of RT treatment for these patients does not seem very appropriate given their very limited survival, and so poorer prognosis patients should be offered hypofractionated RT without any chemotherapy [13].

Pancreatic and biliary tract cancer

Pancreatic cancer is among the most fatal cancers worldwide, with a 5-year survival rate not exceeding 5% [14,15]. A patient's final months after diagnosis may be dominated by symptoms such as anorexia, nausea, vomiting, pain, itching, and fatigue. CRT may be given for locally advanced disease as a definitive treatment or as a neoadjuvant treatment with the hope of making the tumor resectable, though the cumulative survival rates are still poor and the side effects of therapy may be significant [16]. So while these patients may potentially receive treatment aimed at cure of their disease plus palliation of symptoms, for most patients the administered RT should be thought of as being given solely for palliative purposes.

Similarly, locally advanced inoperable cholangiocarcinomas are a challenge for oncologists since they cause significant symptoms, the treatment may cause toxicity, and therapeutic options are even more limited than is true for those with pancreatic cancer. While the use of RT has been shown to help palliate symptoms of cholangiocarcinoma, it would seem to be a misnomer to categorize the treatment as "curative" when survival often does not exceed one year [17,18].

Lung cancer

Lung cancer is the leading cause of cancer death in the world inasmuch as over 1.35 million new cases are diagnosed each year and between 85% and 90% of patients diagnosed with lung cancer die of their disease [19]. Lung cancer is subdivided into small cell lung cancer (SCLC) which constitutes about 20% and non-small cell lung cancer (NSCLC) which constitutes approximately 80% of all lung cancers. The majority of cases of NSCLC are diagnosed in advanced stages with correspondingly poor survival rates, even in countries that have ease of availability to health care and diagnostic scanners [20]. Patients with locally advanced disease (Stage III) may suffer symptoms such as cough, shortness of breath, hemoptysis, chest pain, post-obstructive pneumonia, dysphagia, and superior vena cava syndrome. These Stage III patients are not normally good candidates for surgical resection, and even with advanced CRT techniques their survival may just reach beyond one year [21–23]. Care must be taken to limit curative intent treatment to circumstances where the volume of lung in the high-dose RT volume is not so large as to place the patient at risk for severe or even life-threatening toxicity in the form of radiation pneumonitis.

Patients with limited stage SCLC who can receive curative intent CRT have 2-year survival rates that exceed those with locally advanced NSCLC. RT plays a significant role in those successes through treatment of the primary disease in the lung as well as prophylactic treatment of the brain [24–26]. Still, the same caveats regarding the choice for curative RT plus PC versus palliative RT plus PC apply to this patient group. For patients whose performance status does not allow for concurrent CRT, sequential treatment offers an alternative approach. Furthermore, patients who have significant fatigue after initial CRT should weigh the potential benefits of prophylactic cranial irradiation with the drawback of an additional transient decrease in energy level and potential detriment in cognition. Overall, in spite of recent improvements in the survival rates of patients with SCLC, the majority of those diagnosed with even the most favorable disease will succumb to their illness. As such, early and aggressive PC is vital for this group.

Esophageal cancer

Esophageal carcinomas are common worldwide and can result in symptoms such as pain, cough, hemoptysis, and dysphagia. More than 50% of patients with esophageal cancer have inoperable disease with 5-year survival limited to less than 20% [27]. While a subset of patients with the most favorable prognosis can benefit from aggressive concurrent CRT their long-term prognosis is often still poor [28–30]. For the majority of patients, palliative RT can improve symptoms such as dysphagia, especially when combined with stenting procedures.

Gynecologic malignancies

Gynecologic malignancies have been decreasing in incidence in developed countries, but they remain highly prevalent throughout many of the most populous countries of the world. Women with locally advanced gynecologic tumors may suffer from symptoms such as pain, bleeding, foul smelling discharge, and hydronephrosis. RT is the mainstay of treatment for those seeking cure plus PC or for those needing purely palliative RT plus PC. Therefore, the decision to be made for the poorest prognosis patients is whether they may tolerate and benefit from a lengthy course of CRT or whether they should simply receive a course of hypofractionated RT instead, with the sole aim of palliation of their symptoms [31].

Genitourinary cancer

Locally advanced prostate or urinary bladder cancer can cause pain, hematuria, infection, urinary frequency, and urinary retention. RT can improve all of these symptoms, including hematuria associated with locally advanced disease [32,33]. While CRT may be substituted for radical cystectomy in those who are unwilling or unable to undergo surgery, many such patients have significant comorbidities that limit the use of aggressive non-surgical therapy. RT has also proved to be effective in the management of pain in patients with locally advanced hormone resistant prostatic carcinomas [34]. In general, there are very limited data regarding the delineation between therapy which may relieve symptoms and still provide a chance for cure versus treatment that is meant to provide palliation of local symptoms for patients in these situations.

Gastric cancer

For patients with resectable gastric cancer the indicated treatment with curative intent is radical surgery followed by combined post-operative radiochemotherapy [35]. In patients with unresectable gastric tumors, bleeding, pain, and obstructive symptoms are a major concern. RT can achieve palliation of bleeding, dysphagia, and pain with doses that are equivalent or lower than might be offered in curative situations [36].

Colorectal cancer

Locally advanced or recurrent unresectable rectal cancer can cause bleeding, pain, obstruction, and discharge, any of which have a negative impact on the patient's quality of life. Different RT schemes have been implemented either as monotherapy or in combination with chemotherapy providing acceptable rates of symptom alleviation. The dividing line between predominately curative therapy versus palliative therapy is again based on extent of disease and the patient's fitness to tolerate more toxic CRT [37–40].

Advanced head and neck cancers

Head and neck cancers constitute about 2–3% of all cancers in the United States and account for 1–2% of all cancer deaths [41]. Patients with locally advanced disease are usually treated with aggressive/radical (high dose) CRT regimes aiming for cure of their disease and because a higher total dose of RT is needed to maximize the chance of obtaining local control. Patients who fail to gain local control may suffer symptoms such as dysphagia, odynophagia, otalgia, shortness of breath, hoarseness of voice, cough, and weight loss. Patients with significant comorbidities, poor PS, or even metastatic disease merit a more palliative approach or a less demanding RT fractionation [42,43].

Special considerations in developing countries

A major concern regarding RT availability worldwide is that a significant portion of the rise in cancer incidence is occurring in parts of the world where the availability of RT is quite limited [44]. It is estimated that in 2020, approximately 70% of the world cancer incidence will occur in countries of moderate or low income, and that these cases will typically be diagnosed at an advanced stage with most patients in need of palliative treatment [45,46]. In addition to increased RT demand, limited RT capacity due to lack of investment in RT services, lack of organization of health-care systems, lack of screening initiatives, geographic isolation, and other factors in developing countries create a situation where the chances for cure of these tumors are lower and the needs for PC are higher than in developed countries. So, while in developed countries one may debate about which patients with locally advanced tumors are likely to benefit from curative RT, in developing countries the debate may relate to who gets treated and who does not [46]. There is an urgent need for both an expansion of RT facilities in developing countries and a more efficient use of limited resources to avoid circumstances where patients are denied access even to palliative RT treatment.

Conclusion

Patients who are treated with RT commonly have disease circumstances with no clear distinction between curative and palliative goals, especially when factors such as comorbidity, performance status, organ reserve, and prognosis are taken into account. In this chapter, we have highlighted tumor sites where patients with locally advanced disease are offered radical RT despite the knowledge that the chance of cure is going to be low, and hence the treatment is often in essence palliative. Equally, we have highlighted circumstances where radical RT may not be feasible due to either tumor or patient factors, and palliative RT is offered instead. It is also important to emphasize that while treating those with heavy disease burden with curative intent, they also require PC treatment that helps to quell disease symptoms and minimize treatment-related toxicity. Subsequent chapters in this textbook will focus on the details of dose and fractionation for patients whose clinical circumstances demand palliative radiotherapy.

References

1. Kirkbride P, Bezjak A. Therapies with palliative intent. In: Berger AM, Portenoy RK, Weissman DE (eds.) *Principles and Practice of Palliative Care and Supportive Oncology.* Philadelphia: Lippincott Williams & Wilkins, 1998, pp. 685–697.
2. World Health Organization. Cancer pain relief and palliative care: a report of a WHO expert committee. *World Health Organ Tech Rep Ser* 1990; **804**: 1–75.
3. Foley KM, Gelband H. *Improving Palliative Care for Cancer.* Washington, DC: National Research Council. 2001. Available at: http://www.nap.edu/openbook.php?isbn= 0309074029 (accessed August 4, 2012).
4. Smith TJ, Temin S, Alesi ER, *et al.* American society of clinical oncology provisional clinical opinion: the integration of palliative care into standard oncology care. *J Clin Oncol* 2012; **10**(30): 880–887.
5. ASTRO. Scope of Radiation Oncology Practice. 2012. Available at: http://www.astro.org (accessed June 20, 2012).
6. Lutz S, Korytko T, Nguyen J, *et al.* Palliative radiotherapy when is it worth it and when is it not? *Cancer J* 2010; **16**: 473–482.
7. Louis DN, Ohgaki H, Wiestler OD, *et al. WHO Classification of Tumours of the Central Nervous System.* Lyon: IARC, 2007.

8. Gurney JG, Kadan-Lottick N. Brain and other central nervous system tumours; rates, trends, and epidemiology. *Curr Opin Oncol* 2001; **13**: 160–166.

9. De Angelis L, Loeffler JS, Mamelak AN. Primary brain tumours. Chapter 28. In: Pazdur R, Coia LR, Hoskins WJ, Wagman L (eds.) *Cancer Management: A Multidisciplinary Approach*, 8th edn. CMP Healthcare Media, Oncology Publishing Group: Manhasset, NY, 2004, pp. 591–606.

10. Laws ER, Parney IF, Huang W, *et al.* Survival following surgery and prognostic factors for recently diagnosed malignant glioma: data from the Glioma Outcomes Project. *J Neurosurg* 2003; **99**: 467–473.

11. Chan JL, Lee SW, Fraass BA, *et al.* Survival and failure patterns of high grade gliomas after 3-dimensional conformal radiotherapy. *J Clin Oncol* 2002; **20**: 1635–1642.

12. Hegi M, Diserens A, Gorlia T, *et al.* MGMT gene silencing and benefit from temozolomide in glioblastoma. *N Engl J Med* 2005; **352**: 997–1003.

13. McAleese JJ, Stenning SP, Ashley S, *et al.* Hypofractionated radiotherapy for poor prognosis malignant glioma: matched pair survival analysis with MRC controls. *Radiother Oncol* 2003; **67**: 177–182.

14. Evans DB, Abbruzzese JL, Rich TA. Cancer of the pancreas. In: DeVita VT Jr, Hellmann S, Rosenberg SA (eds.) *Cancer, Principles and Practice of Oncology*, 5th edn. Philadelfia: Lippincott William & Wilkins, 1997, pp. 1054–1087.

15. Wichert GV, Seufferlein T, Adler G. Palliative treatment of pancreatic cancer. *J Dig Dis* 2008; **9**: 1–7.

16. Ogawa K, Ito Y, Hirokawa N, *et al.* Concurrent radiotherapy and gemcitabine for unresectable pancreatic adenocarcinoma. Impact of adjuvant chemotherapy on survival. *Int J Radiat Oncol Biol Phys* In press.

17. Golfieri R, Giampalma E, Renzulli M, *et al.* Unresectable hilar cholongiocarcinoma: multimodality approach with prersutaneous treatment associated with radiotherapy and chemotherapy. *In Vivo* 2006; **20**: 757–760.

18. Takamura A, Saito H, Kamada T, *et al.* Intraluminal low-dose-rate 1921r brachytherapy combined with external beam radiotherapy and biliary stenting for unresectable extrahepatic bile duct carcinoma. *Int J Radiat Oncol Biol Phys* 2003; **57**: 1357–1365.

19. Parkin DM, Bray F, Ferlay F, *et al.* Global cancer statistics, 2002. *CA Cancer J Clin* 2005; **55**: 74–108.

20. Kamangar F, Dores GM, Anderson WF. Patterns of cancer incidence, mortality, and prevalence across five continents: defining priorities to reduce cancer disparities in different geographic regions of the world. *J Clin Oncol* 2006; **24**: 2137–2150.

21. Curran WJ Jr, Paulus R, Langer CJ, *et al.* Sequential vs. concurrent chemoradiation for stage III non-small cell lung cancer: randomized phase III trial RTOG 9410. *J Natl Cancer Inst* 2011; **103**: 1452–1460.

22. Albain KS, Swann RS, Rusch VW, *et al.* Radiotherapy plus chemotherapy with or without surgical resection for stage III non-small-cell lung cancer: a phase III randomised controlled trial. *Lancet* 2009; **374**: 379–386.

23. Van Meerbeeck JP, Kramer GW, Van Schil PE, *et al.* Randomized controlled trial of resection versus radiotherapy after induction chemotherapy in stage IIIA-N2 non-small-cell lung cancer. *J Natl Cancer Inst* 2007; **99**: 442–450.

24. Turissi A, Kim K, Blum R, *et al.* Twice-daily compared with once daily thoracic radiotherapy in limited small cell lung cancer treated concurrently with cisplatin and etoposide. *N Engl J Med* 1999; **340**: 265–271.

25. Auperin A, Arriagada R, Pignon J-P, *et al.* Prophylactic cranial irradiation for patients with small cell lung cancer in complete remission: prophylactic Cranial Irradiation Overview Collaborative Group. *N Engl J Med* 1999; **341**: 476–484.

26. Slotman B, Faivre-Finn C, Kramer G, *et al.* Prophylactic cranial irradiation in extensive small-cell lung cancer. *N Engl J Med* 2007; **357**: 664–672.

27. Pisani P, Parkin DM, Bray F, *et al.* Estimates of the worldwide mortality from 25 cancers in 1990. *Int J Cancer* 1999; **83**: 18–29.

28. Ikeda E, Kojima T, Kaneko K, *et al.* Efficacy of concurrent chemoradiotherapy as a palliative treatment in stage IVB esophageal cancer patients with dysphagia. *Jpn J Clin Oncol* 2011; **41**: 969–972.

29. Wong SK, Chiu PW, Leung SF, *et al.* Concurrent chemoradiotherapy or endoscopic stenting for advanced squamous cell carcinoma of esophagus: a case-control study. *Ann Surg Oncol* 2008; **15**: 576–582.

30. Harvey JA, Bessell JR, Beller E, *et al.* Chemoradiation therapy is effective for the palliative treatment of malignant dysphagia. *Dis Esophagus* 2004; **17**: 260–265.

31. Van Lonvhuijzen L, Thomas G. Palliative radiotherapy for cervical carcinoma, a systematic review. *Radiother Oncol* 2011; **98**: 287–291.

32. Scholten AN, Leer JW, Collins CD, *et al.* Hypofractionated radiotherapy for invasive bladder cancer. *Radiother Oncol* 1997; **43**: 163–169.

33. Duchesne GM, Bolger JJ, Griffiths GO, *et al.* A randomized trial of hypofractionated schedules of palliative radiotherapy in the management of bladder carcinoma: results of a Medical Research Council trial BA09. *Int J Radiat Oncol Biol Phys* 2000; **47**: 379–388.

34. Din O, Thanvi N, Ferguson C, *et al.* Palliative prostate radiotherapy for symptomatic advanced prostate cancer. *Radiother Oncol* 2009; **93**: 192–196.

35. Macdonald JS, Smalley SR, Benedetti J, *et al.* Chemoradiotherapy after surgery compared with surgery alone for adenocarcinoma of the stomach or gastroesophageal junction. *N Engl J Med* 2001; **345**: 725–730.

36. Kim MM, Rana V, Janjan NA, *et al.* Clinical benefit of palliative radiation therapy in advanced gastric cancer. *Acta Oncol* 2008; **47**: 421–427.

37. Bal SH, Park W, Choi DH, *et al.* Palliative radiotherapy in patients with symptomatic pelvis mass of metastatic colorectal cancer. *Radiat Oncol* 2011; **6**: 52.

38. Wong CS, Cummings BJ, Brierley JD, *et al.* Treatment of locally recurrent rectal carcinoma results and prognostic factors. *Int J Radiat Oncol Biol Phys* 1998; **40**: 427–435.

39. Lingareddy V, Ahmad NR, Mohiuddin M. Palliative reirradiation for recurrent rectal cancer. *Int J Radiat Oncol Biol Phys* 1997; **38**: 785–790.

40. Ajani JA, Winter KA, Gunderson LL, *et al.* Intergroup RT06 98-11. A phase III randomised study of 5-fluorouracil (5-FU), mitomycin and radiotherapy versus 5FU, cisplatin and radiotherapy in carcinoma of the anal canal. *Proc Am Soc Clin Oncol* 2006; **24**: 4009.

41. Ridge JA, Glisson BS, Horwitz EM, *et al.* Head and Neck tumours. Chapter 4. In: Pazdur R, Coia LR, Hoskins WJ, Wagman L (eds.) *Cancer Management: A Multidisciplinary Approach*, 8th edn. CMP Healthcare Media, Oncology Publishing Group: Manhasset, NY, 2004, pp. 39–86.

42. Al-Mamgani A, Tans L, Van P, *et al.* Hypofractionated radiotherapy denoted as the "Christie scheme": an effective means of palliating patients with head and neck cancers not suitable for curative treatment. *Acta Oncol* 2009; **48**: 562–570.

43. Porcedd SV, Rosser B, Burmeister BH, *et al.* Hypofractionated radiotherapy for the palliation of advanced head and neck cancer in patients unsuitable for curative treatment–"Hypo Trial". *Radiother Oncol* 2007; **85**: 456–462.

44. Barton MB, Frommer M, Shafiq J. Role of radiotherapy in cancer control in low income and middle income countries. *Lancet Oncol* 2006; **7**: 584–595.
45. Mellstedt H. Cancer Initiatives in developing countries. *Ann Oncol* 2006; **17**(suppl): v11124–v11131.
46. Wagner H. Just enough palliation: palliation dose and outcome in Patients with Non Small Cell Lung Cancer. *J Clin Oncol* 2008; **26**: 3920–3922.

CHAPTER 5

Side effects of palliative radiotherapy

Alysa Fairchild

Department of Radiation Oncology, Cross Cancer Institute, University of Alberta, Edmonton, AB, Canada

Introduction

A good palliative intervention should be non-invasive, simple to administer, have a high probability of timely and durable symptom control, little toxicity, minimal patient inconvenience, and be cost-effective [1–3]. Secondary aims include tumor regression and short recovery time [4]. Palliative radiotherapy (RT) should meet all of these criteria, and it additionally may prophylactically address an area with a high likelihood of becoming symptomatic in the near future [3]. RT can positively impact several symptoms simultaneously, such as dyspnea, dysphagia, chest pain, and hemoptysis from an intrathoracic malignancy [5].

The selection of the optimal palliative RT dose depends on individualized considerations of symptom burden, extent of disease, life expectancy, performance status (PS), comorbidities, risk of toxicity, prior treatment, and patient wishes [3,6]. The best schedule balances administration of a sufficient dose to achieve the desired treatment goal while minimizing the risk of side effects [7]. There are many circumstances where single fractions have been proven efficacious; without assurances of improved outcomes, multi-fraction RT in these settings increases the burden of toxicity, time, and transportation on patients and caregivers [8]. If insufficient dose is delivered, disease progression (and its attendant symptoms) will almost always occur.

Factors that contribute to RT toxicity include volume of tissue irradiated, total dose, dose per day (fraction size), concurrent systemic therapy, and radiosensitivity of neighboring normal tissues [9]. Functional comorbidities may also affect the rate of toxicity (e.g. ageing-associated decreases in bone marrow reserve). The predictable side effects of RT, similar to those of chemotherapy, should probably not be described as "complications". This term does

Radiation Oncology in Palliative Cancer Care, First Edition. Edited by Stephen Lutz, Edward Chow, and Peter Hoskin.
© 2013 John Wiley & Sons, Ltd. Published 2013 by John Wiley & Sons, Ltd.

apply, however, if side effects are significant enough to interfere with planned treatment, or are unexpected [9].

Tumors do not have to be completely eradicated in order to improve symptoms, and therefore doses lower than that required for total lesion ablation are used in palliative situations [10]. Additionally, not all known and potential sites of disease are necessarily encompassed within a palliative RT field; small, asymptomatic sites may be excluded to decrease toxicity [11]. The use of an effective, but lower, total dose has several advantages: the risk of acute side effects is minimized; RT can be delivered over fewer days; it is more convenient; there is decreased discomfort with positioning and travel; and it frees resources for treatment of other patients [10].

Acute RT side effects are influenced by the total dose and overall treatment time [8]. They tend to be cumulative, may peak after the RT is finished, and are self-limited. The time frame of acute side effects is generally taken to mean 3 months or less after completion of treatment, although they are most commonly experienced over a period of days or weeks immediately following RT. The toxicity profile of RT has an advantage over systemic therapy in that the deleterious effects are limited to the site of treatment, whereas chemotherapy causes toxicity in several organ systems repetitively after each dose and in an additive fashion after each cycle [8].

Generally, palliative RT is delivered using a higher dose per fraction than would be used in a curative-intent course, and that higher fraction size correlates with risk of late, rather than acute, damage to normal tissues [8]. Large fraction sizes may provide faster onset of relief for some indications, such as tumor-related bleeding [3]. RT dose schedules are chosen to limit the risk of long-term side effects to <5%. By definition, "late" is taken to mean 3 months or more after completion of RT; however, they may in fact occur 6–12 months or longer afterwards. Late side effects are almost always permanent. Although the possibility of late toxicity must be considered in patients with incurable malignancy, many will not live long enough to manifest this [12].

There is no evidence that incidence or severity of side effects correlate with eventual response. Likewise, degree of toxicity does not usually correlate with pre-RT symptom burden, and acute toxicity does not correlate with incidence of late effects.

Issues with interpreting palliative radiotherapy toxicity data

In comparison to curative-intent regimens, there are often less data available on optimization of palliative treatment [11,13]. Retrospective, single-institution chart audits with small patient numbers form much of the available literature, with well-known biases [8]. There is a lack of sound prospective studies examining optimal palliative RT, particularly those reporting toxicity from standard fractionation schedules.

One of the main challenges in interpreting palliative RT toxicity data is determining the methodology of its measurement. Was it reported by the patient or clinician? Was the instrument validated in that population? Was there documentation of baseline symptoms on the same scale to enable comparison? The incidence of toxicity is sensitive to methods used to measure it. For example, dysphagia due to esophageal RT occurred in one study in 13% of patients' quality of life (QoL) questionnaires, 18% of weekly physician ratings, and in 28% of patients' weekly descriptions [6]. Published toxicity data are often derived retrospectively using non-standardized scales [8,14,15], when in fact it can be difficult to distinguish the etiology of post-RT adverse events in patients with significant comorbidities and progressive tumor [16].

There are no specific criteria which can reliably distinguish between symptoms related to tumor progression versus the same ones due to treatment [9]. This uncertainty in causation can result in under- or over-reporting of toxicity depending on interpretation by individual clinicians [6]. Patients, especially those who have exhausted all systemic therapy options, are at risk of disease progression or new sites of disease which may cause symptoms that mimic RT toxicity [17]. Some authors automatically attribute complications to tumor if present at the symptomatic site, while others score all adverse outcomes following RT as treatment-induced, regardless of tumor status [3]. Tumor progression must be ruled out before ascribing worsening symptoms post-treatment to RT toxicity.

What was the median follow-up of the population in relation to the median survival? The incidence of late effects will depend on the proportion of patients still alive and at risk, and whether they are evaluated routinely, investigated based on symptoms, or not followed at all [11].

Finally, RT from different eras is not directly comparable in terms of likelihood of toxicity: older techniques using 2D planning and lower energy machines such as cobalt-60 are much more likely to cause side effects than modern technologies [18].

This chapter will focus on toxicity related to external beam RT only, the most common RT technique used for palliation. Radiopharmaceuticals and brachytherapy are addressed in other chapters.

Acute side effects

General

As it is a localized treatment modality, potential RT side effects are site-specific; the only exception to this is fatigue [12]. Acute side effects of RT are generally mild, self-limited, and controllable with conservative measures (Tables 5.1 and 5.2). Most begin after 1–2 weeks of treatment, although some, such as nausea, may begin within hours of the first fraction. Most will resolve 2–6 weeks after RT is stopped.

Fatigue

Up to 80% of patients undergoing RT describe fatigue, the causes of which are poorly understood [19,20]. RT-related fatigue may be exacerbated by

Table 5.1 Acute and subacute side effects.

Acute

Irradiated Site	Symptom	Incidence %	References
Bone	Pain flare	SF – 7–39 MF – 3–41	[28,57]
Bone	Various	SF – 5–12 MF – 11–18	[57,58]
Bone	Emesis	30–32	[59]
Head & Neck	Skin erythema	Mild – 37§–52*	[4,11]
Head & Neck	Mucositis	Mild or moderate – 44*–63§	[4,11]
Head & Neck	Xerostomia	Mild or moderate – 74*–88§	[4,11]
Head & Neck§	Dysphagia	Mild or moderate – 75	[11]
Head & Neck^	Various	79	[60]
Breast	Moist desquamation	14	[61]
Esophagus‡	Various	Anorexia – 25; Esophagitis – 18; Nausea – 13	[6]
Gastric	Nausea/emesis	Mild or moderate – 12–28	[18]
Gastric	Hepatic enzyme abnormalities	Mild – 3	[7]
Gastric	Anemia	Mild – 73; Moderate – 14	[7,18]
Gastric	Anorexia	Mild or moderate – 12–57	[7,18]
Lung€	Esophagitis	Mild – 34 Moderate or severe – 10	[14]
Bladder	Various	48	[62]
Prostate	Various	Mild – 13; Moderate – 9	[15]

Subacute

Irradiated Site	Symptom	Incidence	References
Whole brain	Somnolence syndrome	Not specified	[21]
Lung	Pneumonitis	2–4	[34]

*Quad Shot = 14 Gy/4 fractions BID for 2 days repeated at 4-weekly intervals a maximum of 3 times.
^Split course with concurrent chemotherapy.
§Hypo trial = 30 Gy/5 twice per week, ≥3 d apart with an optional further 6 Gy boost.
‡40 Gy/20 fractions BID 5 d/week.
€High-dose palliation delivered via split course. Sites irradiated with multi-fraction courses unless indicated. Abbreviations: MF, multi-fraction; SF, single fraction.

Table 5.2 Management of acute side effects.

Symptom/Sign	Management Suggestions	Reference
Fatigue	• Supervised exercise program	[63]
Desquamation	• Good hygiene • Dressings • Topical steroids • Silver sulfadiazine	[12]
Mucositis	• Dietary modifications • Oral rinses – sodium bicarbonate • Anti-fungals – mycostatin • Analgesics in elixir form, viscous xylocaine, "Pink Lady," benzydamine mouthwash • Sucralfate suspension • Fluid supplementation & electrolyte correction	[12,24]
Esophagitis	• Similar to mucositis • Analgesics in elixir form • Treatment of associated acid reflux • Fluid supplementation & electrolyte correction	[1,9]
Pneumonitis	• Prednisone 60–100 mg/day in divided doses	[9]
Nausea/Emesis	• Anti-emetics • H2 blockers • Fluid supplementation & electrolyte correction	[1]
Gastritis	• Antacids • H2 blockers • Anti-emetics • Fluid supplementation & electrolyte correction • Analgesics	[1]
Enteritis	• Fluid supplementation & electrolyte correction • Anti-diarrheals once C difficle ruled out • Anti-emetics • Dietary modifications (low residue, low fat, lactose-free) • Octreotide • Steroids	[1,40]
Proctitis	• Sitz baths • Local measures – hydrocortisone acetate, zinc sulfate, phenylephrine hydrochloride	[12]
Increased intracranial pressure	• Dexamethasone 4–16mg/day in divided doses	[21]

anemia, sleep disorders, psychologic issues, chemotherapy, or hormonal disturbances [19] . Fatigue may occur with treatment of any site and generally improves on its own after a variable and unpredictable time interval. No agent has yet been validated against cancer-related fatigue, although many have been tried, including methylphenidate, modafinil, and guarana [19,21–23].

Hematologic

Hematologic side effects are usually mild and transient, but myelosuppression may occur if the treatment portals are large, the total dose is moderate to high, and a significant proportion of marrow is included, especially in patients who have already received myelosuppressive systemic treatments [24]. Even after hemi-body irradiation (HBI), pancytopenia is transient and not of clinical significance. Thrombocytopenia, leucopenia, and anemia reach a nadir at day 10, but counts can remain low for weeks [20]. Approximately 1/4 of patients will require transfusion support after HBI. Blood counts should be monitored until recovery, however, as patients will be at risk of neutropenic sepsis until the end of that time frame [20].

Skin and bone

Skin toxicity may also occur with treatment of any site, but is limited to the RT fields and usually consists of mild erythema, pruritis, or dry skin [25]. Higher dose to skin may result in desquamation which should be treated similar to sunburns [12]. Alopecia will occur in the irradiated area usually 1–2 weeks after the first dose is delivered. Regrowth of hair in the treated area may take several months, and the texture, color, and amount of hair might not return to normal when it does regrow.

Pain flare is a self-limited worsening of pain in a treated bone metastasis occurring within a week of commencing RT. Its incidence varies from 3–44% and it lasts for a median of 3 days [26]. In order to distinguish pain flare from disease progression, pain scores and analgesic intake must return to baseline after the increase [27]. Pain flare is usually managed by adjusting analgesic dosing. Corticosteroids have shown promise in early phase trials at decreasing pain flare incidence [28]. A large phase III trial investigating the utility of dexamethasone in preventing pain flare is underway (ClinicalTrials.gov identifier NCT01248585).

Although reossification does occur, bone weakened by disease will not be strengthened immediately by RT. It may in fact be temporarily weakened [29]. Post-RT fractures within the treatment field have been reported in up to 18% of patients [24] . In the three bone pain metastases meta-analyses, there were no significant differences in pathologic fracture rates after single- versus multi-fraction regimens (2–3%) [30–32]. However, van der Linden *et al.* suggest that patients with significant axial cortical involvement of the femur be treated with surgery or fractionated radiotherapy rather than a single 8 Gy fraction to diminish the risk of late fracture, based upon the results of the Dutch bone metastases study [33].

Acute toxicity other than pain flare or fracture after bone metastasis RT is mild; there is conflicting evidence as to whether nausea, emesis, and diarrhea are worse after higher dose treatment.

Head and neck

Radiotherapy to the mucosa of the head and neck may induce mucositis which can be associated with odynophagia, dysphagia, dry mouth, taste changes, and pain [25]. Mucosal surfaces should be monitored frequently for secondary infections, with prompt treatment initiated at the earliest sign of bacterial infection or fungal overgrowth.

Thorax

A meta-analysis of 13 randomized controlled trials evaluating different dose-fractionation schedules for palliation of incurable lung cancer included 3473 patients [34]. Dysphagia secondary to esophagitis was the most common acute side effect described, but timing and method of assessment varied. Physician-assessed dysphagia was more common after higher versus lower RT dose (20.5% vs 14.9%; $P = 0.01$), yet pooling of patient self-report data could not be performed [34]. Dysphagia can lead to complications such as malnutrition, dehydration, and aspiration [6].

Palliative thoracic RT may also cause pneumonitis, typically occurring 4–12 weeks after treatment completion [9]. Pneumonitis affected 3.6% of patients after higher dose RT compared with 1.8% of patients who received lower dose in the meta-analysis [34]. Symptoms include acute worsening of dyspnea, cough, and low grade fever, with signs of wheeze, rub, or consolidation. Chest X-ray typically reveals diffuse haziness, loss of the vascular pattern, confluent consolidation or pleural effusion in the RT field. A post-treatment computed tomography scan (CT) of a patient with radiation pneumonitis commonly demonstrates patchy or generalized consolidation [9].

Other acute toxicities of thoracic RT include anorexia, nausea, and lethargy, all of which tend to resolve by 8 weeks after completion of treatment [6]. Pericarditis or pericardial effusion may occur, but are often asymptomatic [9].

Abdomen and pelvis

Irradiation of the liver, stomach, intestine, or pancreas may induce nausea and emesis within hours of the first RT fraction [1]. Malaise and anorexia are very common, affecting up to three-quarters of patients receiving gastric RT [7]. Approximately one-third of patients experience some degree of nausea, especially with large RT volumes [20]. Prophylactic oral anti-emetics (e.g. ondansetron) should be offered 45–60 minutes prior to each fraction and continued on an as-needed basis between fractions.

Gastric RT can result in abdominal pain from gastritis and less commonly reduces acid secretion resulting in dyspepsia and ulcers [1]. RT-induced gastrointestinal (GI) bleed or perforation is very uncommon, although abnormalities of hemoglobin or hepatic enzymes may be seen [7].

Diarrhea related to enteritis can occur when the small or large intestine or rectum are in the radiation path [25]. Enteritis is manifested by abdominal cramping, pain, frequent loose stools, and occasionally bleeding [24]. The risk may be lessened if patients are already receiving high dose opioids. In fact, some patients on opioids welcome enteritis to help their medication-induced constipation. If patients experience RT-induced diarrhea, their stool softeners and laxatives should be held temporarily and patients should be counseled about the use of anti-diarrheal medications.

Along with enteritis, patients receiving RT to the prostate or rectum may experience hematuria, hematochezia, tenesmus, or urgency [1,15]. RT cystitis often responds to increased fluid intake and analgesics, but coexistent infection should be ruled out and actively treated, if present [12].

Central nervous system (CNS)
Partial or whole brain radiation therapy (WBRT)-induced edema often exacerbates pre-existing neurologic symptoms and increases intracranial pressure, if not prevented by corticosteroids [21]. Patients experience mental status or level of consciousness alterations, headache, nausea, emesis, weakness, hearing impairment from otitis media, and possibly seizures [21,35]. In a 2005 meta-analysis, rates of aggregate acute toxicity varied from 8–45% depending on the study, but definitive conclusions were not made because of heterogeneity of data [36]. Anti-epileptic medications are not used prophylactically due to the required dose monitoring and additional side effects.

Subacute somnolence syndrome is infrequent, but patients should be warned that it may occur 2–6 months after RT [35]. This syndrome is characterized by drowsiness, anorexia, and irritability without new focal deficits. It is thought to be due to demyelination, and this constellation of symptoms usually resolve within 2–5 weeks [21].

Late side effects

General
Serious late effects are uncommon after palliative RT, but they should be managed by the treating radiation oncologist [12]. Evaluation and reporting of long-term toxicity is often limited by the short median survival of patients with incurable malignancy [7,18] (Table 5.3).

Fatigue
Up to 60% of patients continue to experience fatigue after RT or chemotherapy has been completed, which may be associated with confusion, inability to concentrate, inability to organize daily activities, neurobehavioral impairment, memory loss, and decreased mental clarity [21,37].

Table 5.3 Late side effects.

Irradiated Site	Symptom	Incidence %	Timeline	References
Bone	Fracture	SF – 2–5 MF – 0.5–18	Median time to fracture: SF – 7 weeks; MF – 20 weeks	[58,59,64,65]
Bone	Various	SF – 4–5 MF – 4–11	NS	[57,58,66]
Head & Neck	Various	Severe to life-threatening – up to 11	NS	[11,67]
Breast	Skin (cosmetic effects)	11	NS	[61]
Esophagus‡	Dysphagia*	5	NS	[6]
Thorax	Pneumonitis	2	NS	[68]
Thorax	Osteoradionecrosis	2	NS	[68]
Thorax	Myelopathy	0.7–3	NS	[68–70]
Large Pelvic fields – SF repeated 3× q3–4 wks	Various	7–45*^	In 1 study, most occurred ≥10 months after RT	[71–74]
Large Pelvic fields – BID split course (q3–6 wks)§	Various	7	NS	[75]
Whole Brain	RT necrosis	Not specified	6 – 24 months	[21]
Whole Brain	Dementia**	0–11*	At 12 months	[38]

*Not related to tumor progression/recurrence.
^Highest incidence from concurrent RT + misonidazole.
**All patients with dementia received non-standard RT due to either fraction size or concurrent radiosensitizer. §44.4 Gy/12 (3.7 Gy BID x 2 days with 3–6 week breaks).
§Hypo trial = 30 Gy/5 2× per week, ≥3 d apart ± further 6 Gy boost (optional).
‡40 Gy/20 fractions BID, ≥6 hrs apart, 5 d/week. Sites irradiated with multi-fraction courses unless indicated. Abbreviations: MS, multi-fraction; NS, not specified; SF, single fraction.

Skin and bone

Late toxicity after palliative bone metastasis RT is rare regardless of dosing schedule. Increased or decreased skin pigmentation may be seen within RT fields. Late fibrosis or dermal atrophy can lead to scarring and telangiectasia. Rarely, alopecia can be permanent.

Thorax

RT delivered to any tubular structure, such as the esophagus, can result in perforation, submucosal fibrosis, mucosal atrophy, stenosis, ulceration, or fistula [1,9]. Pulmonary fibrosis evolves over 6–24 months, causing worsening dyspnea and cough. Chest X-rays show streaky opacification, volume loss, and pleural thickening; historically, demarcation of RT field borders was seen on follow-up radiographic studies. Treatment of pulmonary fibrosis is supportive with no intervention of proven benefit [9]. Cardiomyopathy due to progressive interstitial pericardial fibrosis can decrease ejection fraction, cause conduction defects and coronary artery disease. Cardiomyopathy is virtually never seen following post-palliative RT as it requires 10–20 years to develop [9].

Abdomen and pelvis

Similar to intrathoracic structures, RT to abdominal or pelvic viscera may result in bleeding, ulcers, strictures, fibrosis, ischemia, or fistula [1]. For rectal side effects, as an example, analgesics, suppositories, steroid enemas, and surgical and endoscopic procedures can be considered [1]. RT-induced liver disease is rarely seen after palliative RT.

Central nervous system

Fear of significant toxicity surrounding whole brain radiation therapy stems from historical data from pediatrics and primary brain tumors, neither of which is generalizable to adults with brain metastases [17]. A commonly cited publication from 1989 described 47 patients alive without recurrence 1 year post-WBRT, of which 11% had dementia. However, all of those patients received non-conventional treatment with fraction sizes of >5 Gy or concurrent systemic therapy [38].

Late complications after brain RT can manifest as neurologic deterioration, dementia, or both [35]. Focal post-RT neurologic deficits may be related to perilesional edema, demyelination, radionecrosis, or blood-brain barrier disruption [21]. Necrosis occurs between 6 months and 2 years after treatment, and its presence is suggested by irregular enhancement and surrounding high signal on MRI. Its diagnosis may be difficult to separate from persistent tumor, and therefore it is often made retrospectively after a trial of steroids and/or surgical resection [21]. Diffuse white matter injury can cause lassitude, memory loss, personality change, ataxia, dysarthria, and confusion possibly due to microangiopathy. Magnetic resonance imaging in this setting shows diffuse white matter high signal areas, ventricular dilatation, and cortical atrophy [21]. Neurocognitive changes and endocrine dysfunction may also be seen [8,17,39].

Another symptom related to reversible demyelinating injury is transient myelopathy causing L'hermitte's sign (paresthesias) within 6 months of RT to the cervical or thoracic spinal cord. Paraplegia from late RT myelitis is an irreversible complication secondary to demyelination, necrosis, and vasculopathy [9]. In the palliative thoracic RT meta-analysis, three trials reported confirmed cases of myelopathy. Estimates of incidence rates were <0.5% and did not correlate with RT dose [34].

Second malignancies

The risk of a second cancer after a first diagnosis of lung cancer is 1–2% per patient per year [9]. The risk of a radiation-induced second cancer is <1% and may take up to 20 years to occur.

Additive toxicity

Exacerbation of baseline symptoms due to RT-induced edema may transiently worsen QoL during treatment. Fatigue as a side effect of RT can be additive with that induced by chemotherapy, adrenal insufficiency, or anemia from bone marrow replacement [21]. In some settings, concurrent chemoradiotherapy has been investigated to augment palliation. However, the combination unequivocally worsens toxicity and therefore has not been pursued if there is no improvement in outcomes, such as in WBRT [36]. In esophageal cancer, for example, symptomatic toxicity occurs on average one week earlier when RT is given in conjunction with systemic therapy [1]. Higher proportions of patients cannot complete planned treatment with the concurrent treatment approach, and there is a higher risk of treatment-related death [5]. Even two treatments (e.g. erlotinib plus short course bone metastasis RT) that separately have innocuous side effects can result in fatal toxicity if given concurrently, despite prophylactic supportive medications [40].

Clinical advice

1. Select Appropriate Patients
   Patients who are not likely to benefit from palliative RT, especially those who are not likely to complete the prescribed course, should not be offered treatment [26]. In one retrospective series of 153 patients, 12% discontinued RT prematurely due to clinical deterioration, lack of efficacy, or death [41]. It may take 3–6 weeks to see maximal benefit in many circumstances [8]. So, if a patient has an expected lifespan of <1 month, he or she will not likely live long enough to benefit, but may still experience acute toxicity which can worsen QoL. The only absolute way to prevent RT toxicity is not to give RT. There are clinical settings in which RT should be omitted entirely in favor of supportive care, described in a review by Lutz *et al.* [26]. However, disease progression causing worsening of symptoms should be expected.
2. Prevent Toxicity When Possible
   The RT treatment position is, with few exceptions, supine. Supportive care should be provided to maximize comfort with both transportation and RT positioning, such as pre-medication for breakthrough pain, oxygen for

orthopnea, and anxiolytics for anxiety. Medical management of baseline symptoms should be maximized prior to RT start.

Patients should be warned about the incidence and timeline of predictable RT side effects, and toxicity should be prevented when possible. This approach includes pre-treatment consultations to optimize baseline status and QoL, such as clinical nutrition. For example, Kassam *et al.* recommend prophylactic insertion of feeding tubes prior to esophageal RT for patients who can only swallow liquids [6]. Occupational therapy can provide customized comfort measures such as a sling or a walker.

Up to 40% of patients will experience pain flare subsequent to RT for bone metastasis. In general, patients informed of this possibility are not concerned by this experience. Otherwise, pain flare can have a pronounced effect both physically and psychosocially, and patients overwhelmingly prefer prophylaxis to management with increased pain medications [42].

Dexamethasone has been used to prevent RT-induced side effects including nausea, emesis, and worsening of neurologic symptoms. It should be strongly considered for symptomatic patients just prior to the first fraction for brain metastases, spinal cord compression, and RT to the abdomen. It is presently being investigated for prevention of pain flare after single fraction RT for bone metastasis. The half-life of dexamethasone is at least 36 hours, and it has analgesic and anti-emetic properties. It also has an extensive side effect profile which must be taken into account, and routine concurrent gastric protection should be considered when initiating dexamethasone. The goal should be to maintain patients on the lowest effective steroid dose possible, avoiding concurrent medications such as nonsteroidal anti-inflammatory drugs which increase the risk of gastrointestinal toxicity. A dose taper should start within 2–3 days after RT is completed, presuming stable symptoms.

3. Monitor Ongoing Need for Supportive Care

   Measurement of post-RT toxicity, especially when identical to pre-existing tumor-induced symptoms, is challenging. Best post-treatment response must be compared with symptom burden at baseline. To obtain a complete picture of the impact of RT, one should measure symptom control, toxicity, QoL, PS, and analgesic requirements [11]. The same scale should be utilized prior to and following treatment. Another option is to employ a composite endpoint such as percent net symptom relief; the ratio between the duration of symptom relief and survival × 100 represents the proportion of remaining life spent with relief of the index symptom [18]. Patients should be monitored for evolution of RT response and resolution of side effects so that analgesics and other medications can be appropriately titrated.

4. Monitor Disease Progression *versus* Radiation Toxicity

   Do not assume that symptom worsening after treatment is due to RT toxicity. For example, while pneumonia may be related to RT, it may also be a consequence of airways obstructed by disease, due to chronic obstructive pulmonary disease (COPD), or neutropenia related to chemotherapy [9]. Worsening quality of life after WBRT is more likely to be related to poor tumor control than to therapy [8,43].

New technologies

Careful treatment planning using modern three-dimensional techniques allows precise tumor coverage while limiting the volume of normal tissue irradiated. A Canadian study recently compared patients treated after 2D (historical) versus 3D CT-guided planning for bone metastases [44]. There was no statistical difference in post RT symptom scores although more patients reported improved pain and fatigue after 3D RT. The proportion of patients agreeing that RT was worthwhile was identical in both groups [44].

There are few studies investigating advanced RT delivery such as intensity-modulated RT (IMRT), tomotherapy, stereotactic radiosurgery (SRS), and stereotactic body RT (SBRT) for palliative indications. Most hypothetical gains with newer technologies relate to decreased volumes of critical tissue irradiated, decreasing side effect severity and frequency [1,15]. One series of 57 patients treated with IMRT with median dose of 20 Gy/5 reported more homogeneous tumor doses and less irradiation of adjacent normal tissues [12]. SRS for brain metastases is well-tolerated with little toxicity, and may avoid the need for surgery and its complications [17,45]. Single- and multiple-fraction SBRT have been used for spinal and paraspinal lesions, liver metastases, and re-irradiation, with promising results [16,46,47]. Tomotherapy utilized for the treatment of bone metastases produced no acute toxicity in a series of 20 patients [48].

The potential gains in side effects, however, may be outweighed by cost, resource use, need for specialized equipment, and laborious set-up and treatment. A steep institutional learning curve does affect toxicity rates, especially initially [16]. The additional advantages of newer technologies may not be relevant in palliative settings [8].

Challenges in developing countries

In developing countries, a higher priority may be given to basic health-care needs such as antibiotics, vaccines, clean water, and adequate nutrition [49,50]. Limited resources may translate into high patient loads, long waits for therapy, and inadequate numbers of physicians [51,52]. These challenges may preclude institution of definitive-intent treatment for many cancers. In practical terms, therefore, the main clinical problem is often palliation of symptoms rather than cure [50,53,54].

Symptoms from disease and toxicity from treatment may be more difficult to manage in countries where supportive care lags. Health-care provider knowledge varies with geographic location [49,50]. Deandrea *et al.* reviewed 26 studies investigating adequacy of cancer pain management. After adjusting for potential confounders, year of publication, low gross national income per capita, and setting of care were each associated with a higher proportion of undertreatment [55]. Barriers to adequate symptom control are reviewed by Mitera *et al.* [56].

An International Atomic Energy Agency publication illustrates differences in management in resource-poor countries [53]. This prospective multi-center randomized clinical trial accrued 219 patients from Brazil, China, Croatia, India, South Africa, and Sudan to investigate palliation of esophageal obstruction. Lack of available radiology infrastructure resulted in patients being relatively understaged at study entry, and symptom progression was not radiologically investigated. Discovery of toxicity was incidental at the time of follow-up endoscopy. RT was delivered with cobalt-60 in 85% of patients and 98% were planned two dimensionally. Actuarial dilatation rate was 20% at 400 days' follow-up, with a 25% rate of fistula, 15% stent placement and 10% rate of stricture. There were 3% treatment-related deaths [53].

Conclusion

Incidence and severity of acute and late toxicity are important components in evaluating whether an intervention provides good palliation. Concerns regarding RT-related morbidity must be weighed against baseline deficits, and likelihood and timeline of disease progression. Acute side effects are generally mild, reversible, and self-limited, while late side effects, although permanent, are less common in a patient population with a limited expected survival.

References

1. Howell D. The role of radiation therapy in the palliation of gastrointestinal malignancies. *Gastroenterol Clin North Am* 2006; **35**: 125–130.
2. Chow E, Wong R, Hruby G, *et al.* Prospective patient-based assessment of effectiveness of palliative radiotherapy for bone metastases in an outpatient radiotherapy clinic. *Radiother Oncol* 2001; **61**: 77–82.
3. Smith S, Koh WJ. Palliative radiation therapy for gynaecological malignancies. *Best Pract Res Clin Obstet Gyne* 2001; **15**: 265–278.
4. Corry J, Peters L, D'Costa I, *et al.* The 'QUAD SHOT': a phase II study of palliative radiotherapy for incurable head and neck cancer. *Radiother Oncol* 2005; **77**: 137–142.
5. Harvey J, Bessell J, Beller E, *et al.* Chemoradiation therapy is effective for the palliative treatment of malignant dysphagia. *Dis Esophagus* 2004; **17**: 260–265.
6. Kassam Z, Wong R, Ringash J, *et al.* A phase I/II study to evaluate the toxicity and efficacy of accelerated fractionation radiotherapy for the palliation of dysphagia from carcinoma of the esophagus. *Clin Oncol* 2008; **20**: 53–60.
7. Sun J, Sun YH, Zeng ZC, *et al.* Consideration of the role of radiotherapy for abdominal lymph node metastases in patients with recurrent gastric cancer. *Int J Radiat Oncol Biol Phys* 2010; **77**: 384–391.

8. Lutz S, Chow E, Hartsell W, *et al.* A review of hypofractionated palliative radiotherapy. *Cancer* 2007; **109**: 1462–1470.

9. Spiro S, Douse J, Read C, Janes S. Complications of lung cancer treatment. *Semin Respir Crit Care Med* 2008; **29**: 302–318.

10. Kirkbride P, Barton R. Palliative radiation therapy. *J Palliat Med* 1999; **2**: 87–97.

11. Porceddu S, Rosser B, Burmeister B, *et al.* Hypofractionated radiotherapy for the palliation of advanced head and neck cancer in patients unsuitable for curative treatment – "Hypo Trial." *Radiother Oncol* 2007; **85**: 456–462.

12. Samant R, Gooi A. Radiotherapy basics for family physicians: potential tool for symptom relief. *Can Fam Physician* 2005; **51**: 1496–1501.

13. Hodson D, Bruera E, Eapen L, *et al.* The role of palliative radiotherapy in advanced head and neck cancer. *Can J Oncol* 1996; **6**: 54 60.

14. Metcalfe S, Milano M, Bylund K, *et al.* Split-course palliative radiotherapy for advanced non-small cell lung cancer. *J Thorac Oncol* 2010; **5**: 185–190.

15. Din O, Thanvi N, Ferguson C, *et al.* Palliative prostate radiotherapy for symptomatic advanced prostate cancer. *Radiother Oncol* 2009; **93**: 192–196.

16. Gomez D, Hunt M, Jackson A, *et al.* Low rate of thoracic toxicity in palliative paraspinal single-fraction stereotactic body radiation therapy. *Radiother Oncol* 2009; **93**: 414 418.

17. Oldenburg N. The role of palliative radiation in the management of brain, spinal cord, and bone metastases. *Med Health R I* 2006; **89**: 59–62.

18. Tey J, Back M, Shakespeare T, *et al.* The role of palliative radiation therapy in symptomatic locally advanced gastric cancer. *Int J Radiat Oncol Biol Phys* 2007; **67**: 385–388.

19. Miranda V, Trufelli D, Santos J, *et al.* Effectivness of guarana (Paullinia cupana) for postradiation fatigue and depression: results of a pilot double-blind randomized study. *J Altern Complement Med* 2009; **15**: 431–433.

20. Bashir F, Parry J, Windsor P. Use of a modified hemi-body irradiation technique for metastatic carcinoma of the prostate: report of a 10-year experience. *Clin Oncol* 2008; **20**: 591–598.

21. Taillibert S, Delattre J-Y. Palliative care in patients with brain metastases. *Curr Opin Oncol* 2005; **17**: 588–592.

22. Bruera E, Driver L, Valero V, *et al.* Patient controlled methylphenidate for cancer-related fatigue: a randomized controlled trial. *Proc Am Soc Clin Oncol* 2005; **23**: 740S.

23. Morrow G, Gillis L, Hickok J, *et al.* The positive effect of the psychostimulant modafinil on fatigue from cancer that persists after treatment is completed. *Proc Am Soc Clin Oncol* 2005; **23**: 732S.

24. Frassica DA. General principles of external beam radiation therapy for skeletal metastases. *Clin Orthop Relat Res* 2003; **415S**: S158–S164.

25. Tanner C. Palliative radiation therapy for cancer. *J Palliat Med* 2011; **14**: 672–673.

26. Lutz S, Korytko T, Nguyen J, *et al.* Palliative radiotherapy: when is it worth it and when is it not? *Cancer J* 2010; **16**: 473–482.

27. Chow E, Ling A, Davis L, *et al.* Pain flare following external beam radiotherapy and meaningful change in pain scores in the treatment of bone metastases. *Radiother Oncol* 2005; **75**: 64–69.

28. Hird A, Chow E, Zhang L, *et al.* Determining the incidence of pain flare following palliative radiotherapy for symptomatic bone metastases: results from three Canadian cancer centres. *Int J Radiat Oncol Biol Phys* 2009; **75**: 193–197.

29. Dijkstra S, Wiggers T, van Geel BN, *et al.* Impending and actual pathological fractures in patients with bone metastases of the long bones. A retrospective study of 233 surgically treated fractures. *Eur J Surg* 1994; **160**: 535–542.

30. Chow E, Harris K, Fan G, *et al*. Palliative radiotherapy trials for bone metastases: a systematic review. *J Clin Oncol* 2007; **25**: 1423–1436.

31. Sze WM, Shelley M, Held I, *et al*. Palliation of metastatic bone pain: single fraction versus multifraction radiotherapy – a systematic review of randomized trials. *Clin Oncol* 2003; **15**: 345–352.

32. Wu J, Wong R, Johnston M, *et al*. Meta-analysis of dose-fractionation radiotherapy trials for the palliation of painful bone metastases. *Int J Radiat Oncol Biol Phys* 2003; **55**: 594–605.

33. Van Der Linden YM, Kroon HM, Dijkstra SP, *et al*. Simple radiographic parameter predicts fracturing in metastatic femoral bone lesions: results from a randomised trial. *Radiother Oncol* 2003; **69**: 21–31.

34. Fairchild A, Harris K, Barnes E, *et al*. Palliative thoracic radiotherapy for lung cancer: a systematic review. *J Clin Oncol* 2009; **26**: 4001–4011.

35. Hoegler D. Radiotherapy for palliation of symptoms in incurable cancer. *Curr Probl Cancer* 1997; **21**(3): 134–183.

36. Tsao MN, Lloyd NS, Wong RK, *et al*. Radiotherapeutic management of brain metastases: a systematic review and meta-analysis. *Cancer Treat Rev* 2005; **31**: 256–273.

37. Lower E, Fleishman S, Cooper A, *et al*. A phase III randomized placebo-controlled trial of the safety and efficacy of d-MPH as new treatment of fatigue and 'chemobrain' in adult cancer patients. *Proc Am Soc Clin Oncol* 2005; **23**: 551S.

38. DeAngelis L, Delattre JY, *et al*. Radiation-induced dementia in patients cured of brain metastases. *Neurology* 1989; **39**: 789–786.

39. Schultheiss T, Kun L, Ang K, *et al*. Radiation response of the central nervous system. *Int J Radiat Oncol Biol Phys* 1995; **31**: 1093–1112.

40. Silvano G, Lazzari G, Lovecchio M, *et al*. Acute and fatal diarrhea after erlotinib plus abdominal palliative hypofractionated radiotherapy in a metastatic non-small cell lung cancer patient: a case report. *Lung Cancer* 2008; **61**: 270–273.

41. Van Oorschot B, Schuler M, Simon A, *et al*. Patterns of care and course of symptoms in palliative radiotherapy. *Strahlenther Onkol* 2011; **187**: 461–466.

42. Presutti R, Hird A, DeAngelis C, *et al*. Pain flare following palliative radiotherapy of bone metastases. In: Sahgal A, Chow E, Merrick J (eds.) *Bone and Brain Metastases: Advances in Research and Treatment*. London England: Nova Publishers, 2010, pp. 105–115.

43. Yaneva M, Semerdjieva M. Assessment of the effect of palliative radiotherapy for cancer patients with intracranial metastases using EORTC-QOL-C30 questionnaire. *Folia Med* 2006; **98**: 23–29.

44. Pope K, Bezjak A, McLean M, *et al*. Do modern radiotherapy techniques impact on the effectiveness and toxicity of palliative radiotherapy? *Support Care Cancer* 2010; **18**(Suppl 3): S85, Abstr 03-016.

45. Papaleo A, Russo D, Adriana P, *et al*. Stereotactic radiotherapy for the treatment of brain metastases. *Radiother Oncol* 2011; **99**: S377.

46. Ambrosino G, Constantin G, Polistina F, *et al*. Stereotactic body radiotherapy in patients with unresectable hepatocellular carcinoma. Preliminary results and comparison with other palliative treatments. *J Hepatol* 2011; **54**: S259.

47. Nelson J, Yoo D, Sampson J, *et al*. Stereotactic body radiotherapy for lesions of the spine and paraspinal regions. *Int J Radiat Oncol Biol Phys* 2009; **73**: 1369–1375.

48. Franco P, Sciacero P, Catuzzo P, *et al*. TomoDirect: an efficient mean to deliver palliative radiotherapy with discrete angles tomotherapy for skeletal metastases. *Radiother Oncol* 2011; **99**: 378.

49. Davis M, Walsh D. Epidemiology of cancer pain and factors influencing poor pain control. *Am J Hosp Palliat Med* 2004; **21**: 137–142.

50. Koshy R, Rhodes D, Devi S, *et al*. Cancer pain management in developing countries: a mosaic of complex issues resulting in inadequate analgesia. *Support Care Cancer* 1998; **6**: 430–437.

51. Potter V, Wiseman C, Dunn S, *et al*. Patient barriers to optimal cancer control. *Psychoon-cology* 2003; **12**: 153–160.

52. Randall-David E, Wright J, *et al*. Barriers to cancer pain management: home-health and hospice nurses and patients. *Support Care Cancer* 2003; **11**: 660–665.

53. Rosenblatt E, Jones G, Sur R, *et al*. Adding external beam to intra-luminal brachytherapy improves palliation in obstructive squamous cell esophageal cancer: a prospective multi-centre randomized trial of the International Atomic Energy Agency. *Radiother Oncol* 2010; **97**: 488–494.

54. De Lima L. Advances in palliative care in Latin America and the Caribbean: ongoing projects of the Pan American Health Organization. *J Palliat Med* 2001; **4**: 228–231.

55. Deandrea S, Montanari M, Moja L, *et al*. Prevalence of undertreatment in cancer pain A review of published literature. *Ann Oncol* 2008; **19**: 1985–1991.

56. Mitera G, Zeiadin N, Kirou-Mauro A, *et al*. Retrospective assessment of cancer pain management in an outpatient palliative radiotherapy using the pain management index. *J Pain Symptom Manage* 2010; **39**: 259–267.

57. Roos D, Turner S, O'Brien P, *et al*. Randomized trial of 8Gy in 1 versus 20Gy in 5 fractions of radiotherapy for neuropathic pain due to bone metastases (Trans-Tasman Radiation Oncology Group, TROG 96.05). *Radiother Oncol* 2005; **75**: 54–63.

58. Hartsell W, Konski A, Scott C, *et al*. Randomized trial of short versus long-course radiotherapy for palliation of painful bone metastases. *J Natl Cancer Inst* 2005; **97**: 798–804.

59. Bone pain Trial Working Party. 8Gy single fraction radiotherapy for the treatment of metastatic skeletal pain: randomised comparison with a multifraction schedule over 12 months of patient follow-up. *Radiother Oncol* 1999; **52**(2): 111–121.

60. Minatel E, Gigante M, Granchin G, *et al*. Combined radiotherapy and bleomycin in patients with inoperable head and neck cancer with unfavourable prognostic factors and severe symptoms. *Oral Oncol* 1998; **34**: 119–122.

61. Dulley L, Li S, Ah-See M. Efficacy of hypofractionated palliative radiotherapy in locally advanced breast cancer. *Clin Oncol* 2011; **23**: S35–S36, Abstr P29.

62. Spagnoletti G, De Nobili G, Marchese R, *et al*. Palliative radiotherapy for bladder cancer: a small retrospective study. Proceedings of the Italian Society of Uro-Oncology 2010; 1515, Abstr 243.

63. Rorth M, Andersen C, Quist M, *et al*. Health benefits of a multidimensional exercise program for cancer patients undergoing chemotherapy. *Proc Am Soc Clin Oncol* 2005; **23**: 731S.

64. Tong D, Gillick L, Hendrickson F. The palliation of symptomatic osseous metastases: final results of the study by the Radiation Therapy Oncology Group. *Cancer* 1982; **50**(5): 893–899.

65. Steenland E, Leer JW, van Houwelingen H, *et al*. The effect of a single fraction compared to multiple fractions on painful bone metastases: a global analysis of the Dutch Bone Metastasis Study. *Radiother Oncol* 1999; **52**(2): 101–109.

66. Kaasa S, Brenne E, Lund J-A, *et al*. Prospective randomised multicenter trial on single fraction radiotherapy (8Gy x 1) versus multiple fractions (3Gy x 10) in the treatment of painful bone metastases. *Radiother Oncol* 2006; **79**: 278–284.

67. Erkal H, Mendenhall W, Amdur R, *et al.* Squamous cell carcinomas metastatic to cervical lymph nodes from an unknown head and neck mucosal site treated with radiation therapy with palliative intent. *Radiother Oncol* 2001; **59**: 319–321.
68. Quddus A, Kerr G, Price A, Gregor A. Long-term survival in patients with non-small cell lung cancer treated with palliative radiotherapy. *Clin Oncol* 2001; **13**: 95–98.
69. Macbeth F, Wheldon T, Girling T, *et al.* Radiation myelopathy: estimates of risk in 1048 patients in three randomized trials of palliative radiotherapy for non-small cell lung cancer. *Clin Oncol* 1996; **8**: 176–181.
70. Harrington C, James M, Wynne C. Radiation myelopathy after 36Gy in 12 fractions palliative chest radiotherapy for squamous cell cancer of the lung: case report and review of published studies. *Clin Oncol* 2010; **22**: 561–563.
71. Boulware R, Caderao J, Delclos L, *et al.* Whole pelvis megavoltage irradiation with single doses of 1000 rad to palliative advanced gynecologic cancers. *Int J Radiat Oncol Biol Phys* 1979; **5**: 333–338.
72. Halle J, Rosenman J, Varia M, *et al.* 1000cGy single dose palliation for advanced carcinoma of the cervix or endometrium. *Int J Radiat Oncol Biol Phys* 1986; **12**: 1947–1950.
73. Spanos W, Wasserman T, Meoz R, *et al.* Palliation of advanced pelvic malignant disease with large fraction pelvic radiation and misonidazole: final report of RTOG phase I/II study. *Int J Radiat Oncol Biol Phys* 1987; **13**: 1479–1482.
74. Spanos W, Clery M, Perez C, *et al.* Late effects of multiple daily fraction palliation schedule for advanced pelvic malignancies (RTOG 8502). *Int J Radiat Oncol Biol Phys* 1994; **29**: 961–967.
75. Spanos W, Perez C, Marcus S, *et al.* Effect of rest interval on tumor and normal tissue response–a report of phase III study of accelerated split course palliative radiation for advanced pelvic malignancies (RTOG-8502). *Int J Radiat Oncol Biol Phys* 1993; **25**(3): 399–403.

General principles of palliation and symptom control

CHAPTER 6

A history of hospice and palliative medicine

Michelle Winslow[1], Marcia Meldrum[2]
[1]Academic Unit of Supportive Care, University of Sheffield, South Yorkshire, UK
[2]Center for Health Services and Society, University of California, Los Angeles, CA, USA

Introduction

Organized care for the dying is centuries old, yet hospice care as we understand it today is relatively new. Modern hospice care began to take shape in England in the late 1950s, and Dame Cicely Saunders is recognized as the pivotal figure in the growth of the modern hospice, both in the UK and worldwide. However, the seeds of the modern hospice movement go further back in time and have been shaped by multiple influences. This chapter considers the historical development of end-of-life care, focusing on the two countries most influential in its development, the United Kingdom and United States.

Before the modern movement

Traditional hospices date back to early Christianity and led to the development of the first European hospitals in the Middle Ages. Medieval hospices, run by religious orders, were places of shelter and care for the poor, the sick, and the friendless traveler; care of the dying was part of a spectrum of care. Until the late 19th century, the dying most often received care at home, rather than in hospices. Clare Humphries, in her study of the development of English hospices in England 1878–1914, proposed that late 19th-century homes dedicated to the care of the dying were precursors to the modern hospice. For the first time, qualified people in an institutional setting provided specialized care to the dying. Humphries highlights Christian commitment as the major influence in the development of hospices and terminal care [1].

The 1905 opening of St. Joseph's Hospice for the Dying in Hackney, East London, highlighted a shift in attitudes; for the first time, the dying poor were

Radiation Oncology in Palliative Cancer Care, First Edition. Edited by Stephen Lutz, Edward Chow, and Peter Hoskin.
© 2013 John Wiley & Sons, Ltd. Published 2013 by John Wiley & Sons, Ltd.

perceived as needing special medical, nursing, and spiritual care. A few Victorian physicians and a fragile institutional commitment supported the new model, also exemplified by three other London homes: The Friedenheim and the House of God, both run on Anglican principles; and St. Luke's House, a Methodist home [2]. Humphries argues that these hospices were small, isolated attempts to perpetuate a tradition of pastoral care at risk of erosion by wider social, medical, and religious changes. Yet they laid the foundations of modern hospice [1].

St. Joseph's Hospice, in particular, grew from its modest origins in 1905 into a modern facility for hospice and palliative care, education, and research, which inspired global interest and was the setting for Cicely Saunders' early pain research [2]. For 7 years in Hackney, Saunders developed her ideas and strategies for palliative care, recording conversations with patients about matters that concerned them, and using these as the basis for a revolutionary new practice and philosophy. She coupled an emphasis on pain prevention rather than alleviation, exemplified by the regular giving of relief, with a thorough understanding of available analgesia. She advocated the use of heroin and the Brompton Cocktail mixture of morphine and gin to treat pain and maintain quality of life until its end. By 1964, Saunders introduced her concept of "total pain," which integrated physical symptoms, mental distress, social problems, and emotional difficulties [3].

The Second World War had created an unprecedented opportunity for a few clinicians on both sides of the Atlantic to advance pain management. The Harvard anesthesiologist Henry Beecher argued that pain was a combination of physical sensation and cognitive and emotional reaction, while at Memorial Sloan-Kettering in New York, Raymond Houde and Ada Rogers used crossover trials to individualize analgesic research with cancer patients [4,5]. In Washington State, John Bonica's interest in the clinical management of pain also developed from his work with soldiers injured in war, who presented complex pain problems difficult to solve with existing tools [6]. Bonica's definitive work *The Management of Pain* (1953) brought together information about its etiology, diagnosis, and treatment [7]. As a practitioner, Bonica promoted the use of therapeutic nerve blocks, enabling physicians to manage difficult pain problems without the need for surgery; he supported regular opiate giving and dismissed the idea that addiction was an obstacle to prescribing in late stage disease. William Livingston in Oregon, Duncan Alexander in Texas, and Mark Swerdlow in Manchester (UK) were also working with these methods [4].

Within this pioneering pain research environment, Cicely Saunders planned her model of hospice care and defined a holistic concept of management focused on the individual patient's "total pain."

St. Christopher's and the modern hospice

Although several individuals contributed to the development of the modern hospice movement in the UK, it was Cicely Saunders who emerged as the catalyst. Beginning outside the formal structure of the National Health Service, hospice expanded relatively quickly into mainstream service provision. In the 1960s, the three leading causes of death in the UK were circulatory disease, respiratory disease, and cancer. Twenty percent of the population died before age 65, most while being cared for at home [8].

In 1967, Saunders and her collaborators opened the first modern hospice, St. Christopher's in Sydenham. In its early days, St. Christopher's carried out major studies that changed the nature of palliative care, demonstrating better methods of pain control and the safety and efficacy of strong opioids [9]. Saunders and her team also developed new strategies for action in service delivery, with major involvement of volunteers and fundraisers. St. Christo pher's brought hospice into mainstream medicine. Clark and colleagues note that, within a decade of its opening, health professions had come to accept that the principles of hospice could be practiced in acute hospital units, as well as in specialist facilities and by home and day care services [10].

The St. Christopher's model inspired a wave of local hospice development in the UK in the 1970s and 1980s, characterized by adherence to Saunders' principles, extensive use of volunteers, and dynamic fundraising. Proponents asserted that the public wanted a more personalized, less institutionalized approach to end-of-life care [11]. The second modern hospice, St. Luke's in Sheffield, opened in 1971 [10]. Its first Medical Director, Eric Wilkes, later opened the UK's first day hospice, a model replicated throughout the country, and in the 1990s the multi-disciplinary Trent Palliative Care Centre – a research and educational unit attached to St. Luke's. During the 1980s, new hospices, funded by local communities, appeared at a rate of 10 a year. However, new hospices grew in a haphazard manner, without cohesion or uniformity. Medical cover was mostly provided by GPs who were committed but who lacked skills in end-of-life care.

Eric Wilkes expressed concern about this rapid and uncoordinated growth spurt in the famous "Wilkes Report" [12]; themes later developed in "No Second Chance: A discussion document for the Trent Regional Health Authority on the development of terminal care services" [13]. In 1984, with the Duchess of Norfolk, Peter Quilliam, and Cicely Saunders, Eric Wilkes founded Help the Hospices, a national charity that stressed the need for better symptom management and communication skills within hospices. With the support of the Minister of Health, he organized meetings between independent hospices, NHS units, and major charities, uniting them in the National Council for Palliative Care [14].

In 1986, the Association for Palliative Medicine (APM) of Great Britain and Ireland was established to support the development of specialty training in palliative care [15], and this was the probable catalyst for the growth of other British and Irish professional associations in the field [10]. In 1987, the United Kingdom became the first country in the world to recognize palliative medicine as a medical specialty. Shortly afterwards, a 4-year training program in the new discipline was established for senior registrars [15]. Since then, community palliative care services, hospital palliative care teams, and day-hospice units have forged new links between community, hospice, and hospital care, and between the NHS and the voluntary sector. All medical and nursing schools in the UK now have dedicated palliative care teaching and an End-of-Life Care Strategy has been announced by the Department of Health. Since 1995, the development of cancer services following the publication of the Calman–Hine Report has given further impetus to specialist palliative care integrated with cancer services. In particular, this has led to a rapid and continuing expansion in consultant posts.

The extent to which the hospice movement has progressed in the UK since the opening of St. Christopher's Hospice in 1967 can be seen in figures for palliative care provision 2011–2012, presented by Help the Hospices. Today there are 220 hospice and palliative care inpatient units; 3175 hospice and palliative care beds; 288 home care services; 127 Hospice at Home services; 272 day care centres; 343 hospital support services. Services for children are also developing – 42 hospice inpatient units have been established with 334 hospice beds [16].

Palliative care in the United States

Terminal-care homes under religious auspices have existed in the United States since the 19th century; examples include Calvary Hospital in New York, Youville Hospital in Cambridge, Massachusetts, and the seven homes of the Order of Sister Rose Hawthorne [17]. By the 1970s, however, most patients died in hospitals or in nursing homes, where the standard of care was extremely varied. The nursing home was often understaffed and tried to keep patients clean and well-fed, but had inadequate standards for pain management and rarely provided spiritual or psychosocial services. Skilled nursing facilities offered a higher standard of technical care, but not necessarily other services.

The first modern US hospice was founded in 1974 in New Haven by Florence S. Wald (1917–2008), associate clinical professor of nursing at Yale, who had begun studying the British hospice movement after Cicely Saunders' visit there in 1963. Wald began an interdisciplinary study group, which sent many visitors to St. Christopher's after it opened in 1969. She launched a home palliative care program in March 1974 and raised funds to build a 44-bed inpatient facility, The Connecticut Hospice, in Branford [18,19]. By 1975, her work and Saunders' had inspired three other home-based hospice services and one inpatient palliative care service (St. Luke's in New York) in the United States. Drawing on Saunders' concepts, Wald described palliative care as positive, not a last resort, quoting one patient: "Even when you're dying, you fight all the more to live [17]."

Some of the first US articles on St. Christopher's Hospice appeared in nursing journals in 1974–1975, and nurses were pioneers in the hospice movement nationally. In 1976, the National Cancer Institute (NCI) requested proposals for 3-year contracts to build demonstration hospices, including a free-standing facility and home care. By 1978, Wald was able to identify four different "models" and one quasi-model of palliative care operating in the United States: 1) a free-standing open system with home care (Hospice Inc.); 2) a home health agency offering both home and inpatient care (Hospice of Marin, California); 3) a hospital-based interdisciplinary team providing day care in both hospital and home (St. Luke's, New York City); 4) an inpatient unit based on Canada's Royal Victoria Model, using volunteers and nurses from the Visiting Nurse Association (Green Bay, Wisconsin). The quasi-model was Elizabeth Kubler-Ross' teaching center, Shanti Nilaya, in Escondido, California, founded in 1977, which provided "special programs" for dying patients and their families [20]. Osterweis and Champagne identified two other models in 1979: hospitals providing home care services and special nurse "advocates." "Each of these has evolved out of the needs and resources of the local community [21]." Funding for these programs came largely from private foundations, with some support from NCI. A few hospitals were able to negotiate Blue Cross coverage to provide home care for terminal patients.

By 1979, the National Hospice Organization (NHO) had developed a set of "widely accepted" standards of care. Soon after, in 1984, the JCAH (Joint Commission for the Accreditation of Hospitals, the national accrediting body) developed a set of "measurable outcome" standards and a voluntary accreditation process for hospices. In 1988, the Academy of Hospice Physicians was founded and soon began offering certifying exams in palliative care. By the 1980s, "the hospice movement" was receiving a good deal of media attention. There was considerable debate over the high costs of labor-intensive palliative care; the British model made extensive use of volunteers, but US hospices relied more on professionals. Critics also questioned the "exclusion" of patients from "mainstream medicine" and their primary care physicians. American medicine traditionally placed a high value on aggressive measures to preserve life as long as possible; patients transferred to hospice were seen as being denied both hope and the highest quality care [22]. Some US programs, notably the Pain and Palliative Care Unit at the NIH Clinical Center, established by Dr. Ann Berger in 2000, expanded the concept to provide symptom relief, patient and family education, and "humanistic, not cellular" care to patients undergoing stressful experimental treatments for life-threatening and chronic diseases [23].

US hospice growth increased exponentially when the Federal Medicare program, following 2-year demonstration projects begun in 1978, added hospice benefits for eligible patients. Evaluation of the demonstrations was not yet complete when a bipartisan hospice benefit bill was introduced in Congress in 1981 by Representative Leon Panetta of California and Senator Robert Dole of Kansas. The Reagan administration would not allow Medicare staff overseeing the demonstration projects to participate in drafting the bill; however, Congress saw the hospice benefit as popular and cheap, and the bill passed as part of the Tax Equity and Fiscal Responsibility Act (TEFRA) of

1982. The new benefit allowed a relatively low $6500 for the care of each patient, with no more than 20% for inpatient care. Patients were only eligible if they had a life expectancy of less than 6 months and would not receive significant inpatient care or aggressive treatments; this accentuated the difficulty of the decision to transfer a patient to hospice and deny possible curative or lifesaving measures. Benefits included 80% of outpatient medication cost, home care visits and other home services, and bereavement counseling for the family. But hospice care expanded rapidly with the new funding; there were 1500 US programs in 1985, and 3000 by 1997 [24].

By 2010, there were 5150 hospice programs in the United States (including all 50 states, the District of Columbia, Puerto Rico, Guam, and the US Virgin Islands), ranging from small voluntary agencies caring for 50 patients or fewer per year to large, national chains with a daily census in the thousands. Fifty-eight percent (58%) of these were free-standing, 21% hospital-based, 19% home health-agency programs, and the remainder were based in nursing homes. Most US hospice care today (80%) is provided in homes and nursing homes. Medicare covers 84% of hospice care, and health entrepreneurs have taken full advantage: the majority of US hospice programs are for-profit companies; (36%, including homes run by religious groups, are non-profit, and 6% are state or city government-run). This figure represents a major shift in the last decade; in 1998, 76% of hospice programs were non-profit [25].

Global development of hospice and palliative care

The work of Saunders and Wilkes inspired palliative care movements throughout the world. In 2011, 136 of the world's 234 countries (58%) were identified as having established hospice-palliative care services; this represents an increase of 21 countries (+ 9%) since 2006. The most significant gains have been made in Africa. The World Health Organization (WHO) Analgesic Ladder for the use of opioids to relieve the pain of advanced cancer and other terminal illnesses, based on work done at St. Christopher's and introduced in 1986, has become a tool recognized, although often modified, worldwide [26]. However, a report by the Worldwide Palliative Care Alliance concludes that despite interest expressed by many nations, the advanced integration of palliative care with wider health services has been achieved in only 20 countries (8.5%): Australia, Austria, Belgium, Canada, France, Germany, Hong Kong, Iceland, Ireland, Italy, Japan, Norway, Poland, Romania, Singapore, Sweden, Switzerland, Uganda, UK, and United States [27]. Palliative care leaders identify the ongoing challenges as lack of public recognition and understanding, indifference by health and social-care providers, lack of funding, poor recognition of palliative care by health policymakers, underdeveloped training programs, and inadequate evidence bases for palliative care and cost-effectiveness in delivering it. Current provision of hospice and palliative care reaches only a fraction of those who need it [28].

Continuing challenges

Palliative care today encompasses a wide range of specialist services and is available throughout the United States and the UK, as well as other developed countries. However, as Jonathan Koffman has argued, end-of-life care is not readily accessible to all groups in society. Those who are likely to have unmet palliative care needs include: poor, black and minority ethnic groups; asylum seekers and refugees; the homeless; those in the penal system; drug users; those who abuse alcohol; and travelling communities [29]. Moreover, the population is aging, as more and more individuals live past the age of 65 and medicine is able to prolong life expectancy for illnesses such as cancer and AIDS. Pain, the major issue in palliative care, is difficult to treat in such illnesses, even by trained specialists, and more so when facilities are limited. Worldwide, an estimated 67–80% of cancer patients, for example, suffer from undertreated pain [30,31]. The financial burden on both government and charitable funding will become heavier as demand for palliative services increases and hospices face pressure to provide more varied services [32].

In 1980, Eric Wilkes proposed access to palliative care for all, through the provision of effective services at home. Research has documented that most individuals would prefer to die in their homes, and there is growing recognition of community care as an option for the future of palliative care. However, according to ONS figures, less than 20% of deaths in the UK in 2007 occurred in the home [33].The United States has developed more home-based palliative care programs, yet these are only available to a subset of the population. In 2005, nearly 70% of deaths took place in acute-care hospitals or long-term care nursing facilities [34]. Modern hospice has made "the good death" a reality, but for many it remains a mirage.

References

1. Humphries C. "Waiting for the last summons": the establishment of the first hospices in England 1878-1914. *Mortality* 2001; **6**: 146–166.
2. Winslow M, Clark D St. Joseph's Hospice, Hackney: documenting a centenary history. *Prog Palliat Care* 2006; **14**: 68–74.
3. Winslow M, Clark D. Partnerships in care. In: Winslow M, Clark D (eds.) *St. Joseph's Hospice, Hackney: A Century of Caring in East London*. Lancaster: Observatory Publications, 2005, pp. 43–71.
4. Meldrum M. A capsule history of pain management. *JAMA* 2003; **290**: 2470–2475.
5. Meldrum M. The property of euphoria: research and the cancer patient. In: Meldrum M (ed.) *Opioids and Pain Relief: A Historical Perspective*. Seattle: IASP Press, 2003, pp. 193–211.
6. Seymour J, Winslow M. Pain and palliative care: the emergence of new specialties. *J Pain Symptom Manage* 2005; **29**: 2–13.
7. Bonica JJ. *The Management of Pain: With Special Emphasis on the Use of Analgesic Block in Diagnosis, Prognosis and Therapy*. Philadelphia: Lea & Febiger, 1953.

8. Small N. The modern hospice movement: "Bright lights sparkling" or "a bit of heaven for a few"? In: Bornat J, Perks R, Thompson P, Walmsley J (eds.) *Oral History, Health and Welfare*. London: Routledge, 2000, pp. 288–308.
9. Clark D. From margins to centre: a review of the history of palliative care in cancer. *Lancet Oncol* 2007; **8**: 430–438.
10. Clark D, Small N, Wright M, *et al*. Hospice teamwork. In: Clark D, Small N, Wright M, *et al*. (eds.) *A Bit of Heaven for the Few: An Oral History of the Modern Hospice Movement in the United Kingdom*. Lancaster: Observatory Publications, 2005, p. 43.
11. Porter R. Medicine and the people. In: Porter R (ed.) *The Greatest Benefit to Mankind: A Medical History of Humanity from Antiquity to the Present*. London: Fontana Press, 1999, pp. 699–700.
12. Wilkes E. *Report of the Working Group on Terminal Care*. The Standing Medical Advisory Committee. London: DSS, 1980.
13. No second chance: a discussion document for the Trent Regional Health Authority on the development of terminal care services. Trent Regional Health Authority, 1987.
14. Winslow M, Ostrovskis-Wilkes R, Noble B. Homage to Eric Wilkes. *Eur J Palliat Care* 2010; **17**: 252–253.
15. Scott J, Macdonald N. Education in palliative medicine. In: Doyle D, Hanks G, Macdonald N (eds.) *Oxford Textbook of Palliative Medicine*. Oxford: Oxford University Press, 1993.
16. Help The Hospices. *Hospice and Palliative Care Directory 2011-2012*. London: Help the Hospices, 2011, Available at: http://www.helpthehospices.org.uk/about-hospice-care/facts-figures (accessed November 16, 2012).
17. Craven J, Wald FS. Hospice care for dying patients. *Am J Nurs* 1975; **75**: 1816–1822.
18. Wald FS. Hospice care in the United States: a conversation with Florence S. Wald. Interview by MJ Friedrich. *JAMA* 1999; **281**: 1683–1685.
19. Sullivan P, Florence S. Wald, 91: hospice pioneer. Washington Post, Nov 13, 2008. Available at: http://www.washingtonpost.com (accessed February 26, 2012).
20. Foster Z, Wald FS, Wald HJ. The hospice movement: a backward look at its first two decades. *New Physician* 1978; **27**: 21–24.
21. Osterweis M, Champagne DS. The US hospice movement: issues in development. *Am J Public Health* 1979; **69**: 492–496.
22. Connor SR. The development of hospice and palliative care in the United States. *Omega* 2007–2008; **56**: 89–99.
23. Berger A, Baker K, Bolle J, Pereira D. Establishing a palliative care program in a research center: evolution of a model. *Cancer Invest* 2003; **21**: 313–320.
24. Miller PJ, Mike PB. The Medicare hospice benefit: ten years of federal policy for the terminally ill. *Death Stud* 1995; **19**: 531–542.
25. National Hospice and Palliative Care Organization. NHPCO Facts and Figures: Hospice Care in America. 2011. Available at: http://www.nhpco.org (accessed February 26, 2012).
26. Vargas-Schaffer G. Is the WHO analgesic ladder still valid? Twenty-four years of experience. *Can Fam Physician* 2010; **56**: 514–517.
27. Lynch T, Clark D, Connor S. Mapping levels of palliative care development: A global update 2011. Worldwide Palliative Care Alliance, 2011. http://www.thewpca.org/resources/ (accessed November 16, 2012).
28. Clark D, Graham F. Evolution and change in palliative care around the world. *Medicine* 2011; **39**: 636–638.
29. Koffman J. Social inequalities at the end of life. In: Cohen J (ed.) *A Public Health Perspective on the End of Life*. Oxford: Oxford University Press, 2012, pp. 183–191.

30. Winslow M, Paz S, Clark D, *et al.* Pharmacogenetics and the relief of cancer pain. *Int J Technol Knowl Soc* 2007; **2**: 7.

31. Mori M, Elsayem A, Reddy S, *et al.* Unrelieved pain and suffering in patients with advanced cancer. *Am J Hosp Palliat Care* 2011; doi: 10.1177/1049909111415511.

32. Theodosopoulos G. Voluntary hospices in England: a viable business model? *Account Forum* 2011; **35**: 118–125.

33. Department of Health. End of Life Care Strategy: First Annual Report. Department of Health, London, UK, 2008. http://www.dh.gov.uk/en/Publicationsandstatistics/Publications/PublicationsPolicyAndGuidance/DH_086277 (accessed November 26, 2012).

34. Frontline: Facing Death: How We Die. PBS. http://www.pbs.org/wgbh/pages/frontline/facing-death/facts-and-figures (accessed March 30, 2012).

CHAPTER 7

Radiation therapy and hospice care

Charles F. von Gunten[1], Frank D. Ferris[2], and Arno J. Mundt[3]
[1]Hospice and Palliative Medicine, OhioHealth, Columbus, OH, USA
[2]Research and Education, OhioHealth, Columbus, OH, USA
[3]Center for Advanced Radiotherapy Technologies (CART), Department of Radiation
Medicine and Applied Sciences, University of California, San Diego, CA, USA

Introduction

An estimated 7.6 million people die from cancer each year in the world; 70%
of those deaths occur in low and middle-income countries [1]. The World
Health Organization (WHO) has consistently advocated that palliative care
should be a part of the national cancer plans for each of its member countries
as a way to address that suffering [2]. Yet, only a tiny fraction of patients
receive such care. There are a variety of reasons for this including lack of
training of physicians and other health-care professionals, unavailability of
opioids, and lack of government policy providing palliative care as part
of the country's health-care plan [3]. As part of its advocacy, the WHO has
promoted a strategic framework for a country to use to make palliative care
available to its people. Palliative care should begin at the time of the cancer
diagnosis and be combined with standard cancer care. Hospice care has been
demonstrated to be the best approach to providing palliative care in the last
months of life [4].

Hospice care around the world

The term hospice shares the same Latin root with the words hospital and
hospitality. In the Middle Ages in Europe, religious institutions provided
health care to travelers and those without homes in inpatient facilities. Care
was provided until the patient recovered or died. By the 12th century, hospitals had emerged as places where patients were expected to recover, while
hospices were places to care for the dying. These institutions were dissolved
during the Protestant Reformation. However, in the 19th century, a few
reemerged in France, England, and the United States.

Radiation Oncology in Palliative Cancer Care, First Edition. Edited by Stephen Lutz,
Edward Chow, and Peter Hoskin.
© 2013 John Wiley & Sons, Ltd. Published 2013 by John Wiley & Sons, Ltd.

In the 1940s, Cicely Saunders, trained first as a nurse then as a social worker, observed poor care of the dying in hospitals in London. In order to be more effective in improving care of the dying in hospitals or existing hospices she trained as a physician. She founded St. Christopher's Hospice in a southern suburb of London, England in 1967 as the culmination of nearly 20 years of direct observation of the care of terminally ill people. The principles she articulated and demonstrated have come to be known as modern hospice care.

In most of the world, the term hospice continues to refer to an inpatient facility that cares for patients near the end of life. They may have associated home care support teams or outpatient facilities. Worldwide variation in drug availability, the standards of practice for physicians and nurses, the availability of counselors like social workers or psychologists, and the availability of chaplains and other health-care professionals makes broad statements about the actual care delivered impossible. Nevertheless, all are united in trying to provide the best quality of life in Cicely Saunders' dimensions of physical, emotional, social (practical), and spiritual domains for the patient and his or her family.

Hospice care in the United States

In contrast with the rest of the world, the term hospice care in the United States refers to a primarily home-based approach to providing care. Although there are inpatient hospice units, they are few in number and in bed capacity. Box 7.1 describes what a patient enrolled in hospice care in the United States can expect [5]. In the hospice programs around the world, a very similar set of services is likely to be in place, although the qualifications, scope of practice, and medications and supplies available may vary greatly.

In 1982, the US Congress enacted the Medicare Hospice Benefit (MHB) legislation authorizing payment for hospice care to everyone over the age of 65 who met three criteria. First, the patient must have a prognosis of less than 6 months (later changed to less than 6 months if the disease follows its normal course) as determined by two physicians. Table 7.1 summarizes some prognostic criteria for cancer. Second, the patient must elect hospice care, rather than "standard care," for the care of the terminal illness. Third, the patient must be enrolled in Medicare.

Once a patient is eligible and elects hospice care, the hospice agency receives a fixed amount of money per patient per day for care, in the order of $120 per day at the time of this writing. In the United States, this was the first federal example of a managed care plan where the hospice agency carried the "risk" for caring for the population of patients rather than being reimbursed on a cost basis as was the standard for Medicare coverage.

Once enrolled in hospice care, the patient and his or her family are assigned to a team that is usually comprised of a nurse, social worker, chaplain, and nurse's aide. The team meets at least every other week to discuss the care of

---

Box 7.1 Medicare hospice benefit

Covered Services (100%–No Copay)
- Nursing care: to provide intermittent (usually 1–3 times/week) assessment, support, skilled services, treatments, and case management services
- 24-hour availability for assessment and management of changes, crises, and other acute needs
- Social work: supportive counseling, practical aspects of care (other community services), and planning (health-care surrogates, advance directives)
- Counseling services, including chaplaincy
- Home health aide and homemaker services
- Speech therapy, nutrition, physical therapy, and occupational therapy services
- Bereavement support to family after the death
- Medical oversight of the plan of care by the hospice medical director
- All medications and supplies for management and palliation of the advanced illness (hospices may collect a small co-pay for medications)
- Durable medical equipment (e.g., hospital bed, commode, wheelchair, etc.)
- Short-term general inpatient care for problems that cannot be managed at home, such as pain, dyspnea, delirium, acute needs requiring skilled care
- Short-term respite to permit family caregivers to take a break
- Continuous care at home for short episodes of acute need

Services Not Covered by the Medicare Hospice Benefit
- Continuous nursing or nurse aide care
- Medications unrelated to the advanced illness
- Physician visits for direct medical care (billed to Medicare separately)
- Residential (non-acute) care in a facility

---

the patient and his or her family. The frequency and duration of the visits to the patient and family are determined by the team and the circumstances.

The most common complaint from patients and families about hospice care is that they weren't informed about the practical benefits; there was too much talk about the philosophy of care and not enough about who would help and how [6]. While the management of symptoms and ensuring physical comfort is important, patients and families frequently experience multiple issues that cause suffering that are outside the physical domain and lie in the emotional, practical, and spiritual domains.

When patients elect coverage using the MHB, the hospice agency becomes responsible for coordinating and paying for all treatments and medications related to the primary hospice diagnosis. Patients can continue to receive care for diseases unrelated to the advanced illness (e.g. dialysis for renal failure if

Table 7.1 Cancer: prognostic factors, median survival assuming maximal medical therapy.

Factor		Median Survival
Karnofsky performance status	50–60	90 days
Karnofsky performance status	20–30	50 days
Karnofsky performance status	10–20	17 days
ECOG / Zubrod / WHO Score	3	3 months
ECOG / Zubrod / WHO Score	4	1 month
Hypercalcemia		1 month
Brain mets (multiple)	No Rx	1 month
Brain mets (multiple)	Corticosteroids	3 months
Brain mets (multiple)	Radiation therapy	6 months
Malignant pleural effusion		4 months
Serum albumin	<2.5 mg/dl	<6 months
Unintentional weight loss	10%	<6 months
Dyspnea		<6 months
Anorexia		<6 months
Delirium		6 weeks

ECOG, Eastern Cooperative Oncology Group; WHO, World Health Organization.

the patient is dying of cancer, cataract removal) using regular Medicare coverage. Most Medicaid and commercial insurers use the MHB as a model to guide their coverage of hospice care.

To be eligible for federal payment for hospice care, both the attending physician and hospice physician certify that the patient has a life expectancy of 6 months or less if the disease or condition runs its normal course. The standard for certainty is "more likely than not"; in other words, a 51% chance or more of dying in the next 6 months. If patients improve or resume disease-directed therapy with the primary goal of extending life expectancy, they can be discharged and have their care paid for under the usual Medicare Part A, Part B, and Part D benefits. They can resume hospice services later without penalty. One way to begin the process of determining eligibility is to ask oneself "would I be surprised if the patient died in the next 6 months?" If the answer is no, refer for hospice care.

Individual patients can continue to be eligible if they live longer than 6 months as long as the hospice medical director believes death is more likely than not within 6 months. The patient does not need a Do Not Resuscitate (DNR) order to be eligible for hospice care. There is no limit to the number of days a patient can receive hospice care. There is no penalty if the patient outlives the initial prognosis. For example, one of the authors had a patient with refractory breast cancer live for 6 years while enrolled in hospice care. At each recertification period, it was clear that the patient was more likely than not to die within 6 months because of her underlying disease. It was unforeseeable that this particular patient would live much longer than average.

Prognosis

Physicians overestimate prognosis when compared with actual survival by a factor of three or greater [7]. Though the survival of cancer patients can be difficult to predict, the prognostications for this patient group are commonly more accurate than for patients with other life-limiting diagnoses such as congestive heart failure or chronic obstructive pulmonary disease. The performance status of cancer patients remains a reliable shorthand estimate of survival of cancer patients, though more complex measures have been developed and may be useful.

Plan of care (POC)

The hospice program approves, coordinates, and pays for services that are reasonable and necessary for palliation and for management of the advanced illness. The POC is based on the patient's diagnosis, prognosis, functional status, needs, goals of care, orders of the attending physician, and, as necessary, collaboration with the hospice medical director. It includes education and support for the patient and family as the unit of care. It is surprising to many physicians that the hospice team can spend more time with the patient's family members than with the patient when those issues are the most important to the well-being of the patient.

The plan of care is quite specific to individual hospice programs. Some will include chemotherapy, radiotherapy, blood transfusions, antibiotics, laboratory testing, radiological imaging, total parenteral nutrition (TPN), etc. when they are likely to make the patient feel better. Other, usually small, hospice programs will not be able to provide these as part of the plan of care. The MHB includes no rules about what may or may not be included in the plan of care.

Physician role

The attending physician is indicated by the patient at the time of enrollment. This can be the oncologist. Sometimes the patient will select a hospice physician for this role. Sometimes the oncologist will request that the hospice physician be the attending physician for the purposes of hospice enrollment in order to deal with the issues of ordering and renewing medications; others prefer to retain this role.

The attending physician is responsible for working with the hospice team to determine appropriate care. Direct patient care services by the attending physician are billed to Medicare in the usual fashion using the standard Evaluation and Management codes [8].

Places of care

Home: The majority (95%) of hospice care days take place in the home because that is where patients say they want to be. Hospice team members visit the patient and family on an intermittent basis. Care continues as long as the patient remains eligible and wants the care. Medicare rules do not require a primary caregiver in the home; many patients live alone and like it that way.

Nursing home or other long-term care facility: This is the patient's home, and the patient's "family" frequently includes the staff. Hospice care is specialty care provided in addition to usual nursing home care.

Hospice inpatient unit: Dedicated units that are free-standing or within other facilities such as nursing homes or hospitals are sometimes available. Permitted length-of-stay varies as some are for residential care and others for short term acute palliative care.

Hospital: Occasionally pain and other symptoms or other conditions related to the advanced illness cannot be managed at home and the patient is admitted to an inpatient hospital or other contracted inpatient facility for more intensive management. The inpatient facility must have a contract with the hospice program.

Payment to the hospice

Medicare pays for covered services using a per diem capitated arrangement in one of four categories:

• Routine home care: care at home or nursing home.

• Inpatient respite care: care in an inpatient setting (usually a nursing home or inpatient hospice unit) for up to 5 days to give family caregivers a break when the patient is otherwise clinically stable.

• General inpatient care: Acute inpatient care for conditions related to the advanced illness (e.g. pain and symptom control, caregiver breakdown, impending death and the patient does not want to die at home).

• Continuous home care: Provides short-term acute care at home with around-the-clock care for a crisis that might otherwise lead to inpatient care. Many hospice programs find this challenging to provide due to the staffing requirements.

Palliative radiation and hospice

It has been widely noted that about 50% of a radiation oncologist's practice is composed of giving radiation for palliative intent. However, what the word "palliative" means in radiation oncology compared with its use in a hospice setting may lead to misunderstanding and conflict.

Many in radiation oncology view curative- and palliative-intent treatment as mutually exclusive rather than concurrent goals. In contrast, in hospice care, palliative-intent treatment strives to make the patient and family unit feel better in physical, emotional, practical, or spiritual terms. In other words, if the radiation won't change how the patient feels, it is not palliative. Further, if it makes the patient feel worse, it is anathema. The radiation oncologists who deliver the most effective care take into account potential adverse effects of therapy including fatigue, skin irritation, time spent in traveling to and from the treatment, and physical discomfort getting on and off the treatment table.

> **Vignette 1**: A patient has pain in the left leg. Evaluation shows a lytic lesion with less than 30% loss of cortical bone in the left femur from metastatic lung cancer, Eastern Cooperative Oncology Group (ECOG) performance level 4 (bedbound with a prognosis of about one month) and lives about 30 miles (48 kilometers) from the radiation center. What is the role of radiation therapy for this patient?

As is discussed extensively in Chapter 20, data show that 8 Gy in a single fraction, where evaluation, simulation, and treatment occur in a single session, is as efficacious as any other fractionation scheme [9]. Similarly, whether it is an "old" cobalt machine or a new linear accelerator does not influence the treatment plan or outcome. The treatment can be expected to fully relieve the pain for up to 80% of patients by 4–6 weeks after treatment; pain relief will begin 5–7 days after treatment. If the patient lives longer than expected, and the pain returns, he can be retreated.

There are no conclusive data to show that a more extended course (20 Gy over 5 days, or 30 Gy over 10 days, or 60 Gy over 30 days) will be more durable. Even if such an approach added to the durability of response, a patient would need to have a prognosis of >3 months to consider the time commitment. For the patient in vignette 1, such a course would likely be unnecessarily lengthy and expensive, causing the patient and family to spend most of their remaining life traveling to and from radiation treatment prior to death.

> **Vignette 2**: A 48-year-old woman has widely metastatic breast cancer refractory to maximal chemotherapy with numerous new brain metastases. She has a performance status of 4. There has been no improvement since initiating dexamethasone 20 mg daily. She has just begun a course of 3 Gy of radiation in 10 fractions. She has been referred for hospice care. Her prognosis is less than one month.

One of the challenges for hospice programs is the therapy plans that have been initiated by radiation oncologists seemingly removed from the clinical circumstance of the patient as the hospice team encounters it in the home. In vignette 2, where there is no improvement in function with high dose corticosteroids, it is difficult to imagine what palliative benefits the radiation will bring to the patient or family. Because of cost, many hospice programs will not admit patients who are receiving such a treatment plan. Some hospice programs will want to initiate a discussion with the radiation oncologist to address the purpose of the treatment plan. Sometimes, the treating radiation oncologist is not aware of the short prognosis, or is reluctant to address this with the patient or the referring medical oncologist. Consequently, treatment is administered that no one wants. Although the patient can tolerate the therapy, it is difficult to characterize the radiation for this case as anything other than useless, expensive, and wasteful of resources. In this vignette 2, the right choice is either to change the fractionation scheme or to stop the radiation entirely.

> **Vignette 3**: A 69-year-old man with slowly progressive widely meta-static non-small cell lung cancer has a left thigh metastasis that is growing through the skin. The skin wound is oozing blood. His ECOG performance status is 4.

This is a case where a single fraction, aimed at the skin, may palliate the blood loss. While it won't change the prognosis, it will dramatically change the experience of the patient, his family, and his caregivers to not cope with progressive bleeding that makes it look like he is bleeding to death.

Conclusion

Hospice care has been proven to be the best approach to providing palliative care for patients with cancer and their families. There is a role for radiation therapy in hospice care for the palliation of pain and symptoms. However, to contribute to the total plan of care for the patient and family, the radiation oncologist must evaluate the radiation therapy for its ability to contribute to how the patient feels, and what the patient and family unit define as their goals of care. For many radiation oncologists, this challenges their paradigms for how they do radiation oncology.

References

1. Jemal A, Bray F, Center MM, *et al.* Global cancer statistics. *CA Cancer J Clin* 2011; **61**: 69–90.
2. Ventafridda V. According to the 2002 WHO definition of palliative care. *Palliat Med* 2006; **20**: 159.
3. Gomes B, Harding R, Foley KM, Higginson IJ. Optimal approaches to the health economics of palliative care: report of an international think tank. *J Pain Symptom Manage* 2009; **38**: 4–10.
4. Teno JM, Clarridge BR, Casey V, *et al.* Family perspectives on end-of-life care at the last place of care. *JAMA* 2004; **291**: 88–93.
5. Harold JK, von Gunten CF. Hospice approach to palliative care, including Medicare Hospice Benefit. In: Yennurajalingam S, Bruera E (eds.) *Oxford American Handbook of Hospice and Palliative Care.* New York: Oxford University Press, 2011, pp. 229–240.
6. Casarett D, Crowley R, Stevenson C, *et al.* Making difficult decisions about hospice enrollment: what do patients and families want to know? *J Am Geriatr Soc* 2005; **53**: 249–254.

7. Christakis N, Lamont E. The extent and determinants of error in physicians' prognosis for terminally ill patients. *BMJ* 2000; **320**: 469–473.
8. von Gunten CF, Ferris FD, Kirschner C, Emanuel LL. Coding and reimbursement mechanisms for physician services in hospice and palliative care. *J Palliat Med* 2000; **3**: 157–164.
9. Lutz S, Berk L, Chang E, *et al.* Palliative radiotherapy for bone metastases: an ASTRO evidence-based guideline. *Int J Radiat Oncol Biol Phys* 2011; **79**: 965–976.

CHAPTER 8

The current status of palliative care and radiotherapy

Thomas Smith, Susannah Batko-Yovino
Department of Radiation Oncology, and Program of Palliative Medicine, John Hopkins University, Baltimore, MD, USA

What *is* palliative care?

The World Health Organization (WHO) defines palliative care as "an approach that improves the quality of life of patients and their families facing the problem associated with life-threatening illness, through the prevention and relief of suffering by means of early identification and impeccable assessment and treatment of pain and other problems, physical, psychosocial and spiritual." Box 8.1 provides other definitions of palliative care provided by practitioners.

Who can benefit from palliative care?

We will define palliative care, enumerate the benefits and risks of such care, discuss the standards for palliative treatment, and suggest ways in which palliative care can fit into a typical radiation oncology practice. We would like to note that palliative care is obviously not restricted to cancer patients and can be immensely valuable for individuals with chronic heart or lung disease, traumatic injuries, neurodegenerative diseases, and many other serious medical problems. Because this text is directed towards oncology providers, we will focus primarily on the role that palliative care can play in the care of patients with cancer. First, we would like to present a few case vignettes illustrating the diverse types of cancer patients who might be able to benefit from palliative care interventions.

Jane V. is a 64-year-old woman with breast cancer. Three years ago, she was diagnosed with a locally advanced, estrogen-receptor-positive tumor of the left breast. She received chemotherapy, had a mastectomy, and received adjuvant radiation and hormonal therapy. She has newly diagnosed bone-only metastatic disease with a painful vertebral compression fracture.

Radiation Oncology in Palliative Cancer Care, First Edition. Edited by Stephen Lutz, Edward Chow, and Peter Hoskin.
© 2013 John Wiley & Sons, Ltd. Published 2013 by John Wiley & Sons, Ltd.

Box 8.1 Definition of palliative care

Palliative care is specialized medical care for people with serious illnesses. This type of care is focused on providing patients with relief from the symptoms, pain, and stress of a serious illness – whatever the diagnosis. The goal is to improve quality of life for both the patient and the family. Palliative care is provided by a team of doctors, nurses, and other specialists who work with a patient's other doctors to provide an extra layer of support. Palliative care is appropriate at any age and at any stage in a serious illness, and can be provided together with curative treatment.
Diane Meier, MD, Director, Center to Advance Palliative Care, July 1, 2011

Palliative care is open and honest communication, medically appropriate goal setting, and the best symptom management.
Thomas J. Smith MD

Ralph K. is a 55-year-old man with a history of hepatitis C and heavy alcohol use. He lives alone in a third-floor walkup apartment. He was recently admitted for jaundice and progressive ascites. Imaging showed multiple liver tumors and several large lung nodules. His serum alpha-fetoprotein level is above 20,000 ng/mL. He has severe abdominal pain, itching, nausea, and dyspnea in addition to symptoms of alcohol withdrawal.

Marlene B. is a 38-year-old woman with an HPV-positive, locally advanced, squamous cell carcinoma of the tonsil. She has completed two-thirds of her prescribed course of intensive, curative-intent chemoradiation therapy and has developed intractable pain due to mucositis as well as a twenty-pound weight loss. She has been unable to work or to take care of her three young children.

Each of these patients presents a complex set of medical issues, and the cases illustrate several important points about the nature of palliative care. First, and perhaps most importantly, each of these three patients is at a different stage of illness. Palliative care is often mistakenly confused with hospice or end-of-life care, and many patients receiving curative-intent or life-prolonging treatment are not considered for palliative care services. Hospice care is end-of-life care as described in Chapter 7. However, current recommendations suggest that palliative care should be considered early in the course of disease for any patient with metastatic cancer or significant disease-related symptoms [1]. Additionally, like many cancer patients, all three patients have "non-medical" issues that can cause significant distress and suffering. As described by Cecily Saunders, "suffering" includes physical symptoms such as pain and nausea as well as psychological, social, and spiritual distress caused by changes in physical abilities, social role, and life plans that are triggered by the diagnosis of serious illness [2]. Palliative care patients want their health-care providers to be aware of all their issues, even if they may want someone else to address specific aspects such as spirituality [3].

What are the goals of palliative care and what features of a palliative care program help to accomplish these goals?

The overarching goal of palliative care is to alleviate suffering, which can occur at any stage of a serious illness. This goal is simple to understand but frequently can be difficult to fully realize in daily practice. In addition to physical symptoms such as pain, nausea, constipation, and dyspnea, many patients have social issues (such as difficulties with transportation, lack of assistance at home, or problems affording medication) that significantly affect care. Although psycho-social and cultural issues impact care for all patients, such issues often are spotlighted in patients requiring palliative care. Furthermore, the diagnosis of a life-threatening illness creates psychologic and emotional turmoil for patients and their families. Many patients experience depression or spiritual crises. To maximally relieve suffering, patient-centered, interdisciplinary care is necessary as it is impossible for any single physician to adequately address all the medical, social, psychologic, and spiritual needs of a patient [4]. Palliative care programs are designed to ensure that a multi-disciplinary team of professionals are available to individually manage the complex needs of each patient. Although the exact composition of a palliative care program can vary, a typical team includes physicians, advanced practice nurses, pharmacists, social workers, mental health professionals, nutritionists, chaplains, and physical/occupational therapists.

Palliative care is comprised of several essential elements [5]. It is important to note that these elements should be integrated into each interaction, as the patient's condition and goals for care can change with each visit. The first is a detailed assessment of patient symptoms and concerns. Several validated instruments are available to facilitate and standardize such assessments including the Edmonton Symptom Assessment Scale, which evaluates nine physical and mental symptoms on a Likert scale [6]; the more detailed Memorial Symptom Assessment scale, with 32 items [7]; and the Condensed Memorial Symptom Assessment Scale (CMSAS), which takes 2–4 minutes to complete at the bedside [8]. As shown recently in a randomized trial, just identifying concerns without integrating those concerns into the care of the patient does not improve the quality of care [9]. It is essential that clinicians use such a scale in their daily rounds and be directly involved in the care of the patient if they are to uncover fixable symptoms. For our most recent research intervention, we used an even shorter version of the CMSAS, which we have continued in usual practice, as shown in Figure 8.1. This approach is an excellent way to identify physical symptoms for which there may be fixes.

The next key component of the palliative care process is to inquire what the patient wants to know about their diagnosis and prognosis and to

Reported by: Patient Caregiver RN MD									
Able to respond: Yes No Reason _____									
Delirium: Yes No									
Pain: 0–10 Usual ___ Worst ___ Best ___ Neuropathic component Yes__ No__									
	Tiredness	Nausea	Depression	Anxiety	Drowsiness	Anorexia	Constipation	Dyspnea	Secretions
0									
1									
2									
3									
4									
7									
Enter: 0=none, 1=a little bit, 2=somewhat, 3=quite a lot, 4=very much, 7=refused									

Figure 8.1 An abbreviated symptom assessment scale for use in everyday practice.

establish the goals of treatment and decision-making regarding care. In this context, decisions can range from a simple alteration in the dosage of a pain medication to plans for transitioning from possibly life-prolonging treatment to hospice, or discussions regarding advance directives and end-of-life care. Once care has been provided, frequent and detailed follow-up is necessary to ensure that the patient's goals are being met and to adapt plans for care as the patient's needs change over time. Close communication on the part of the palliative care team with the patient and his or her family is key throughout all phases of the assessment and care process. We strongly endorse the "ASK, TELL, ASK" method to ensure that the patient and family understand [10].

The optimal way to perform or integrate a palliative care consultation into usual care has not been determined, but there are some overarching principles. We use the National Consensus Palliative Care Guidelines Project template to pattern our approach (Box 8.2).

What is the evidence regarding the benefits and risks of palliative care? When should palliative care be introduced to a patient?

Oncologists rely on evidence from clinical trials to provide data regarding optimal patient care. Formal studies regarding the effectiveness of palliative care interventions in cancer patients are somewhat scarce partly because less than 1% of the national research budget is dedicated to palliative care [11]. Seven clinical trials randomizing patients to a palliative care intervention versus usual care have been published. Table 8.1 summarizes the five most significant studies. Of the seven trials, only three were restricted to cancer

---

Box 8.2 Suggested components for goals of care discussion (*with suggested phrases*)

Illness understanding
- Ask permission. *"What do you want to know about your situation? "Would you like to discuss what might happen to you?"*
- Inquire about illness and prognostic understanding. *"What do you <u>want</u> to know about your illness? What <u>do</u> you know about your situation?"*
- Offer clarification of treatment goals – after checking with the other members of the treatment team to make sure the goals are the same.
  - Patient perception
  - Reality
  - Understanding after discussion of reality
- Address adapting to changed goals and likely death from cancer. Offer clarification of adaptation to changed goals and foreseeable death on several visits.
- Oncologists tend to think of this conversation as a one-time event, but the existential threat of death and loss of meaning continues from diagnosis. This should be discussed monthly, or at least offered.
- Inquire about life goals. *"What is important to you? What do you plan to do with the time you have (whether 3 days or 3 years)?"*

Symptom Management
- Focus on symptom management as a part of the goals of care.
- Always use a Symptom Assessment Tool such as Edmonton or Memorial Symptom Assessment Scales.
- Inquire about common uncontrolled symptoms with a focus on:
  - *Always ask "What is bothering you the most?"*
  - Pain
  - Pulmonary symptoms (cough, dyspnea)
  - Fatigue and sleep disturbance
  - Mood (depression and anxiety) Use the single question *"Are you depressed?"*[29]
  "Are there things you are looking forward to doing?"
  - Gastrointestinal (anorexia, weight loss, nausea & vomiting, constipation)

Decision-Making
- Inquire about mode of decision-making. *"Are you a person who likes to make decisions by her/himself? Do you like to share that decision-making with your family? With your doctors? Who helps you with your decision-making?"*
- Assist with treatment decision-making, if necessary. *"How can we be helpful to you?"*

(Continued)

- Assess coping with life-threatening illness by patient and family *"This must be hard on you and your family. How are you coping with this illness?"*
- Enlist help. *"Are there family or spiritual issues that are important to you? Would you like to see our chaplain or our social worker?"*

Other
- Referrals and note new prescriptions
- Identify care plan for future appointments
- Indicate referrals to other care providers, and communicate directly by fax, email, or electronic medical record

*Modified from the National Palliative Care Consensus Guidelines [4].

---

patients; the other four included patients with a variety of serious illnesses, and the percentage of patients with cancer ranged from 22 to 47%. Significant variability in terms of outcome measurements, palliative care interventions provided, and patient populations may also limit the generalizability of the results of these trials.

However, in a landmark study published in 2010, 151 patients with newly diagnosed, metastatic non-small cell lung cancer were randomized to an early palliative care intervention (within 3 weeks of diagnosis and continuing throughout treatment) versus "standard palliative care" (meaning that palliative care interventions occurred only at the request of the patient, his/her family, or treating physician) [12]. This study found that patients in the early palliative care group had significantly improved quality of life scores and lower rates of depression. Patients receiving palliative care were also less likely to receive "aggressive end-of-life care," defined as receiving chemotherapy within 2 weeks of death, entering hospice care fewer than 3 days before death, or not receiving hospice care at all. Yet, patients in the early palliative care group had significantly longer survival (11.6 vs 8.9 months, $P = 0.02$) than patients in the usual care group. Better survival was associated with better understanding of the disease and goals of care [13], less intravenous chemotherapy in the last 60 days of life [14], and expanded use of hospice. Of note, the intervention took only about 1 hour for the initial consultation [15].

Based on the strongly positive results of this study, evidence of improvement in quality of life and mood in other trials [16–18], and a lack of evidence that palliative care interventions harm patients, the American Society for Clinical Oncology (ASCO) has issued new guidelines recommending that palliative care be considered "early in the course of illness" for any patient with metastatic cancer or with severe symptoms related to a cancer diagnosis [1]. Some apprehension on the part of the physician may accompany the process of suggesting that a patient consider seeing a palliative care specialty team. Difficult questions regarding the patient's prognosis and expectations

Table 8.1 Trials of palliative care in oncology.

Author (year)	Study design	Main findings
Rabow et al. (2004) [30]	• Outpatient clinic • Advanced cancer in 33% • Interdisciplinary PC team (SW, RN, chaplain, pharmacist, psychologist, art therapist, volunteer coordinator, 3 physicians) • 7 component interventions (e.g. home visits, phone calls) • PC team consultants, not responsible for care	• Service had minimal impact • Only improved outcome was decreased dyspnea • Consult-only service • Recommendations were only followed in 10–20% of situations
Brumley et al. (2007) [17]	• Home-bound terminally ill patients (life expectancy <1 year) with ≥1 visit to ER or hospitalization in last year • 47% with cancer • Interdisciplinary home-based care health-care program designed to enhance comfort and improve QOL (hospice model with MD, RN, SW) • PC team responsible for care	• Patient satisfaction improved ($P < 0.05$) • Home death more likely (OR = 2.20, $P < 0.001$) • Hospital days reduced by 4.36 ($P < 0.001$) • ED visits reduced by 0.35 ($P = 0.02$) • Cost decreased ($12,670 vs $20,222, $P = 0.03$)
Gade et al. (2008) [16]	• Patients hospitalized with life-limiting illnesses • 34% with cancer in PC arm • Interdisciplinary PC consult service (MD and RN, hospital SW and chaplain) • Home service continued with local resources • PC team responsible for care	• Satisfaction improved ($P = 0.04$) • Providers' communication improved ($P = 0.0004$) • Net cost savings of $4,855 per patient ($P < 0.001$) • Longer median hospice stays (24 days versus 12 days, $P = 0.04$)
Cassel et al. (2010) [31]	• PC specialist shares clinic space with oncologists	• Satisfaction high among patients, families, staff, referring physicians, oncologists. • Physician can earn a reasonable income: billings $59,070, collections $29,604 (50%) for about 15 hours a week. • Hospital saves about $400 a day on inpatients, $80–$130,000 yearly.
Muir et al. (2010) [32]	• PC attending and fellow share clinic space with oncologists and receive referrals from oncologists within the practice	• Oncologist saved 170 minutes per PC consultation • Patient symptom burden decreased by 21% • PC consultation requests increased by 87% • Oncologist overall satisfaction with PC consultants was 9/10

MD, medical doctor; RN, registered nurse; SW, social worker.

for the future often arise. However, we would like to emphasize that patient and family satisfaction appears to increase when patients receive palliative care [16,17]. Furthermore, a large number of resources are available to help physicians learn techniques for communication with patients in such difficult situations. A selection of such resources available online is shown in Table 8.2.

Palliative care should be introduced early, as should the concept of hospice care. ASCO recommends a "hospice information visit" when patients have 3 to 6 months to live, in order to smooth the transition later. Most radiation and other oncologists prefer to wait until "there are no more treatment options left" before discussion of advance medical directives, resuscitation, and even hospice [19]. This partly explains why half of lung cancer patients reach 60 days before death with none of their doctors ever mentioning hospice [20]. The average "end of life" conversation comes with just 33 days left to live and was documented by the oncologists in only 27% of cases [21]. This does not allow time for appropriate planning. All the available studies have reported longer – not shorter – survival with hospice use and better spouse survival if hospice was used [22–24].

Are there standards for palliative care? If so, what are the defining measures?

Palliative care has generated a significant amount of academic interest within the past 10 years and has recently been recognized as an independent specialty by the American Council on Graduate Medical Education (ACGME). In the United States, trainees receive a year of specific clinical training in pain and symptom control for patients with severe illness, communication techniques with patients and families, and establishment and maintenance of a strong physician–patient relationship. Advanced practice nurses often play a prominent role in palliative care programs and are required to have at least master's level training in their area of specialization [25].

A task force including the American Academy of Hospice and Palliative Medicine (AAHPM), the Center to Advance Palliative Care (CAPC), the Hospice and Palliative Nurses Association (HPNA), and the National Hospice and Palliative Care Organization (NHPCO) developed general guidelines for palliative care programs in the National Consensus Project for Quality Palliative Care [4]. The Consensus Project guidelines focus on the philosophies, structures, and processes that should underlie palliative care programs and do not enumerate specific techniques of medical management. However, the National Comprehensive Cancer Network (NCCN) and many professional organizations, including ASCO, have published detailed guidelines for pain and symptom management in cancer patients, as shown in Table 8.2. More than any other measure, palliative care is defined by a focus on alleviating suffering through evidence-based, patient- and family-focused, interdisciplinary care. Empathetic and clear communication with patients and their families, respecting cultural differences, and elucidating psychosocial and spiritual

Table 8.2 Online palliative care resources and clinical guidelines.

Title (with Web address as of March 2012)	Topics discussed
Oncotalk: Improving Your Communication Skills http://depts.washington.edu/oncotalk/learn/modules.html	General communication skills, delivering bad news, discussing advance directives, conducting family meetings, discussing discontinuation of ineffective "treatments."
The University of Sydney's Question Prompt Lists (for patients) http://www.ncbi.nlm.nih.gov/pmc/articles/PMC2376858/	List of questions for patients and their families to discuss with physicians regarding palliative and end-of-life care issues and decision-making.
EPEC-O (Education in Palliative and End-of-Life Care for Oncology) http://www.cancer.gov/cancertopics/cancerlibrary/epeco	Palliative care education materials from the U.S. National Cancer Institute. Online self-study modules discussing patient evaluation, communication skills, symptom management, end-of-life planning. Also available on CD-ROM.
City of Hope Pain and Palliative Care Resource Center http://prc.coh.org	Clearinghouse of materials on a wide range of palliative care topics.
NCCN Guidelines for Supportive Care http://www.nccn.org/professionals/physician_gls/f_guidelines.asp#supportive	General palliative care guideline with specific attention to symptom management (e.g. pain, nausea, fatigue, anemia).
Agency for Health Care Research and Quality General Guideline Clearinghouse http://www.guideline.gov/browse/by-topic.aspx	Comprehensive list of cancer care guidelines from both U.S. and international professional societies.
General Guidelines for Palliative Care Interventions http://www.nejm.org/doi/suppl/10.1056/NEJMoa1000678/suppl_file/nejmoa1000678_appendix.pdf	Structure of the palliative care intervention used by Temel *et al.* in the recently published randomized trial of a palliative care intervention in lung cancer patients.
Palliative Radiotherapy for Bone Metastases: an ASTRO Evidence-Based Guideline https://www.astro.org/Clinical-Practice/Guidelines/Bone-Metastases.aspx	Provides guidance regarding the treatment of bone metastases, including fractionation and dosing schemes, treatment margins, and retreatment.
Palliative Radiotherapy in Lung Cancer: an ASTRO Evidence-Based Clinical Practice Guideline https://www.astro.org/Clinical-Practice/Guidelines/Palliative-thoracic.aspx	Provides guidance regarding the treatment of symptomatic, metastatic lung cancers, including dosing and fractionation schemes, the use of brachytherapy, and the use of concurrent chemotherapy.

needs are other critical requirements of an adequate palliative care program. We have used a simple framework for effective palliative consultations, shown in Box 8.2.

The establishment of specific standards of care for palliative radiation therapy (RT) remains a work in progress. The American Society for Radiation Oncology (ASTRO) has issued guidelines regarding the treatment of painful bone metastases and patients with symptomatic, metastatic thoracic malignancies [26,27]. Radiation therapy is also mentioned in the NCCN palliative care guidelines and in guidelines for the treatment of brain metastases, spinal cord compression, and bone metastases issued by other professional organizations. These guidelines were designed to provide guidance regarding appropriate treatment techniques, particularly dosage and fractionation schemes, for patients with symptomatic bony or thoracic lesions. Table 8.2 also highlights a selection of available guidelines.

Overall, however, there is a relative paucity of formal recommendations to guide the care of patients requiring palliative radiation therapy, and the nationwide level of adherence to such guidelines has been questioned. For example, use of a 2-week fractionation scheme for the treatment of bone metastases remains common, despite a national guideline recommending the use of single-fraction treatment in many cases [28]. There is a particular lack of guidance regarding decision-making about which patients need RT and when to institute treatment. Rarely do patients present directly to a radiation oncologist to request care, and early multi-disciplinary assessments of many patients with metastatic disease are infrequent. Instead, radiation oncologists rely on referrals from medical oncologists, surgeons, and occasionally general practitioners (particularly hospitalists). Depending on individual practice patterns, referrals for radiation therapy may be made any time in the course of disease, and clinical practice is highly variable in this regard. Some suggestions for "triggers" for considering palliative radiation therapy are included in Table 8.3. It should be noted that, for most of these situations, little prospective evidence is available to guide treatment, and these recommendations are based primarily on clinical experience. Where applicable, however, citations are provided.

How does palliative care fit in with radiation oncology?

Radiation oncologists are often called upon to manage symptomatic lesions in patients with incurable disease. They are also frequently involved in the care of patients with curable tumors but who have severe symptoms related to the disease itself or to side effects of treatment. Because most patients receive RT on a daily basis, a radiation oncology treatment course provides an excellent opportunity for close monitoring of a patient's clinical status (e.g. responses to changes in medication). Palliative care can therefore be easily integrated across the spectrum of radiation oncology practice, particularly

Table 8.3 Clinical situations where radiotherapy can provide symptom palliation; techniques for improving the therapeutic ratio of radiotherapy.

Diagnosis	When to consider radiotherapy	Techniques to improve radiotherapy therapeutic ratio
Bony metastatic disease or painful soft tissue lesions [26]	• Pain refractory to medication • Unacceptable medication side effects	• Hypofractionation • Stereotactic body RT (spine disease)
Brain metastases	• Symptomatic brain lesions (single or multiple) • After resection of brain metastasis [33]	• Stereotactic radiosurgery [34] • Hypofractionated whole brain radiation • Close attention to steroid dose and avoidance of unnecessary antiepileptic medications
Spinal cord compression	• After decompressive spinal surgery [35] • Patients with SCC not eligible for surgery	• Stereotactic radiotherapy [36]
Thoracic tumors [27]	• Airway obstruction • Hemoptysis • SVC syndrome • Hoarseness/Dysphagia	• Brachytherapy
Gastrointestinal tumors	• Gastric outlet obstruction • Biliary tree obstruction • GI bleeding	• Prophylactic anti-emetic regimens during RT • Brachytherapy
Pelvic tumors	• Existing or impending hydronephrosis or other urinary tract obstruction (due to tumor) • Existing or impending bowel obstruction (due to tumor) • Vaginal or rectal bleeding • Sacral nerve root compression (from posterior pelvic tumors) • Malignant pelvic fistulae	• Hypofractionation • Brachytherapy

because palliative care interventions do not preclude the patient from receiving curative-intent or life-prolonging treatment.

For all patients, but particularly in those with metastatic or end-stage disease, the radiation oncologist must be sensitive to balancing the side effects of a planned treatment with its anticipated benefits. Table 8.3 provides examples of commonly encountered clinical situations where RT can provide symptom palliation and suggests techniques for improving the therapeutic ratio of RT. The duration of a planned radiation therapy treatment (both in terms of time spent on the table and in terms of the overall length of the treatment course) and its anticipated side effects should be carefully considered and balanced with available clinical evidence, the patient's performance status, and his or her preferences for treatment. For example, in many patients, RT for bone metastases may be safely condensed into a single external beam or stereotactic treatment session. Single-fraction palliative RT decreases costs, increases convenience for patients, and has similar outcomes to prolonged fractionated treatment [26]. By weighing an understandable enthusiasm for the latest technology with a careful, individualized assessment of each patient's needs, the radiation oncologist may be able to challenge established pre-conceptions about the costs, efficacy, side effects, and inconvenience of radiation therapy.

References

1. Smith TJ, Temin S, Alesi ER, *et al.* American society of clinical oncology provisional clinical opinion: the integration of palliative care into standard oncology care. *J Clin Oncol* 2012; **30**: 880–887.
2. Saunders C. A personal therapeutic journey. *BMJ* 1996; **313**: 1599–1601.
3. Hills J, Paice JA, Cameron JR, Shott S. Spirituality and distress in palliative care consultation. *J Palliat Med* 2005; **8**: 782–788.
4. National Consensus Project for Quality Palliative Care. Clinical practice guidelines for quality palliative care, second edition [Internet]. Available at: http://www.nationalconsensusproject.org/guideline.pdf (accessed March 20, 2002).
5. National Cancer Institute. EPEC-O palliative care educational materials, self-study guide [Internet]. Available at: http://www.cancer.gov/cancertopics/cancerlibrary/epeco/selfstudy (accessed March 20, 2012).
6. Bruera E, Kuehn N, Miller MJ, *et al.* The edmonton symptom assessment system (ESAS): a simple method for the assessment of palliative care patients. *J Palliat Care* 1991; **7**: 6–9.
7. Portenoy RK, Thaler HT, Kornblith AB, *et al.* The memorial symptom assessment scale: an instrument for the evaluation of symptom prevalence, characteristics and distress. *Eur J Cancer* 1994; **30A**: 1326–1336.
8. Chang VT, Hwang SS, Kasimis B, Thaler HT. Shorter symptom assessment instruments: the condensed memorial symptom assessment scale (CMSAS). *Cancer Invest* 2004; **22**: 526–536.
9. Scandrett KG, Reitschuler-Cross EB, Nelson L, *et al.* Feasibility and effectiveness of the NEST13+ as a screening tool for advanced illness care needs. *J Palliat Med* 2010; **13**: 161–169.
10. Schapira L, Tulsky J, Buckman R, Pollak J. Communication: what do patients want and need? *J Oncol Pract* 2008; **4**: 249–253.
11. Gelfman LP, Morrison RS. Research funding for palliative medicine. *J Palliat Med* 2008; **11**: 36–43.
12. Temel JS, Greer JA, Muzikansky A, *et al.* Early palliative care for patients with metastatic non-small-cell lung cancer. *N Engl J Med* 2010; **363**: 733–742.

13. Temel JS, Greer JA, Admane S, *et al*. Longitudinal perceptions of prognosis and goals of therapy in patients with metastatic non-small-cell lung cancer: results of a randomized study of early palliative care. *J Clin Oncol* 2011; **29**: 2319–2326.

14. Greer JA, Pirl WF, Jackson VA, *et al*. Effect of early palliative care on chemotherapy use and end-of-life care in patients with metastatic non-small-cell lung cancer. *J Clin Oncol* 2012; **30**: 394–400.

15. Jacobsen J, Jackson V, Dahlin C, *et al*. Components of early outpatient palliative care consultation in patients with metastatic nonsmall cell lung cancer. *J Palliat Med* 2011; **14**: 459–464.

16. Gade G, Venohr I, Conner D, *et al*. Impact of an inpatient palliative care team: a randomized control trial. *J Palliat Med* 2008; **11**: 180–190.

17. Brumley R, Enguidanos S, Jamison P, *et al*. Increased satisfaction with care and lower costs: results of a randomized trial of in-home palliative care. *J Am Geriatr Soc* 2007; **55**: 993–1000.

18. Bakitas M, Lyons KD, Hegel MT, *et al*. Effects of a palliative care intervention on clinical outcomes in patients with advanced cancer: the project ENABLE II randomized controlled trial. *JAMA* 2009; **302**: 741–749.

19. Keating NL, Landrum MB, Rogers SO, *et al*. Physician factors associated with discussions about end-of-life care. *Cancer* 2010; **116**: 998–1006.

20. Huskamp HA, Keating NL, Malin JL, *et al*. Discussions with physicians about hospice among patients with metastatic lung cancer. *Arch Intern Med* 2009; **169**: 954–962.

21. Mack JW, Cronin A, Taback N, *et al*. End-of-life care discussions among patients with advanced cancer: a cohort study. *Ann Intern Med* 2012; **156**: 204–210.

22. Connor SR, Pyenson B, Fitch K, *et al*. Comparing hospice and nonhospice patient survival among patients who die within a three-year window. *J Pain Symptom Manage* 2007; **33**: 238–246.

23. Saito AM, Landrum MB, Neville BA, *et al*. Hospice care and survival among elderly patients with lung cancer. *J Palliat Med* 2011; **14**: 929–939.

24. Christakis NA, Iwashyna TJ. The health impact of health care on families: a matched cohort study of hospice use by decedents and mortality outcomes in surviving, widowed spouses. *Soc Sci Med* 2003; **57**: 465–475.

25. Meier DE, Beresford L. Advanced practice nurses in palliative care: a pivotal role and perspective. *J Palliat Med* 2006; **9**: 624–627.

26. Lutz S, Berk L, Chang E, *et al*. Palliative radiotherapy for bone metastases: an ASTRO evidence-based guideline. *Int J Radiat Oncol Biol Phys* 2011; **79**: 965–976.

27. Rodrigues G, Macbeth F, Burmeister B, *et al*. Consensus statement on palliative lung radiotherapy: third international consensus workshop on palliative radiotherapy and symptom control. *Clin Lung Cancer* 2012; **13**: 1–5.

28. Kachnic L, Berk L. Palliative single-fraction radiation therapy: how much more evidence is needed? *J Natl Cancer Inst* 2005; **97**: 786–788.

29. Chochinov HM, Wilson KG, Enns M, Lander S. "Are you depressed?" screening for depression in the terminally ill. *Am J Psychiatry* 1997; **154**: 674–676.

30. Rabow MW, Dibble SL, Pantilat SZ, McPhee SJ. The comprehensive care team: a controlled trial of outpatient palliative medicine consultation. *Arch Intern Med* 2004; **164**: 83–91.

31. Cassel JB, Webb-Wright J, Holmes J, *et al*. Clinical and financial impact of a palliative care program at a small rural hospital. *J Palliat Med* 2010; **13**: 1339–1343.

32. Muir JC, Daly F, Davis MS, *et al*. Integrating palliative care into the outpatient, private practice oncology setting. *J Pain Symptom Manage* 2010; **40**: 126–135.

33. Patchell RA, Tibbs PA, Regine WF, *et al.* Postoperative radiotherapy in the treatment of single metastases to the brain: a randomized trial. *JAMA* 1998; **280**: 1485–1489.
34. Kocher M, Soffietti R, Abacioglu U, *et al.* Adjuvant whole-brain radiotherapy versus observation after radiosurgery or surgical resection of one to three cerebral metastases: results of the EORTC 22952-26001 study. *J Clin Oncol* 2011; **29**: 134–141.
35. Patchell RA, Tibbs PA, Regine WF, *et al.* Direct decompressive surgical resection in the treatment of spinal cord compression caused by metastatic cancer: a randomised trial. *Lancet* 2005; **366**: 643–648.
36. Cox BW, Spratt DE, Lovelock M, *et al.* International spine radiosurgery consortium consensus guidelines for target volume definition in spinal stereotactic radiosurgery. *Int J Radiat Oncol Biol Phys* 2012; **83**: e597–605.

CHAPTER 9

Palliative care in low and middle income countries: A focus on sub-Saharan Africa

Henry Ddungu[1], Elizabeth A. Barnes[2]
[1]Uganda Cancer Institute, Kampala, Uganda
[2]Department of Radiation Oncology, University of Toronto, Odette Cancer Centre, Toronto, ON, Canada

Introduction

Africa is the second largest and second most populated continent on Earth, with over one billion people residing in over 50 countries. In spite of abundant natural resources, Africa remains the world's poorest continent. As such, it serves as an extreme example of the challenges faced by those who deliver palliative care in low- and middle-income countries (LMC). The region faces a multitude of infectious diseases such as malaria and AIDS that help to limit the overall life expectancy of the population. While the average age of Africans remains only about 25 years, the increasing number of older patients contributes to the 45% of the adult global non-infectious disease burden in LMC facing limited health-care resources.

The need for palliative care

The need for palliative care for cancer patients in developing countries is significant owing to the number who are affected and the propensity for advanced-stage disease at presentation. There were over 700,000 new cancer cases and nearly 600,000 cancer-related deaths in Africa in 2007, and it is expected that cancer rates will grow by 400% over the next 50 years [1]. Treatment options are often limited by the tumor burden at the time of diagnosis, even in comparably affluent LMC countries. The factors that lead to delayed diagnosis are predictable and include the absence of screening for common cancers, lack of awareness and education about cancer amongst the general

Radiation Oncology in Palliative Cancer Care, First Edition. Edited by Stephen Lutz, Edward Chow, and Peter Hoskin.
© 2013 John Wiley & Sons, Ltd. Published 2013 by John Wiley & Sons, Ltd.

population, poor access to physicians and health-care facilities, and distrust of the medical system.

The true incidence and mortality of cancer in LMC is difficult to quantify given the difficulties of obtaining accurate cancer statistics. Cancer cases may not be registered, pathology not obtained on sites difficult to biopsy, and hospital series are biased by the clinical facilities available [2]. Mortality statistics are sparse based on the absence of death registries in many countries. The AIDS epidemic has increased the number of cancers as immunosuppresed patients are more likely to develop malignancy. Rapid population growth and better control of other infectious disease will also increase the incidence of cancer, along with lifestyle changes associated with economic development such as sedentary work and nutritional preferences. There is enormous geographical diversity in the incidence of cancer between different countries in Africa. Overall, cancers with the highest incidence are cervix, breast, and AIDS-associated Kaposi sarcoma (KS) in women; and Kaposi sarcoma, liver, bladder, prostate and non-Hodgkin lymphoma in men [2]. As many as 36% of cancers in Africa are infection-related, double the world average.

The burden of symptoms amongst cancer patients is huge, with only very few being able to access quality palliative care services. In a study carried out in two African countries to determine the symptom prevalence and burden amongst advanced cancer patients, pain and psychologic problems were the most common symptoms and the mean number of symptoms was far higher than reported in other global studies [3]. The etiology of symptoms is usually multi-dimensional, hence the need for holistic approaches to patient assessment and management.

Radiotherapy

Radiotherapy has an essential role in cancer treatment, in both the curative and palliative setting. In high-income countries it is estimated that 52% of new cancer cases should receive radiotherapy at least once, and up to 25% might receive a second course [4]. Patients in LMC countries may have an even greater need given the types of cancer and advanced stage of disease at presentation [5]. Access to radiotherapy services in Africa is extremely limited. Of the 56 African countries, 33 have none or only orthovoltage facilities, resulting in 21% of the population having no access to radiotherapy [6]. A multitude of barriers exist preventing access to quality radiotherapy [5]. There is a need for trained physicians, radiation therapists, and physicists, as well as technicians for machine maintenance. Opportunities for continuing medical education and links with high-income countries to facilitate knowledge transfer would be beneficial. Patients also need to be referred by primary care and palliative care physicians who recognize the role of radiotherapy in cancer management. Radiotherapy facilities are typically located in large urban cancer centers, meaning that patients from rural settings need assistance with travel and accommodation. Given that radiotherapy is one of the most cost-effective forms of cancer treatment, the financial and manpower investment would seem to be a worthwhile endeavor.

Specific clinical indications for palliative radiotherapy in Africa

Kaposi sarcoma

Radiation therapy is a known treatment option for Kaposi sarcoma, especially the endemic type that typically affects the foot and which is common in African countries. The etiology of this affliction seems perhaps to be associated with soil exposure and oncogenes that lead to chronic inflammation, and this typically affects elderly men [7]. Such patients usually experience severe discomfort that makes it difficult to ambulate or even wear shoes. Response to radiotherapy treatment is often dramatic, with 80–90% of the patients reporting complete resolution of symptoms by the end of treatment [8]. AIDS-associated KS (epidemic KS) is widely spread in sub-Saharan Africa where HIV prevalence is still relatively high [9]. Like endemic KS, epidemic KS is radiosensitive, and radiation therapy is considered to be the palliative treatment of choice for localized disease. A South African trial demonstrated an objective response rate of 96% using 20 Gy in 5 fractions [10]. Single fractions of 8 Gy can also be utilized, although that approach may be more appropriate for patients with limited survival as the duration of response is thought to be shorter, of the order of a few months [11].

Cervical cancer

More than 85% of cervix cancer cases worldwide are found in LMC. Recent advances in cervix cancer management, such as the introduction of the HPV vaccine for disease prevention and incorporation of concurrent chemoradiation for definitive treatment, have not been extended to the vast majority of women who live in countries with limited resources [12,13]. Routine screening is not available to the vast majority of the population, and as a result many women present with advanced stage disease. Radiotherapy is the mainstay of treatment for these patients, either in the curative or purely palliative setting. There is a lack of information in the literature on the optimal palliative radiation schedule [14]. Vaginal bleeding and pelvic pain are among the most common symptoms, and these can be alleviated with the use of palliative radiotherapy with response rates of 45–100% and 0–83% respectively [15]. Various hypofractionated regimes have been reported, and the use of large single fractions repeated monthly up to 3 times can provide durable and effective palliation.

Cervical cancer is the most common cancer in young woman in sub-Saharan Africa, and 1 in 6 women of reproductive age in South Africa is HIV positive [16]. HIV-associated disease is characterized by a rapid progression to more advanced stages and lower rates of completing radical chemoradiotherapy treatment [17]. Higher rates of treatment failures and recurrence have been reported in the HIV compared to the non-HIV population [18,19].

Challenges of palliative care delivery

Cancer treatment modalities such as radiotherapy and chemotherapy are available to less than 20% of the population in Africa, and consequently a cancer diagnosis is almost a sentence to a painful and distressing death [20]. Access to holistic care aimed at improving the quality of life of a cancer patient is a right yet to be realized in most parts of Africa. The reasons why patients with life-threatening illnesses unduly suffer include a lack of: a) national policies that would enable palliative care development; b) education of health workers and the general public about this important aspect of care; c) access to essential pain medicines, particularly opioids; and d) implementation at all levels of service delivery. These are the fundamentals for an effective palliative care program, and their coexistence is rare in most parts of the African continent.

Over 80% of cancer patients in need of pain relief in Africa are not able to access effective pain medicines as recommended by the World Health Organization (WHO) because of national policies and regulations that are not well-balanced to enable access to pain control while preventing illicit use. It is only a few countries in LMCs that have reasonable access to medicines that are controlled under international drug conventions, whereas a large percentage of countries have almost no access to drugs such as opioids. In addition to the overly restrictive legislation, physicians have fallen out of practice in prescribing appropriately strong pain medicines even in locales where they are available.

Even in countries that have put emphasis on pain medicine availability and education about best-use policies, they have often not instituted concurrent policies to motivate implementation of appropriate palliative care. The relative lack of legalized prescribers can act as a barrier to appropriate palliative pain interventions in a specific geographic area, leaving medicines to expire on the shelves of pharmacies. Lack of government commitment to funding of palliative care programs can also limit proper pain control measures. Uganda has been one of the African nations that has included palliative care in the basic care package for its populace, allowing trained nurses and clinical officers to prescribe opioids, and including palliative care training in the curriculum of public medical training institutions [21,22].

Addressing challenges to adequate palliative care

Palliative care in medical training curricula

It has been 45 years since modern palliative care came into existence when St. Christopher's Hospice was opened in England. However, due to limitations in education in most LMCs, palliative care is rather "new" and is not taught in medical training institutions. Health professionals in these countries are therefore not aware of palliative care and many interpret it as only applicable when aggressive treatment fails. The general public, as well as policy makers, are also not aware of palliative care and cannot therefore demand this right in health-related policies.

In 1990, a WHO report, *Cancer Pain Relief and Palliative Care*, recommended to all WHO member states that "pain relief and palliative care programs are incorporated into their existing health-care systems..." and that "governments should ensure that health-care workers are adequately trained in palliative care and the relief of cancer pain" [23]. The initiation of successful training in palliative care requires recognition by and enlistment of national opinion leaders in health and allied professional schools that train physicians, pharmacists, and nurses. Only then can one engage the required professionals in the process of incorporating palliative care into existing curricula and subsequently into patient care clinics.

Unfortunately, palliative medicine in Africa has been unable to successfully enter the competition for curriculum space in most medical schools, which are already concerned about information overload. However, it is possible to integrate palliative care courses in the curricula, and this has been seen to work in countries such as Uganda, where education and training were successfully started in two medical schools by delivering palliative care lectures to fourth-year medical students [24]. Furthermore, implementation of useful palliative oncology care will require adequate education of the general public about the advantages of this approach.

Leadership
Another important challenge faced by palliative care development is the general lack of dedicated leaders that are visionary, inspiring, honest, credible, and competent. This lack of palliative care leadership has contributed to the slow growth of palliative care in LMCs. The International Palliative Care Leadership Initiative has been working to develop palliative care leaders for LMCs around the world [25]. The leadership courses are provided by grants and facilitate palliative care education through mentoring by senior palliative care professionals as well as local and peer palliative care mentors. The overarching goal of the program is to facilitate proper palliative care techniques to countries worldwide.

Further efforts to promote advocacy of worldwide palliative care specifically as related to appropriate pain medicine are underway. These include developing methods and resources to assist governments, oncologists, and pain and palliative care groups to examine national policies and make regulatory changes that would be supportive of access. The African Palliative Care Association (APCA), WHO, and the Pain and Policy Studies Group (PPSG) have developed several resources all geared towards improving access to pain medicine. Other attempts include working with governments and health-care providers to ensure that patients can access pain medicines. In Africa, APCA has been engaged in advocating for increased access to pain medicines throughout the region since its operational formation in 2005. APCA advocates for affordable oral morphine that is reconstituted from morphine sulphate powder to an elixir. Oral morphine can be safely administered from a patient's home, which has been reported as the preferred place to die in a study from Uganda [26]. Home is also where patients are able to actively participate in the control of their own dosing after receiving training on how to administer the medicine.

The International Pain Policy Fellowship (IPPF) is an initiative developed by the Pain and Policy Studies Group (PPSG), a WHO Collaborating Center at the University of Wisconsin, with the goal to develop national leaders from LMCs to improve availability of, and access to, opioid analgesics in their countries for the treatment of pain related to cancer and AIDS. The 2-year Fellowship is intended for mid-career health professionals, health-care administrators, policy experts, and lawyers. The IPPF program has been successful in developing national leaders from LMCs who have engaged with government to identify and remove barriers that block patient access to opioid analgesics. As an example, the program empowered fellows from Sierra Leone, Colombia, and Serbia, with knowledge, skills, and guidance to improve the availability and accessibility of opioids for medical use in their countries, while also making efforts to prevent abuse and diversion [27].

The role of governments

To effectively integrate palliative care into existing health systems, governments need to develop appropriate policies that provide for adequate availability of medicines (particularly opioids), education of health-care workers and the general public, and appropriate implementation of palliative care services at all levels of society.

Governments in developing countries should include palliative care in the national health plan, policies, and related regulations as well as devise a mechanism for funding and/or service delivery models that support palliative care service delivery [28]. Unfortunately, most countries in Africa have not yet included palliative care in their national policies or regulations.

Palliative care research

Evidence generated through well-designed research has contributed to changing policy and clinical practice for patients with life threatening diseases in need of palliative care. The challenge is that most of this evidence has been generated in developed countries and is therefore not generalizable to LMCs. The primary challenges to conducting rigorous palliative care research in LMCs include the scarcity of validated outcome measures; methodologic challenges; inadequate research capacity and skills, plus logistical challenges to data collection and transfer; and the absence of formalized mechanisms for ethical research in some countries.

An African outcome tool, the African Palliative Care Association Palliative Outcome Scale (APCA POS), is a brief 10 item self-report that enables the patient and family to score their problems across domains essential to palliative care [29]. The APCA POS has been validated across diseases, countries, settings, and languages and found to have sound psychometric properties, be well comprehended, and be brief to use [30]. It has resulted in a tool that is widely adopted and has facilitated the measurement and improvement of outcomes in a wide range of settings, and these studies are beginning to be published. This can allow palliative care initiatives in Africa to prove their effectiveness and use this evidence to powerfully advocate for clinical and policy attention [31].

Funding for palliative care research remains a big challenge that has hindered generations of evidence in this area. The cost of conducting clinical trials, the complexity and delays associated with regulatory approval of new products, and the need to ensure ethical research conduct have been cited as major challenges that need to be overcome so that clinical research is effective and efficient in delivering the evidence necessary to improve cancer care. Overcoming these barriers requires global collaborative partnerships sensitive and responsive to both local and global needs [32].

Delivery of palliative care

To effectively reach the person in need, palliative care has to be integrated into existing health structures through a range of care settings and models. Models that are common in LMC include home-based care, facility-based outpatient or inpatient care, outreach services, hospital based palliative care teams providing liaison palliative care, and hospice inpatient care. Details of each of these models are beyond the scope of this chapter. However, before deciding on a model, the care-giving entity must address several important questions.

• Is there a need for a palliative care service?
• What is the geographic locale of the patients?
• What burden can be sustained by the existing health-care infrastructure?
• What are the special needs of the patient group?

To address methodological challenges, Harding recommended the following strategies [33]:

• Collaboration between researchers in resource-abundant and resource-constrained countries of Africa need to be centered on more meaningful sharing of skills aimed at building individual and organizational capacity.

• Existing palliative care training courses should integrate research methods into their existing curricula for all cadres of staff.

• Adequate resources should be provided for ongoing technical support to centers engaged in research, including resources to support research methods, protocol design, data collection, management, and analysis.

• Designated resources from funding organizations should be directed to evaluate direct care allocation to help ensure effective and systematic documentation of lessons learned and to allow for the replication of successful initiatives and interventions.

• Project-specific staff should be dedicated to research to ensure that data collection and management are completed in a timely fashion and in accordance with the study protocol requirements.

• Development and validation of multi-dimensional outcome measures (e.g. the APCA POS) should address domains of importance to LMCs.

Conclusion

The delivery of palliative oncology care in African nations and other LMC countries is complicated by several factors including poverty, lack of education, poorly funded and coordinated health care, and ineffectual government leadership. Patients with cancer in these nations are unlikely to receive adequate medical care and commonly face great suffering and high rates of death. Improvements in the care of these patients will require greater education of the medical community and general populace about palliative care as well as further resource allocation toward patient advocacy and support. Several international organizations have begun to approach these tasks, though the projected increase in the need for palliative oncology services in these geographic settings requires a more dedicated level of attention than has been paid to this important issue.

References

1. Morris K. Cancer? In Africa? *Lancet Oncol* 2003; **4**: 5.
2. Parkin DM, Sitas F, Chirenje M, *et al*. Part I: cancer in Indigenous Africans–burden, distribution, and trends. *Lancet Oncol* 2008; **9**: 683–692.
3. Harding R, Selman L, Agupio G, *et al*. The prevalence and burden of symptoms amongst cancer patients attending palliative care in two African countries. *Eur J Cancer* 2011; **47**: 51–56.
4. Delaney G, Jacob S, Featherstone C, Barton M. The role of radiotherapy in cancer treatment: estimating optimal utilization from a review of evidence-based clinical guidelines. *Cancer* 2005; **104**: 1129–1137.
5. Barton MB, Frommer M, Shafiq J. Role of radiotherapy in cancer control in low-income and middle-income countries. *Lancet Oncol* 2006; **7**: 584–595.
6. Levin CV, El Gueddari B, Meghzifene A. Radiation therapy in Africa: distribution and equipment. *Radiother Oncol* 1999; **52**: 79–84.
7. Ziegler J, Simonart T, Snoeck R. Kaposi's sarcoma, oncogenic viruses, and iron. *J Clin Virol* 2001; **20**: 127–130.
8. Stein ME, Lakier R, Kuten A, *et al*. Radiation therapy in endemic (African) Kaposi's sarcoma. *Int J Radiat Oncol Biol Phys* 1993; **27**: 1181–1184.
9. Mbulaiteye S, Bhatia K, Adebamowo C, *et al*. HIV and cancer in Africa: mutual collaboration between HIV and cancer programs may provide timely research and public health data. *Infect Agent Cancer* 2011; **6**: 16.

10. Singh NB, Lakier RH, Donde B. Hypofractionated radiation therapy in the treatment of epidemic Kaposi sarcoma–a prospective randomized trial. *Radiother Oncol* 2008; **2**: 211–216.
11. de Wit R, Smit WG, Veenhof KH, *et al.* Palliative radiation therapy for AIDS-associated Kaposi's sarcoma by using a single fraction of 800 cGy. *Radiother Oncol* 1990; **19**: 131–136.
12. Waggoner SE. Cervical cancer. *Lancet* 2003; **361**: 2217–2225.
13. Bello FA, Enabor OO, Adewole IF. Human papilloma virus vaccination for control of cervical cancer: a challenge for developing countries. *Afr J Reprod Health* 2011; **15**: 25–30.
14. van Lonkhuijzen L, Thomas G. Palliative radiotherapy for cervical carcinoma, a systematic review. *Radiother Oncol* 2011; **98**: 287–291.
15. Skliarenko J, Barnes EA. Palliative pelvic radiotherapy for gynaecologic cancer. *J Radiat Oncol* 2012; **1**: 239–244.
16. Draper B, Pienaar D, Parker W, Rehle T. Recommendations for Policy in the Western Cape Province for the Prevention of Major Infectious Diseases, Including HIV/AIDS and Tuberculosis. Cape Town, South Africa: Western Cape Department of Health; 2006.
17. Simonds HM, Wright JD, Du Toit N, *et al.* Completion of and early response to chemoradiation among human immunodeficiency virus (HIV)-positive and HIV-negative patients with locally advanced cervical carcinoma in South Africa. *Cancer* 2012; **118**: 2971–2979.
18. Moodley M, Mould S. Invasive cervical cancer and human immunodeficiency virus (HIV) infection in KwaZulu-Natal, South Africa. *J Obstet Gynaecol* 2005; **25**: 706–710.
19. Gichangi P, Bwayo J, Estambale B, *et al.* HIV impact on acute morbidity and pelvic tumor control following radiotherapy for cervical cancer. *Gynecol Oncol* 2006; **100**: 405–411.
20. Ddungu H. Palliative care: what approaches are suitable in developing countries? *Br J Haematol* 2011; doi: 10.1111/j.1365-2141.2011.08764.x.
21. Merriman A, Harding R. Pain control in the African context: the Ugandan introduction of affordable morphine to relieve suffering at the end of life. *Philos Ethics Humanit Med* 2010; **5**: 10.
22. Powell RA, Kaye RM, Ddungu H, *et al.* Advancing drug availability-experiences from Africa. *J Pain Symptom Manage* 2010; **40**: 9–12.
23. World Health Organization. Cancer pain relief and palliative care. Report of a WHO Expert Committee. *World Health Organ Tech Rep Ser* 1990; **804**: 1–75.
24. Jagwe J, Merriman A. Palliative medicine, an urgent public health need in the developing world. *J Public Health Policy* 2007; **28**: 40–41.
25. The Institute for Palliative Medicine at the San Diego Hospice: International palliative care leadership development initiative. Available at: http://www.ipcrc.net/news/wp-content/uploads/2012/02/Leadership-Development-Initiative-LDI-Overview-Nov-2011.pdf (accessed August 16, 2012).
26. Kikule E. A good death in Uganda: survey of needs for palliative care for terminally ill people in urban areas. *BMJ* 2003; **327**: 192–194.
27. Bosnjak S, Maurer MA, Ryan KM, *et al.* Improving the availability and accessibility of opioids for the treatment of pain: the International Pain Policy Fellowship. *Support Care Cancer* 2011; **19**: 1239–1247.
28. Stjernsward J, Foley KM, Ferris FD. Integrating palliative care into national policies. *J Pain Symptom Manage* 2007; **33**: 514–520.
29. Powell RA, Downing J, Harding R, *et al.* Development of the APCA African Palliative Outcome Scale. *J Pain Symptom Manage* 2007; **33**: 229–232.

30. Harding R, Selman L, Agupio G, *et al*. Validation of a core outcome measure for palliative care in Africa: the APCA African Palliative Outcome Scale. *Health Qual life Outcomes* 2010; **8**: 10.

31. Harding R, Gwyther L, Mwangi-Powell F, *et al*. How can we improve palliative care patient outcomes in low- and middle-income countries? Successful outcomes research in sub-Saharan Africa. *J Pain Symptom Manage* 2010; **40**: 23–26.

32. Lyerly HK, Abernethy AP, Stockler MR, *et al*. Need for global partnership in cancer care: perceptions of cancer care researchers attending the 2010 Australia and Asia Pacific Clinical Oncology Research Development Workshop. *J Oncol Pract/Am Soc Clin Oncol* 2011; **7**: 324–329.

33. Harding R, Powell RA, Downing J, *et al*. Generating an African palliative care evidence base: the context, need, challenges, and strategies. *J Pain Symptom Manage* 2008; **36**: 304–309.

CHAPTER 10

Pain management

Erin McMenamin

Department of Radiation Oncology, Hospital of the University of Pennsylvania, Philadelphia, PA, USA

Introduction

Pain is a common manifestation of cancer, with between half and two-thirds of patients suffering pain at some point in the course of their disease. Given more than 1.6 million Americans and millions more worldwide are diagnosed with cancer each year, the proper management of cancer pain remains a significant health-care priority [1]. Radiation therapy is an effective palliative measure for a variety of cancer-related pain, yet pain medications and adjuvant therapies are often required to augment the positive effects of radiotherapy. Palliative care referral early in the course of a life-threatening cancer can help to optimize pain control [2–5]. Temel reported that it was clinicians trained and skilled in the provision of palliative care that enabled patients to best understand their diagnosis and choose appropriate interventions [5].

Pain assessment

The first and one of the most important aspects of cancer pain management involves the accurate measure of a patient's discomfort. Pain assessment is complex because patients may suffer discomfort that includes a mix of different unpleasant sensations that vary over time. Pain may also exist at several different anatomic sites, any of which may be more problematic depending upon such factors as activity level and time of day. Furthermore, the perception of pain involves cultural, psychologic, and spiritual influences that depend upon a patient's level of understanding and acceptance of the disease.

The first rule of pain management is to perform the assessments frequently enough to evaluate a patient's discomfort and their response to interventions. Any one of several pain scales may be used for these assessments, with the most common ones being those that are one-dimensional in their measurement of pain, alone. Patient-reported, or subjective, pain scales are the most

Radiation Oncology in Palliative Cancer Care, First Edition. Edited by Stephen Lutz, Edward Chow, and Peter Hoskin.
© 2013 John Wiley & Sons, Ltd. Published 2013 by John Wiley & Sons, Ltd.

Table 10.1 Types of pain.

Type of pain	Location	Localized	Description	Treatment
Somatic	Skin, muscle, bone, joints	Yes	Sharp, gnawing, throbbing	Opioids, NSAIDs, topical agents
Visceral	Organs of abdomen and chest	No	Dull, aching, cramping	Opioids, NSAIDs
Neuropathic	Nerves, brain	Yes or No	Hot, burning, shooting, electric-like	Opioids, anti-epileptics, anti-depressants, steroids, topical agents

effective means by which to measure discomfort. Care-givers or health-care workers can act as surrogates for the patient when their performance status does not allow them to document their own pain, though the accuracy of those estimates are less likely to represent reality than would a subjective scale.

Pain assessment measures may be formatted as a numeric rating scale (NRS) or a word scale. Whichever type of scale is used, it is imperative that the patient is able to understand the questions being asked. For instance, one must be aware of a patient's reading capabilities and native language when employing a word scale. The assessment of the pain also needs to take into account its characteristics, such as whether the discomfort is more consistent with somatic, visceral, or neuropathic pain. While cancer pain commonly presents with a mix of these types of characteristics, understanding the nature of the pain allows for improved decision-making when choosing pain medications (Table 10.1). The National Comprehensive Cancer Network (NCCN) describes that the assessment of pain should include: words to describe the sensory aspect of the pain, the time course of the pain, factors that aggravate or alleviate the pain, previous treatments delivered for the pain [2].

Analgesia ladder

The World Health Organization (WHO) has developed a three-step ladder to help clinicians choose the best class of pain medication for a given clinical circumstance [6]. Pain that is minor in severity and which has not yet been treated with medication should first be addressed with non-opioid medications such as non-steroidal anti-inflammatory drugs (NSAIDs) unless there is a medical contraindication to do so. Pain that persists or increases in spite of the drugs given on the first rung of the ladder progress to treatment with low to moderate strength opioids associated with the second step of the ladder. Further persistence of pain leads to movement to stronger and higher dose opioids associated with the third step of the ladder. Adjuvant medications may be added to NSAIDs or opioids at any point on the analgesia ladder, and NSAIDs themselves can serve as adjuvants by decreasing opioid requirements 30–50% when combined [7].

Primary pharmacologic interventions

Non-steroidal anti-inflammatory drugs

NSAIDs have effects that are analgesic, anti-inflammatory, and anti-pyretic. Their functioning involves inhibition of prostaglandins through effects on the cyclooxygenase pathway. Patients with a propensity for bleeding should not receive ibuprofen while those with liver failure should only be given acetaminophen with great care. Other side effects of NSAID therapy can include gastrointestinal problems through direct absorption of the medication through the mucosa, alteration of gastric acid production and blood flow to the stomach. They may also decrease renal perfusion and therefore alter kidney function [8].

Opioids

Opioids function by competitively binding with opiate receptors in the brain and spinal cord as well as by altering mood to diminish psychologic response to pain [9]. Opioids may be prescribed intermittently for episodic pain or around the clock for pain that is present most of the day. A starting dose of 5–15 mg of oral morphine or an equivalent dose of another opioid should be used, with conversion from a short-acting to sustained-release medication possible once adequate anesthesia is established [2]. Sustained release opioids are available in oral, intravenous, or transdermal forms. Opioids commonly cause constipation and their use should be accompanied by a bowel regimen that includes a laxative from the time they are first prescribed. Also, the metabolites formed from morphine may accumulate in the setting of renal insufficiency. Morphine should be avoided or given in altered schedules in that setting [10]. The accumulation of toxic metabolites from other opioids such as hydromorphone usually only become problematic in settings where the drug is delivered intravenously over an extended length of time [11].

Flares of pain during the course of a day are referred to as breakthrough pain (BTP), and they necessitate adequate doses of short-acting pain medication as needed. Episodes of BTP may occur several times per day, they last an average of about 30 minutes, and they are commonly moderate to severe in intensity [12]. BTP medication recommendations include choosing a medicine similar to the patient's long acting opioid at a dose of about 10% of the total 24-hour dose requirement initially, but may be increased as indicated [13]. Equianalgesic dose charts are available to calculate the proper amount of BTP medication or when switching between opioid analgesics. Opioids have incomplete cross-tolerance, making it necessary to decrease doses by 25–50% when switching medicines unless the change is being made for uncontrolled pain [14,15].

In general, opioid prescribers should keep several factors in mind:
- Most opioids do not have a ceiling dose
- Efficacy may be improved by increasing dose rather than switching drugs
- Equianalgesic dose charts can help with dosing BTP or opioid switches
- Side effects between different opioids may be similar but not exactly the same
- Side effect profiles can be predicted and prevented in many cases
- Oral dosing is the least complex and most desirable route of delivery
- More complex delivery routes should be reserved for special circumstances

Adjuvant medications

Adjuvant medications are an important addition to opioids for many patients with complex or refractory cancer pain. The characteristics of the pain often dictate the most appropriate adjuvant medication based upon the cause of the pain and the mechanism of the drug. One must take into account the comorbidities of the patient and the potential overlapping side effects with other pain medicines when choosing adjuvant drugs. For instance, patients with cancer-related fatigue might suffer worsened energy levels when treated with anti-epileptic medication. Alternatively, patients receiving anti-coagulant medications may experience a greater risk of bleeding with the use of NSAIDs due to combined anti-coagulant effects.

Steroids
Tissue edema due to direct tumor effects may contribute to exacerbations of cancer pain. Steroids inhibit phospholipase A2 in the arachidonic acid pathway and relieve pain by diminishing edema and decreasing neural discharges. The ideal dose of steroids in pain settings has not been established, though common sense dictates using the lowest dose that accomplishes the desired results [16]. Steroids are best used on a short-term basis to avoid accumulation of varied and often severe side effects with a more prolonged use. For patients who respond to other pain interventions, steroids should be tapered as quickly as possible to minimize those deleterious effects [17]. Patients who are approaching the end of life may be maintained on steroids to maximize comfort given a lesser relevance of long-term side effects.

Anti-epileptics
Neuropathic pain results from direct tumor invasion of a somatosensory nerve and may be refractory to the most commonly used classes of analgesics [18]. Gabapentin was the first known anti-epileptic medicine proven to be useful in the treatment of neuropathic pain due to interference with the development of $\alpha2\delta1$ thrombospondin [19,20]. Up to 60% of patients with neuropathic pain have some degree of relief with the use of gabapentin, though

side effects of treatment such as fatigue can be dose-limiting, especially in the elderly and other pre-disposed populations. Pregabalin is a second anti-epileptic medication that has been found to improve neuropathic pain syndromes, with the advantage that it is associated with fewer side effects than gabapentin [21,22].

Anti-depressants

Tricyclic anti-depressant medications (TCAs) are useful adjuvant medicines for patients with neuropathic pain, such as might be seen in cases of post-herpetic neuralgia (PHN) and diabetic peripheral neuropathy (DPN). A trial of these medications may also be considered for patients with peripheral neuropathy due to the effects of chemotherapy [23,24]. The side effects of TCAs include anti-cholinergic effects that can be so significant as to preclude their use for many patients.

End-of-life considerations

Many cancer patients suffer a dramatic increase in the severity of pain at the end of life that requires a corresponding increase in pain medicine dosing. Opioid tolerant patients who suffer a moderate increase in pain can often be managed with opioid dosage increases of 25–50%, whereas severe exacerbations or excruciating pain may require larger stepwise increases of 50 to 100% over the previous opioid dose [2]. Patients with pain that progresses beyond control of analgesics at any point during the disease course may require other therapies such as nerve blocks or spinal opioids.

Conclusion

Cancer-related pain is a common yet complex clinical problem that requires aggressive and coordinated multi-disciplinary management. While radiotherapy frequently is successful in palliating cancer-related pain, there is often a lag in time before that relief occurs during which medications are needed to maximize quality of life. Furthermore, there are instances when radiotherapy is ineffective or when pain is too widespread to allow radiotherapy to benefit. A variety of useful pharmacologic interventions are available, and the use of those classes of drugs is guided by approaches such as the pain relief ladder published by the World Health Organization. Proper palliative care demands aggressive management of physical, psychologic, and social pain from the time of cancer diagnosis until death. Additionally, clinicians must realize that concerns regarding addiction or the fear of hastening death are speculative when prescribing appropriately in a population that may otherwise suffer needlessly at a very vulnerable time in their lives. Primary goals should revolve around the comfort of the patient.

References

1. American Cancer Society. *Cancer Facts and Figures 2011*. Atlanta: American Cancer Society, 2011, pp. 1–56.
2. NCCN Guidelines Clinical Practice Guidelines for Quality Palliative Care Version 2. 2011, pp. 1–58.
3. National Consensus Project for Quality Palliative Care. Clinical Practice Guidelines for Quality Palliative Care, Second Edition. 2009, pp. 1–80.
4. Temel JS, Greer JA, Muzikansky A, *et al.* Early palliative care for patients with metastatic non–small-cell lung cancer. *N Engl J Med* 2010; **363**: 733–742.
5. Temel JS, Greer JA, Sodane A, *et al.* Longitudinal perceptions of prognosis and goals of therapy in patients with metastatic non–small-cell lung cancer: results of a randomized study of early palliative care. *J Clin Oncol* 2011; **29**: 2319–2326.
6. World Health Organization: WHO's pain ladder. Available at: http://www.who.int/cancer/palliative/painladder/en/. (accessed August 16, 2012).
7. Khan MA, Walsh D, Brito-Dellan N. Opioid and adjuvant analgesics: compared and contrasted. *Am J Hosp Palliat Care* 2011; **28**: 378–383.
8. Munir MA, Enany N, Zhang JM. Nonopioid analgesics. *Med Clin North Am* 2007; **91**: 97–111.
9. Cleary JF. The pharmacologic management of cancer pain. *J Palliat Med* 2007; **10**: 1369–1394.
10. King S, Hanks GW, Ferro CJ, *et al.* A systematic review of the use of opioid medication for those with moderate to severe cancer pain and renal impairment: a European palliative care research collaborative opioid guidelines project. *Palliat Med* 2011; **25**: 525–552.
11. Thwaites D, McCann S, Broderick P. Hydromorphone neuroexcitation. *J Palliat Med* 2004; **7**: 545–550.
12. Portenoy R, Payne D, Jacobsen P. Breakthrough pain: characteristics and impact in patients with cancer pain. *Pain* 1999; **81**: 129–134.
13. Hagen NA, Fisher K, Victorino C, *et al.* A titration strategy is needed to manage breakthrough cancer pain effectively: observations from data pooled from three clinical trials. *J Palliat Med* 2007; **10**(1): 47–55.
14. American Pain Society. *Principles of Analgesic Use in the Treatment of Acute Pain and Cancer Pain*, 6th edn. Glendale, Illinois: American Pain Society, 4700 Lakeview Avenue, 2008, pp. 19–21.
15. Portenoy R. Treatment of cancer pain. *Lancet* 2011; **377**: 2236–2247.
16. Knotkova H, Pappagallo M. Adjuvant analgesics. *Med Clin North Am* 2007; **91**: 113–124.
17. Soares LG, Chan VW. Review Article: the Rationale for a multimodal approach in the management of breakthrough pain. *Am J Hosp Palliat Care* 2007; **24**: 430–439.
18. Treede RD, Jensen TS, Campbell TS, *et al.* Neuropathic pain. Redefinition and a grading system for clinical and research purposes. *Neurology* 2008; **70**: 1630–1635.
19. Backonja M, Beydoun A, Edwards KR, *et al.* Gabapentin for the symptomatic treatment of painful neuropathy in patients with diabetes mellitus. *JAMA* 1998; **280**: 1631–1636.
20. Eroglu C, Allen NJ, Susman MW, *et al.* The Gabapentin receptor $\alpha 2\delta$-1 is the neuronal thrombospondin receptor responsible for excitatory CNS synaptogenesis. *Cell* 2009; **139**: 380–392.
21. Dworkin RH, Corbin AE, Young JP, *et al.* Pregabalin for treatment of post herpetic neuralgia. A randomized controlled placebo trial. *Neurology* 2003; **60**: 1274–1283.

22. Dooley DJ, Taylor CP, Donevan S, *et al*. Ca2+ channel a2d ligands: novel modulators of neurotransmission. *Trends Pharmacol Sci* 2007; **28**: 75–82.
23. Dworkin RH, O'Connor AB, Backonja M, *et al*. Pharmacologic management of neuro-pathic pain: evidence-based recommendations. *Pain* 2007; **132**: 237–251.
24. Laird B, Colvin L, Fallon M. Management of cancer pain: basic principles and neuro-pathic cancer pain. *Eur J Cancer* 2008; **44**: 1078–1082.

PART 3

Locally advanced or locally recurrent diseases

CHAPTER 11

Primary tumors of the central nervous system

Caroline Chung[1], Eric L. Chang[2]
[1]Department of Radiation Oncology, University of Toronto, Toronto, ON, Canada
[2]Department of Radiation Oncology, Keck School of Medicine at University of Southern California, Los Angeles, CA, USA

Introduction

Incidence/prevalence, at-risk populations

The incidence of primary brain tumors is rising with over 25,000 cases in Canada and the United States in 2012 [1,2]. In adults, the majority of cases are gliomas and meningiomas. Of all malignant gliomas, 60 to 70% are glioblastoma multiforme (GBM), 10 to 15% anaplastic astrocytoma, and 10% anaplastic oligodendroglioma or oligoastrocytoma [3]. Due to the aggressive nature of these tumors and their high likelihood to progress locally following initial therapy, there is a large body of evidence addressing the role of palliative radiotherapy and re-irradiation for malignant gliomas.

There has been no underlying cause identified for the majority of malignant brain tumors, with exposure to ionizing radiation as the only identified risk factor [4]. A family history of malignant gliomas is present in 5% of cases and there are some rare genetic syndromes associated with gliomas including neurofibromatosis types 1 and 2, Li-Fraumeni, and Turcot syndrome [5].

Symptoms

Central nervous system tumors are commonly associated with profound and worrisome symptoms (Box 11.1). Patients can present with signs and symptoms of increased intracranial pressure (ICP), seizures, or focal neurologic symptoms due to both tumor and peritumoral edema. The specific neurologic deficits are typically dependent on the location and size of the tumor(s) and extent of peritumoral edema. These can range from generalized fatigue, headache, cognitive deficits and personality changes, motor or sensory deficits, balance disturbance, speech difficulties, or seizures. The presence of

Radiation Oncology in Palliative Cancer Care, First Edition. Edited by Stephen Lutz, Edward Chow, and Peter Hoskin.
© 2013 John Wiley & Sons, Ltd. Published 2013 by John Wiley & Sons, Ltd.

Box 11.1 Symptoms commonly associated with primary central nervous system tumors

- Generalized fatigue
- Headaches
- Nausea/vomiting
- Seizures
- Cognitive deficits
- Personality changes
- Decreased memory
- Dysphasia/aphasia
- Focal motor deficits
- Sensory deficits
- Visual or auditory disturbance
- Imbalance/dizziness

---

symptoms, performance status, extent of resection and extent of disease may impact management decisions and patient outcome.

Survival

Despite multi-modality therapy including surgery, radiation, and cytotoxic chemotherapy, overall survival continues to be limited for patients with malignant brain tumors. The primary site remains the predominant site of failure and local recurrence greatly impacts patient survival and morbidity [6]. Efforts to improve local tumor control with more aggressive surgical resection, radiation dose escalation, and combined treatment with radiation and systemic therapies have improved outcome. For instance, concurrent and adjuvant temozolomide (TMZ) has improved 2-year survival of patients with newly diagnosed malignant glioma from 11.2% to 27.3% and 5-year survival from 1.9% to 9.8% [7,8] Despite these improvements, nearly all patients (>95%) continue to develop local tumor recurrence with a median time to local recurrence of about 7 months [9,10].

Radiotherapy

Local tumor control improves patients' symptoms, quality of life, and survival. However, the intensity of the treatment can be adjusted based on the primary aim of treatment in terms of the acceptable risk of toxicity for greater potential benefit (Figure 11.1). In patients who may not tolerate aggressive therapy due to their age, performance status, medical comorbidities, or tumor burden (i.e. extent of intracranial disease), a palliative approach to maximize their quality of life is usually favored. Similarly, in patients who have recurrent tumor following prior surgery and radiotherapy, with or without

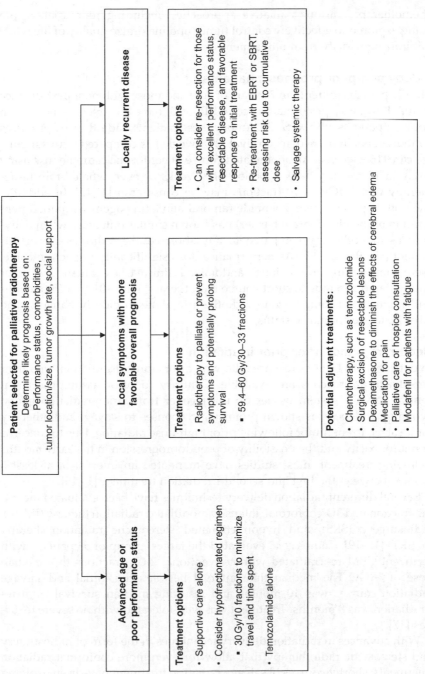

Patient selected for palliative radiotherapy
Determine likely prognosis based on:
Performance status, comorbidities,
tumor location/size, tumor growth rate, social support

Advanced age or poor performance status

Treatment options
- Supportive care alone
- Consider hypofractionated regimen
  - 30 Gy/10 fractions to minimize travel and time spent
- Temozolamide alone

Local symptoms with more favorable overall prognosis

Treatment options
- Radiotherapy to palliate or prevent symptoms and potentially prolong survival
  - 59.4–60 Gy/30–33 fractions

Locally recurrent disease

Treatment options
- Can consider re-resection for those with excellent performance status, resectable disease, and favorable response to initial treatment
- Re-treatment with EBRT or SBRT, assessing risk due to cumulative dose
- Salvage systemic therapy

Potential adjuvant treatments:
- Chemotherapy, such as temozolomide
- Surgical excision of resectable lesions
- Dexamethasone to diminish the effects of cerebral edema
- Medication for pain
- Palliative care or hospice consultation
- Modafenil for patients with fatigue

Figure 11.1 Algorithm for use of palliative radiotherapy for patients with primary central nervous system tumor.

chemotherapy, various palliative approaches, including re-irradiation, are being explored to effectively control tumor and maximize quality of life while minimizing toxicity from retreatment.

Elderly and poor prognosis patients

Elderly patients (older than 70 years of age) and those with poor performance status (Karnofsky performance score, KPS <70) have a worse prognosis than younger patients with KPS >70. Among these patients, radiotherapy produces a modest benefit in median survival (29.1 weeks) as compared with supportive care (16.9 weeks). An abbreviated course of conformal radiotherapy using 40 Gy in 15 fractions over a period of 3 weeks or even whole brain radiotherapy with 30 Gy in 10 fractions may be considered [11,12]. In addition, chemotherapy with temozolomide (an oral alkylating agent with good penetration of the blood–brain barrier) has shown similar outcomes when delivered as monotherapy compared to any short course radiotherapy in this patient population [13]. As performance does significantly impact outcome, there is an ongoing international randomized clinical trial evaluating whether adding temozolomide to short-course radiotherapy with 40 Gy in 15 fractions will improve outcome beyond radiotherapy alone in elderly patients who have better performance status.

Recurrent tumor after prior irradiation

In patients with local recurrence following prior cranial irradiation, a number of salvage approaches are available. Contrary to prior assumptions that central nervous system tissues do not recover from prior radiation injury, evolving evidence has shown promising responses to salvage radiotherapy for local recurrent tumor following prior high-dose radiation. Due to concerns of neurotoxicity and the possibility of pseudoprogression in the early months following treatment, most studies have mandated an interval of at least 6 months between the first and second irradiation treatment [14,15].

Several different radiation delivery techniques have been evaluated including fractionated 3D-conformal, intensity modulated radiation therapy (IMRT), radiosurgery (SRS), and hypofractionated stereotactic radiation therapy (hFSRT) [16–19]. Combs *et al.* evaluated the largest group of 53 patients with recurrent GBM re-irradiated with conventional 2-Gy fractions to a median dose of 36 Gy. The median time interval between the initial and salvage radiation courses was 10 months and resulting median survival from re-irradiation was 8 months. Treatment was well-tolerated with no severe toxicities [17].

With advances in radiation delivery techniques in the form of radiosurgery and stereotactic radiotherapy that allow for even more conformal radiation treatments, shorter courses of salvage radiation treatment have been explored in the salvage setting of focal recurrences. In the palliative setting, it can be appreciated that shortening the time commitment required by the patient to receive treatment may result in better quality of life.

Radiosurgery

Single fraction radiosurgery has been explored as a salvage treatment of small volume recurrences. There are no randomized data to support the use of SRS in the treatment of malignant gliomas, but a growing number of publications support the potential benefit of salvage SRS for recurrent malignant gliomas [18,20–23]. The largest prospective cohort study evaluated 114 patients with grade III and IV gliomas treated with salvage SRS with a median dose of 16 Gy (range 12–50 Gy) delivered to the 50% isodose line with gammaknife or 80% isodose line with a linear accelerator. In this study, the median survival was 23 months for patients with GBM and 37.5 months for patients with grade III gliomas [21]. Other studies have raised concern about the high toxicity of SRS salvage when tumor volumes were relatively large. Hall *et al.* treated 35 patients with large recurrent tumors (median treatment volume 28 cm^3) with a mean dose of 21 Gy (range: 7.5–40 Gy) following prior radiotherapy to a mean dose of 60 Gy and found 7 patients required surgical resection for radionecrosis within several months of radiosurgery treatment [23]. Although it has been recognized that larger volume tumors are associated with higher risk of side effects with single fraction treatment, a clear maximum volume cut-off has not yet been determined for SRS salvage.

Hypofractionated radiotherapy

In an attempt to reduce the toxicity associated with single fraction SRS, particularly for large volume tumors, and to exploit the radiobiologic advantage of fractionation, hypofractionated stereotactic radiation therapy (hFSRT) approaches have also been explored. This approach delivers a highly-targeted dose of radiation around the tumor over a limited number of fractions [14]. A number of different fractionation schedules have been investigated, ranging from 20 to 50 Gy in 3 to 7 Gy fraction sizes. Median survivals in studies have ranged from 6.7 to 11 months and treatments were generally well-tolerated [24–26]. Several studies comparing single fraction SRS to FSRT have reported similar survival outcomes with lower rates of complications for patients who received the fractionated treatments. In patients who are more likely to suffer greater morbidity from radiation toxicity due to the location of the tumor in eloquent brain or those with a higher risk of toxicity due to large volume disease, a fractionated approach may be the better option [27,28].

Recognizing that the intent of salvage radiotherapy for malignant gliomas is palliative, Ernst-Stecken *et al.* reported both survival and quality of life outcomes after hypofractionated stereotactic radiation therapy with a dose of 35 Gy in 5 daily fractions of 7 Gy. A total of 15 patients with recurrent malignant glioma were prospectively evaluated. Progression-free survival (PFS) was 75% at 6 months and 53% at 12 months. Over a median follow-up of 9 months, the quality of life measured using the European Organization for Research and Treatment of Cancer Quality of Life Questionnaire remained stable in two-thirds of patients. Although this was a small study, it suggests that hypofractionated radiotherapy at recurrence is a promising palliative approach that may help maintain quality of life for an acceptable period of time [15]. A subsequent review of quality of life measures in studies of re-irradiation demonstrated that acquisition of this information is highly challenging in this population where disease progression can occur quickly and greatly impact one's ability to participate in quality of life evaluations thereby resulting in data that are biased towards those patients who are well enough to complete the questionnaire [29].

Side-effect risks

Acute
The acute side effects of radiotherapy include fatigue, hair loss, scalp dermatitis, decreased appetite, and possibly increased brain edema requiring increased dexamethasone use. Specific side effects will depend on the particular distribution and dose of radiation delivered.

Late
The possible late side effects of radiotherapy include prolonged fatigue, permanent patchy hair loss in areas that have received higher doses of radiation, neurocognitive decline, and specific neurodeficits associated with high doses to specific neural structures (such as hearing loss and balance difficulties).

With high cumulative doses of radiation, particularly with re-irradiation following prior high-dose radiotherapy, there is a substantial risk of developing symptomatic radionecrosis. Following radiosurgery for various intracranial tumors, 2 to 14% of patients have been reported to develop radionecrosis [30,31]. However, it is appreciated that the difficulty in differentiating recurrent tumor from radionecrosis introduces the potential to over or underestimate the incidence of radionecrosis based on imaging alone. Novel imaging techniques to improve the ability to diagnose radionecrosis and new treatments for this iatrogenic toxicity are under investigation.

Radiotherapy limitations

Radiotherapy can improve tumor control and survival, but local tumor recurrence remains the predominant pattern of progressive disease suggesting that tumor radioresistance is present. Studies of dose escalation up to 84 Gy using various radiotherapy techniques, including the addition of SRS boost, have demonstrated modest improvements in local control and persistent recurrences just outside the high-dose region [32–34]. Therefore, the addition of systemic agents that target tumor cells through non-cross resistant pathways of cell kill or enhance the cell killing effects of radiation appear to show the greatest promise in achieving durable responses.

Adjuvant treatment modalities

Radiotherapy combined with systemic therapy

With recent evidence supporting promising results with re-irradiation, the value of combined chemotherapy and radiation has been tested by several groups. In general, these studies evaluated concurrent chemotherapy with hypofractionated radiation schedules, similar to those investigated for salvage hFSRT alone. Combs *et al.* reported that salvage treatment with temozolomide and radiation was feasible and demonstrated clinical efficacy in 25 patients who were both temozolomide-naïve (n = 19) and pre-exposed (n = 6). Although this was a small study, it reported an impressive 6-month PFS of 48% with low toxicity, suggesting this treatment regimen warrants further investigation [35]. A number of other chemotherapeutic agents have been investigated in combination with radiation including paclitaxel and cisplatin. The median survival reported in these studies ranged from 7 to 13.7 months and these combined chemoradiation treatments were associated with greater toxicity than radiotherapy or chemotherapy alone, as expected. In one of the largest studies by Lederman *et al.*, 11 (12%) patients required a reoperation due to an expanding mass. Pathology was available in 9 of the 11 patients: 7 had pure radionecrosis and 2 had a combination of radionecrosis and tumor identified [36–40].

In addition to conventional cytotoxic chemotherapy, a wide range of molecularly targeted agents are emerging and available for combination with radiotherapy. Agents targeting the vasculature and specifically vascular endothelial growth factor (VEGF) and its pathways have raised particular interest [41]. Bevacizumab, a monoclonal antibody targeting VEGF, has shown promise in early investigations as salvage treatment for recurrent malignant glioma in combination with chemotherapeutic agents [42–46]. Early clinical reports have determined the safety and promising activity of bevacizumab in combination with radiotherapy for malignant gliomas [47]. Torcuator *et al.* have demonstrated that the benefit of combined bevacizumab and SRS or hFSRT is seen even in patients who have progressed on bevacizumab therapy [48]. There are a number of ongoing prospective clinical trials evaluating the role of bevacizumab in combination with radiotherapy for salvage treatment of recurrent malignant glioma, as many unanswered questions remain. These include the optimal timing, dose, and schedule of both bevacizumab and radiation treatment when delivered in combination for salvage therapy. Secondly, due to the radiologic changes in response to bevacizumab, optimal imaging techniques for radiotherapy planning are also evolving.

Promise of newer technologies

Radioimmunotherapy

Radioimmunotherapy (RIT) aims to utilize radioactive isotopes coupled to antibodies in order to increase tumor-specific cell kill. There are several RIT approaches under investigation including antibodies directed against tenascin-C (an extracellular matrix glycoprotein ubiquitously expressed by malignant gliomas), EGFR, and TM-601 (binds to malignant brain tumor cells with high affinity and does not seem to bind to normal brain tissue) [49–51]. These approaches display promising activity in pre-clinical and very early clinical studies, but are still considered highly experimental.

Special considerations in developing countries

As technologic advances allow for more complex radiotherapy delivery with increased use of multi-modal imaging to improve target delineation, variations in practice among different countries can reflect their access to the technologic and educational supports required for these highly advanced treatments. Secondly, the financial burden of more complex radiotherapy treatments as well as newer targeted systemic therapy interventions may dictate the practice in particular countries. Recommendations for future research and palliative practice patterns for CNS tumor patients will require attention to these resource limitations.

Conclusion

Radiotherapy plays an important role in the care of most patients who are diagnosed with primary central nervous system tumors. The particular radiation treatment prescription and technique are commonly determined by the age and performance status of the affected patient, with younger patients undergoing up to 6 weeks of treatment, and frail, elderly patients receiving hypofractionated courses of 1 to 3 weeks in length (Figure 11.1). Ongoing technologic advances in radiotherapy provide hope for further improvement in the therapeutic ratio for initial and salvage treatment. However, at the present time the limited prognosis and high likelihood of early recurrence in patients with high grade disease necessitates early palliative care intervention from the time of diagnosis until the time of death to optimize patient quality of life.

References

1. Siegel R, Naishadham D, Jemal A. Cancer statistics, 2012. *CA Cancer J Clin* 2012; **62**: 10–29.
2. Statistics CCSsSCoC. Canadian Cancer Statistics 2012. Toronto, Canadian Cancer Society, 2012.
3. Wen PY, Kesari S. Malignant gliomas in adults. *N Engl J Med* 2008; **359**: 492–507.
4. Fisher JL, Schwartzbaum JA, Wrensch M, *et al*. Epidemiology of brain tumors. *Neurol Clin* 2007; **25**: 867–890.
5. Farrell CJ, Plotkin SR. Genetic causes of brain tumors: neurofibromatosis, tuberous sclerosis, von Hippel-Lindau, and other syndromes. *Neurol Clin* 2007; **25**: 925–946.

6. Wallner KE, Galicich JH, Krol G, *et al.* Patterns of failure following treatment for glioblastoma multiforme and anaplastic astrocytoma. *Int J Radiat Oncol Biol Phys* 1989; **16**: 1405–1409.

7. Stupp R, Mason WP, van den Bent MJ, *et al.* Radiotherapy plus concomitant and adjuvant temozolomide for glioblastoma. *N Engl J Med* 2005; **352**: 987–996.

8. Stupp R, Hegi ME, Mason WP, *et al.* Effects of radiotherapy with concomitant and adjuvant temozolomide versus radiotherapy alone on survival in glioblastoma in a randomised phase III study: 5-year analysis of the EORTC-NCIC trial. *Lancet Oncol* 2009; **10**: 459–466.

9. Sneed PK, Gutin PH, Larson DA, *et al.* Patterns of recurrence of glioblastoma multiforme after external irradiation followed by implant boost. *Int J Radiat Oncol Biol Phys* 1994; **29**: 719–727.

10. Milano MT, Okunieff P, Donatello RS, *et al.* Patterns and timing of recurrence after temozolomide-based chemoradiation for glioblastoma. *Int J Radiat Oncol Biol Phys* 2010; **78**: 1147–1155.

11. Keime-Guibert F, Chinot O, Taillandier L, *et al.* Radiotherapy for glioblastoma in the elderly. *N Engl J Med* 2007; **356**: 1527–1535.

12. Roa W, Brasher PM, Bauman G, *et al.* Abbreviated course of radiation therapy in older patients with glioblastoma multiforme: a prospective randomized clinical trial. *J Clin Oncol* 2004; **22**: 1583–1588.

13. Glantz M, Chamberlain M, Liu Q, *et al.* Temozolomide as an alternative to irradiation for elderly patients with newly diagnosed malignant gliomas. *Cancer* 2003; **97**: 2262–2266.

14. Combs SE, Debus J, Schulz-Ertner D. Radiotherapeutic alternatives for previously irradiated recurrent gliomas. *BMC Cancer* 2007; **7**: 167.

15. Ernst-Stecken A, Ganslandt O, Lambrecht U, *et al.* Survival and quality of life after hypofractionated stereotactic radiotherapy for recurrent malignant glioma. *J Neurooncol* 2007; **81**: 287–294.

16. Combs SE, Widmer V, Thilmann C, *et al.* Stereotactic radiosurgery (SRS): treatment option for recurrent glioblastoma multiforme (GBM). *Cancer* 2005; **104**: 2168–2173.

17. Combs SE, Gutwein S, Thilmann C, *et al.* Stereotactically guided fractionated re-irradiation in recurrent glioblastoma multiforme. *J Neurooncol* 2005; **74**: 167–171.

18. Biswas T, Okunieff P, Schell MC, *et al.* Stereotactic radiosurgery for glioblastoma: retrospective analysis. *Radiat Oncol* 2009; **4**: 11.

19. Fuller CD, Choi M, Forthuber B, *et al.* Standard fractionation intensity modulated radiation therapy (IMRT) of primary and recurrent glioblastoma multiforme. *Radiat Oncol* 2007; **2**: 26.

20. Kong DS, Lee JI, Park K, *et al.* Efficacy of stereotactic radiosurgery as a salvage treatment for recurrent malignant gliomas. *Cancer* 2008; **112**: 2046–2051.

21. Kondziolka D, Flickinger JC, Bissonette DJ, *et al.* Survival benefit of stereotactic radiosurgery for patients with malignant glial neoplasms. *Neurosurgery* 1997; **41**: 776–783; discussion 783–785.

22. Masciopinto JE, Levin AB, Mehta MP, *et al.* Stereotactic radiosurgery for glioblastoma: a final report of 31 patients. *J Neurosurg* 1995; **82**: 530–535.

23. Hall WA, Djalilian HR, Sperduto PW, *et al.* Stereotactic radiosurgery for recurrent malignant gliomas. *J Clin Oncol* 1995; **13**: 1642–1648.

24. Fokas E, Wacker U, Gross MW, *et al.* Hypofractionated stereotactic reirradiation of recurrent glioblastomas: a beneficial treatment option after high-dose radiotherapy? *Strahlenther Onkol* 2009; **185**: 235–240.

25. Laing RW, Warrington AP, Graham J, *et al*. Efficacy and toxicity of fractionated stereotactic radiotherapy in the treatment of recurrent gliomas (phase I/II study). *Radiother Oncol* 1993; **27**: 22–29.

26. Shepherd SF, Laing RW, Cosgrove VP, *et al*. Hypofractionated stereotactic radiotherapy in the management of recurrent glioma. *Int J Radiat Oncol Biol Phys* 1997; **37**: 393–398.

27. Cho KH, Hall WA, Gerbi BJ, *et al*. Single dose versus fractionated stereotactic radiotherapy for recurrent high-grade gliomas. *Int J Radiat Oncol Biol Phys* 1999; **45**: 1133–1141.

28. Patel M, Siddiqui F, Jin JY, *et al*. Salvage reirradiation for recurrent glioblastoma with radiosurgery: radiographic response and improved survival. *J Neurooncol* 2009; **92**: 185–191.

29. Nieder C, Astner ST, Mehta MP, *et al*. Improvement, clinical course, and quality of life after palliative radiotherapy for recurrent glioblastoma. *Am J Clin Oncol* 2008; **31**: 300–305.

30. Blonigen BJ, Steinmetz RD, Levin L, *et al*. Irradiated volume as a predictor of brain radionecrosis after linear accelerator stereotactic radiosurgery. *Int J Radiat Oncol Biol Phys* 2010; **77**: 996–1001.

31. Flickinger JC, Lunsford LD, Kondziolka D, *et al*. Radiosurgery and brain tolerance: an analysis of neurodiagnostic imaging changes after gamma knife radiosurgery for arteriovenous malformations. *Int J Radiat Oncol Biol Phys* 1992; **23**: 19–26.

32. Piroth MD, Pinkawa M, Holy R, *et al*. Integrated boost IMRT with FET-PET-adapted local dose escalation in glioblastomas. Results of a prospective phase II study. *Strahlenther Onkol* 2012; **188**: 334–339.

33. Monjazeb AM, Ayala D, Jensen C, *et al*. A phase I dose escalation study of hypofractionated IMRT field-in-field boost for newly diagnosed glioblastoma multiforme. *Int J Radiat Oncol Biol Phys* 2012; **82**: 743–748.

34. Tsien C, Moughan J, Michalski JM, *et al*. Phase I three-dimensional conformal radiation dose escalation study in newly diagnosed glioblastoma: Radiation Therapy Oncology Group Trial 98-03. *Int J Radiat Oncol Biol Phys* 2009; **73**: 699–708.

35. Combs SE, Bischof M, Welzel T, *et al*. Radiochemotherapy with temozolomide as reirradiation using high precision fractionated stereotactic radiotherapy (FSRT) in patients with recurrent gliomas. *J Neurooncol* 2008; **89**: 205–210.

36. Lederman G, Arbit E, Odaimi M, *et al*. Recurrent glioblastoma multiforme: potential benefits using fractionated stereotactic radiotherapy and concurrent taxol. *Stereotact Funct Neurosurg* 1997; **69**: 162–174.

37. Lederman G, Wronski M, Arbit E, *et al*. Treatment of recurrent glioblastoma multiforme using fractionated stereotactic radiosurgery and concurrent paclitaxel. *Am J Clin Oncol* 2000; **23**: 155–159.

38. Lederman G, Arbit E, Odaimi M, *et al*. Fractionated stereotactic radiosurgery and concurrent taxol in recurrent glioblastoma multiforme: a preliminary report. *Int J Radiat Oncol Biol Phys* 1998; **40**: 661–666.

39. Glass J, Silverman CL, Axelrod R, *et al*. Fractionated stereotactic radiotherapy with cisplatinum radiosensitization in the treatment of recurrent, progressive, or persistent malignant astrocytoma. *Am J Clin Oncol* 1997; **20**: 226–229.

40. VanderSpek L, Fisher B, Bauman G, *et al*. 3D conformal radiotherapy and cisplatin for recurrent malignant glioma. *Can J Neurol Sci* 2008; **35**: 57–64.

41. Gerstner ER, Sorensen AG, Jain RK, *et al*. Anti-vascular endothelial growth factor therapy for malignant glioma. *Curr Neurol Neurosci Rep* 2009; **9**: 254–262.

42. Vredenburgh JJ, Desjardins A, Herndon JE, 2nd, *et al*. Bevacizumab plus irinotecan in recurrent glioblastoma multiforme. *J Clin Oncol* 2007; **25**: 4722–4729.

43. Kreisl TN, Kim L, Moore K, *et al*. Phase II trial of single-agent bevacizumab followed by bevacizumab plus irinotecan at tumor progression in recurrent glioblastoma. *J Clin Oncol* 2009; **27**: 740–745.

44. Norden AD, Young GS, Setayesh K, *et al*. Bevacizumab for recurrent malignant gliomas: efficacy, toxicity, and patterns of recurrence. *Neurology* 2008; **70**: 779–787.

45. Reardon DA, Desjardins A, Vredenburgh JJ, *et al*. Metronomic chemotherapy with daily, oral etoposide plus bevacizumab for recurrent malignant glioma: a phase II study. *Br J Cancer* 2009; **101**: 1986–1994.

46. Friedman HS, Prados MD, Wen PY, *et al*. Bevacizumab alone and in combination with irinotecan in recurrent glioblastoma. *J Clin Oncol* 2009; **27**: 4733–4740.

47. Gutin PH, Iwamoto FM, Beal K, *et al*. Safety and efficacy of bevacizumab with hypofractionated stereotactic irradiation for recurrent malignant gliomas. *Int J Radiat Oncol Biol Phys* 2009; **75**: 156–163.

48. Torcuator RG, Thind R, Patel M, *et al*. The role of salvage reirradiation for malignant gliomas that progress on bevacizumab. *J Neurooncol* 2010; **97**: 401–407.

49. Mamelak AN, Rosenfeld S, Bucholz R, *et al*. Phase I single-dose study of intracavitary-administered iodine-131-TM-601 in adults with recurrent high-grade glioma. *J Clin Oncol* 2006; **24**: 3644–3650.

50. Popperl G, Gotz C, Gildehaus FJ, *et al*. Initial experiences with adjuvant locoregional radioimmunotherapy using 131I-labeled monoclonal antibodies against tenascin (BC-4) for treatment of glioma (WHO III and IV). *Nuklearmedizin* 2002; **41**: 120–128.

51. Casaco A, Lopez G, Garcia I, *et al*. Phase I single-dose study of intracavitary-administered Nimotuzumab labeled with 188 Re in adult recurrent high-grade glioma. *Cancer Biol Ther* 2008; **7**: 333–339.

CHAPTER 12

The role of palliative care in head and neck cancer

Albert Tiong, June Corry
Peter MacCallum Cancer Centre, Melbourne, Victoria, Australia

Introduction

Head and neck cancers (HNC) include a wide variety of anatomic subsites and histologies. Most commonly, these are (head and neck) squamous cell carcinomas (HNSCC) involving the oral cavity, pharynx, and larynx [1], and so the content of this chapter will be within that context.

Worldwide HNC is ranked as the tenth most common malignancy [2]. Regions of high incidence include much of South East Asia as well as parts of Central and Southern Europe [1]. Globally the most common risk factor is tobacco and alcohol use, so due to behavioral patterns patients are mostly older males [1,3]. While in North America and Western Europe oral cavity and larynx cancers are declining due to improved tobacco control and education, in developing countries the peak of the smoking-related cancer epidemic is yet to be seen due to a lag time in the spread of tobacco use [1,4]. Over the last decade, an interesting phenomenon has been noted with rise in the incidence of human papilloma virus (HPV) related oropharyngeal cancers in Europe, North America, and Australia [5]. These cancers, especially in non-smokers, carry a very good prognosis with high rates of cure, even in locally advanced disease (LAD) [6,7].

Current management of head and neck squamous cell carcinomas

HNSCC patients are a challenge to treat in both the radical (curative) and palliative settings. These are relatively uncommon cancers, occurring in patients who frequently have multiple medical comorbidities and social and financial issues that can all impact on treatment options and results. In addition, tumor and the effects of treatment can impact on vital everyday

Radiation Oncology in Palliative Cancer Care, First Edition. Edited by Stephen Lutz, Edward Chow, and Peter Hoskin.

Box 12.1 Symptoms commonly associated with head and neck cancers

- Neck lump
- Odynophagia
- Dysphagia
- Hoarseness
- Local and referred pain (e.g. otalgia)
- Aspiration and infection
- Bleeding
- Cranial nerve palsies
- Stridor
- Malnutrition and dehydration

---

functions such as eating, breathing, and speaking with the potential for major impact on patient quality of life (Box 12.1, Figure 12.1).

Even in developed countries where there is good access to health care, the majority of HNSCC patients still present with LAD. Over the past two decades there has been a decided shift in the management of HNSCC patients (particularly in the oropharynx and larynx) from a predominantly surgical approach to one of organ preservation. This is most commonly high dose radiotherapy (RT) with concurrent chemotherapy [8]. Whether due to improved staging, improved treatment techniques, rising percentage of HPV cases, or better supportive care during radical treatment, the loco-regional control rates for LAD seem to have risen from the 35–50% rates of the 1990s [9,10] to rates of 60–80% in the next decade [11,12]. Apart from non-smokers with HPV-associated HNSCC, the overall survival rates remain poor largely due to death from other smoking related comorbidities or second malignancies [9–12].

Patient selection for palliative treatment

Selecting the correct treatment intent (radical or palliative) for each individual patient remains one of the most challenging aspects of a head and neck cancer practice. There is the basic clinical priority of not under treating patients who may indeed have curable disease versus the significant side effects of radical treatment (for a duration of 2–3 months), and the small but real risk of treatment related mortality.

Factors that need to be taken into account when using radiotherapy in HNSCC and deciding on the right treatment intent include: the site of disease (e.g. more radiosensitive sites of the oropharynx or larynx versus less sensitive sites of the hypopharynx or oral cavity), performance status, age, stage, volume of disease, previous treatments, and biomarkers such as p16, a

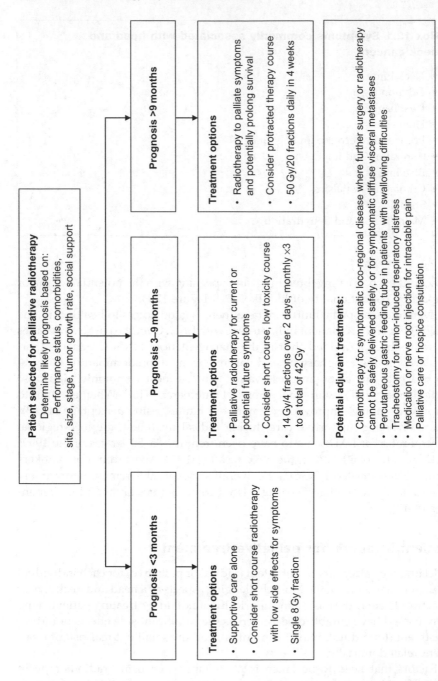

Figure 12.1 Algorithm for use of palliative radiotherapy for patients with head and neck cancer.

surrogate for HPV. Whilst this biomarker is widely utilized clinically, its utility in directing different treatment regimens is still currently confined to clinical trials.

Performance status (PS) is an important and well-recognized factor in oncology that impacts on treatment recommendations and overall survival [13]. PS reflects the overall interplay of a patient's age and medical comorbidities and the impact of their tumor burden. With increased general life expectancy in developed nations, age has become an increasingly common confounding factor in deciding on appropriate treatment for patients. However, the effect of age per se on tumor control appears to be modest. In selected patients who underwent radical radiotherapy or chemoradiotherapy, age did not appear to influence the rate of treatment interruptions, completion of treatment, and treatment related deaths [14]. More important than the biologic age of a patient is the presence of comorbidities in significantly influencing survival of patients [15,16]. In the palliative setting, the importance of comorbidities has also been demonstrated as an important prognostic factor for survival [17]. There are many different indices to measure comorbidities in the head and neck setting and these have been found to be contributory in predicting survival, complications from treatment, functional outcomes, and quality of life [18]. The most commonly used indices are the Adult Comorbidity Evaluation 27 and Charlson Index [19,20].

In general, the higher the stage of disease, the lower the loco-regional control rates. However, volume of tumor, particularly regarding the T classification, may also be important. A large series looking at the impact of tumor volume on local control for radically treated, locally advanced oropharynx, oral cavity, and hypopharynx cancers found that the size of the primary tumor was independently predictive of local control on multivariate analysis [21]. For example, patients with T3 tumors with tumors <30 cm^3 had a 5-year local control of 81.8% compared with 55.1% for patients with patients with tumors >30 cm^3. A lower cut off of 19 cm^3 was found to be prognostic in hypopharyngeal carcinomas [22]. Other studies also note that tumor size can be an independent factor in local control, though cut-off for separating patients into different prognostic groups is variable [23–25]. The caveat to this is patients with HPV-associated disease. Despite advanced disease at presentation (usually by virtue of nodal staging), these tumors have a high complete response rate. The biology of their disease seems more important than their TNM stage [6,7].

In clinical practice there are maneuvers that are not uncommonly used in the attempt to allocate patients with borderline disease and performance status correctly to a radical or palliative treatment regimen. These include the use of 1 to 2 cycles of induction chemotherapy to assess tumor responsiveness as well as patient compliance and tolerance of treatment. A good response can provide greater clinical confidence in the value of pursuing a radical course of concurrent chemoradiotherapy, although this approach has not been validated in prospective studies. Similarly, patients may be commenced on a radical course of chemoradiotherapy with a view to reviewing both tolerance and response at a mid-point in treatment, for example at 30 to 40 Gy, before patients develop significant side effects from treatment. Whilst traditionally this assessment has been done using clinical criteria of disease response and CT scans, use of more sophisticated functional imaging (FDG-PET-CT/F-MISO-PET or diffusion weighted MRI) early in disease treatment may be more accurate in depicting response prior to development of significant treatment toxicity, particularly mucositis [26,27].

Use of palliative radiotherapy in head and neck squamous cell carcinomas

Compared to the extent of clinical research in HNSCC treatments, the published data on palliative radiotherapy regimens are relatively sparse. Palliative radiotherapy [28–38] generally produces higher response rates in HNSCC than chemotherapy [39–47] and thus is the palliative treatment of choice when local or loco-regional disease is the predominant source of a patient's symptoms, whilst chemotherapy is often utilized when distant metastases predominate. The use of RT, however, for non-visceral metastases is well-established but covered in other chapters.

Table 12.1 gives a summary of the current literature for palliative RT in HNSCC. In general, palliative radiotherapy has been shown to be an effective means of improving HNSCC patients' symptoms and potentially their quality of life (QOL). The prospective trials that have been performed measured response to radiotherapy both objectively and subjectively. Quality of life was measured in some of these trials but interestingly none have used QOL as the primary study endpoint. Because treatment was palliative in intent, most trials measured tumor response using only clinical measurements rather than imaging. Response rates (complete and partial) are generally very good, ranging from 54% to 86% [28–38], with complete responses documented in 0% to 45% of patients. These response rates were generally taken as the best response at any time after treatment. Reported median progression-free survival (PFS) ranged from 3.1 to 5.5 months and up to 14 months in complete responders [28–38].

The most commonly reported symptoms responding to palliative radiotherapy were pain (improvement in 56–67% of patients), dysphagia (reduction in 33–53% of patients), and voice quality (improvement in 31–57% of patients). There was a lack of reporting on other potential benefits of radiotherapy on symptoms such as bleeding, upper airway obstruction, and tumor fungation. Only three trials attempted to measure global quality of life using standardized questionnaires including the EORTC QLQ C30, FACT, and UW-QOL. All these trials reported an overall improvement in the quality of life after treatment by somewhere between 44% and 85% of patients [28,29,33].

Which palliative radiotherapy regimen is best is currently unanswered. The ideal palliative regimen is one with a high and durable response rate with

Table 12.1 Studies on palliative radiotherapy for **head and neck squamous cell carcinomas.**

Study	No. of patients	Radiotherapy regime	Overall survival	Objective outcomes	% of patients with subjective outcome improvements	Acute toxicity
Prospective						
Ghoshal et al. 2009 [33]	15	14 Gy/4 fractions over 2 days, monthly × 3	Not specified	PR 67%, SD 13% (RR 67%)	Improved: pain 67, dysphagia 33	Grade 1 mucositis 40%, Grade 2 mucositis 13%, No grade 3 reactions
Agarwal et al. 2008 [32]	110	40 Gy/16 fractions over 3.5 weeks and further RT to 50 Gy if good response	Not specified	CR 10%, PR 63%, (RR 73%) SD 16%	Improved: 74 of patients (individual symptoms not specified)	Grade 3 mucositis 63%, Grade 4 mucositis 3%, Grade 3 skin reaction 14%
Porceddu et al. 2007 [29]	35	30 Gy/5 fractions, 2 per week ± 6 Gy boost	Median 6.1 months	CR 43%, PR 37% (RR 80%) SD 8.6%	Improved: pain 67, dysphagia 33, energy 29	Grade 3 mucositis 26%, Grade 3 skin reaction 11%, Grade 3 dysphagia 11%
Corry et al. 2005 [28]	30	14 Gy/4 fractions over 2 days, monthly × 3	Median 5.7 months	CR 7%, PR 47%, (RR 54 %) SD 23%	Improved: pain 56, dysphagia 33, hoarseness 31	Grade 2 mucositis 11%, Grade 2 xerostomia 37% No Grade 3 toxicities
Mohanti et al. 2004 [31]	505	20 Gy/5 fractions over 1 week (352 patients) and further RT up to biologic equivalent of 70 Gy in responders (153 patients)	Median 6.7 months for lower dose and 13.3 months for high dose	CR 10%, PR 37%, (RR 47%) SD not specified	Improved: pain 57, dysphagia 53, hoarseness 57	Grade 3 skin reaction 56% Grade 3 mucositis 62%, (in higher dose group)
Paris et al. 1993 [34]	37	14.8 Gy/4f over 2 days, every 3 weeks × 3	Average 4.5 months	CR 28%, PR 49%	Improved: 85 of patients (individual symptoms not specified)	Toxicity not graded

(Continued)

Table 12.1 (Continued)

Study	No. of patients	Radiotherapy regime	Overall survival	Objective outcomes	% of patients with subjective outcome improvements	Acute toxicity
Retrospective						
Kancherla et al. 2011 [37]	33	40 Gy/10 fractions over 4 weeks with a 2 week mid-treatment break	Median 9 months	CR 39%, PR 33% (RR 72%)	Improved: 79 of patients (individual symptoms not specified)	Grade 3 skin reaction 3%, Grade 3 mucositis 6%, Grade 3 esophageal toxicity 9%
Stevens et al. 2011 [35]	148	Multiple regimes (50 Gy/20f, 24 Gy/3f, 60 Gy/25f, 30 Gy/10f, 60 Gy/30f, 70 Gy/35f)	Median 5.2 months	"A Response" 82%, "Mixed response" 6%, "No response or progression" 12%	Improved: 85 of patients (individual symptoms not specified and information on only 65 of patients)	Not collected
Al-Mamgani et al. 2009 [30]	158	50 Gy/16 fractions, 5 per week	Median 17 months	CR 45%, PR 25%, (RR 70%) SD 6%	Improved: pain 77, dysphagia 65 (information in only 40 of patients)	Grade 3 mucositis 65%, Grade 3 skin reaction 45%, Grade 3 dysphagia 45%
Chen et al. 2008 [36]	311	Multiple regimes (14 Gy/4f × 3, 70 Gy/35f, 30 Gy/10f 37.5 Gy/15f 20 Gy/5f)	Survival 3 to 8 months depending on regime	Not specified	60–86 of patients had a "palliative response" (no standardized measure)	>Grade 3 reaction varied from 9% with 14 Gy/4f to 38% for 70 Gy/35f
Erkal et al. 2001* [38]	40	30 Gy/10f daily or 20 Gy/2f weekly		CR 12%, PR 76% (RR 86%)	Complete response in symptoms 18, partial response in symptoms 76	Not specified

CR, complete response; PR, partial response; RR, Response Rate (CR + PR); SD, stable disease
* Only included patients with squamous cell carcinoma involving cervical lymph nodes with unknown primary

minimal acute toxicities. In reality the question is which palliative radiotherapy regimen can best approximate this ideal. Across the different prospective trials for palliative radiotherapy in HNSCC there was wide variability in the patient's age, performance status, and disease stage (e.g. the percentage of patients with stage IV disease ranged from 65 to 100%). The method of measuring treatment response varied, as did the method of measuring symptomatic improvements. This makes comparisons between different regimes difficult.

As expected, the studies that used high doses of radiotherapy to achieve high response rates also had the highest rates of significant (grade 2 or 3) mucositis. For example, a regime that used 50 Gy in 16 fractions, 5 fractions per week (of whom 81% had stage IV disease), achieved complete responses in 45% of patients [30]. This was, however, at a cost of grade 3 mucositis in 65% of patients. Similarly, another regime which used 40 Gy in 16 fractions over 3.5 weeks also reported a high (63% grade 3) rate of mucositis [32]. In comparison, lower dose regimes such as 30 Gy in 5 fractions with 2 fractions per week the compete response rate was 42.9%, grade 3 mucositis rates were 26% [29]. The lowest side-effect rate was seen in a regime that was originally used in M.D. Anderson Cancer Center for pelvic radiotherapy, which aims to maximize tumor control whilst minimizing side effects [48]. The dose fractionation used in the current form is 14 Gy in 4 fractions, twice per day, repeated monthly for a maximum of three times. The radiobiology of this fractionation is that each 14 Gy is a dose just below the threshold for development of acute mucositis, and the total dose of 42 Gy gives a late effect equivalent biologic dose of approximately 60 Gy which gives minimal serious late toxicity. Prospective studies using this regime have shown no episodes of grade 3 mucositis, and only around 10% grade 2 mucositis, while delivering an excellent response rate (complete and partial) in the majority of patients (54–67%) [28,33].

In general, patients need to survive more than 6 months in order to develop late treatment side effects. In the study by Al-Mamgani et al., where 50 Gy in 16 fractions was used and median survival was 17 months, late effects reported included feeding-tube dependency in 29% and severe grade 4 toxicity in 4.5% [30]. Severe side effects included esophageal stricture, osteoradionecrosis, and persistent oropharyngeal ulceration. The actuarial rate of grade 2 or worse late side effects was 17% at one year and 8% at 2 years. In the lower dose regimes, Corry et al. (median survival 5.7 months) showed no grade 3 late toxicity, while Porceddu et al. (median survival 6.1 months) reported grade 3 or worse late side effects in only 11.4% patients [28,29].

From the radical setting we know that the addition of chemotherapy increases both tumor response rates and acute treatment toxicities [10,49,50]. Combining chemotherapy with radiotherapy has also been attempted in the palliative setting. Minetal et al. used split course radiotherapy with 50 Gy in 20 fractions with a 2-week break after 25 Gy [51]. Bleomycin was given concurrently in the first 3 weeks of treatment. Sixty-nine percent of patients obtained a partial or complete response and 81% obtained either good or partial symptom relief. The median overall survival of 7 months was similar to radiotherapy alone regimes. As expected, there was a high rate of toxicity with this regime, with 46.6% of patients having grade 3 mucositis.

The value of increased radiotherapy doses and/or the addition of concurrent chemotherapy in the palliative setting are unanswered questions that offer grounds for future research. Incorporated into this research should be measurement of quality of life outcomes and analyses such as time without symptoms or toxicity (TWiST) [52]. TWiST, a measure of the time spent without symptoms of disease or toxicity of treatment, helps quantify the quandary of balancing tumor response and symptom improvement with time spent recovering from treatment related toxicity.

Recurrent disease

The treatment options for recurrent disease depend upon initial treatment modalities and the extent of loco-regional recurrence, the elapsed time from completion of previous treatment, and the presence/absence of distant metastatic disease. Surgery with curative intent is not uncommonly used in patients without distant metastatic disease who have previously been treated with (chemo)radiation. Clearly most published series are in highly selected patients, but there can be a useful duration of progression-free survival and even cure. Because of anatomic location, surgical salvage is much more feasible in certain anatomic locations, for example larynx versus oropharynx. In the RTOG 91-11 larynx cancer trial surgical salvage was feasible in all patients with primary failure [53], while in a series that examined salvage in primary oropharyngeal cancers, surgery was possible in 70% of patients who had local or loco-regional disease recurrence [54]. Five-year survival in patients undergoing laryngectomy after (chemo)radiotherapy was around 50% [53,55] compared with 40% in patients who were operated for recurrent oropharyngeal cancers [54].

Where disease is surgically unresectable, attempting high-dose radiotherapy for loco-regional recurrence in a previously radiated field has also been described. Two phase II trials have been conducted by RTOG [56,57]. Both these trials used high dose radiotherapy in previously radiated fields (60 Gy in 1.5 Gy fractions bid over 5 days given every other week) with concurrent chemotherapy (hydroxyurea and 5-fluorouracil in the first trial and cisplatin and paclitaxel in the second). The median survival in the trials was 8.5 and 12.1 months and 2-year survival rates were 15.2% and 25.9%. Acute grade 4 or worse toxicity developed in a quarter of patients and treatment mortality was reported in 8–10% of patients. Retrospective series in the literature of radical re-irradiation (in conjunction with surgery and chemotherapy in some cases) demonstrate similarly small survival rates with high treatment related toxicity [58–63].

The literature on the palliative benefits associated with surgery or lower doses of re-irradiation is unfortunately sparse. There is anecdotal clinical experience of useful palliation being achieved through re-irradiation, usually following exhaustion of active chemotherapeutic options. When considering re-irradiation the clinician should assess 1) the biologically equivalent dose (BED) delivered in the first course of treatment, 2) the time from initial radical RT, 3) the patient's clinical stigmata of late radiation damage, and 4) the type of tissue that will be undergoing re-irradiation – the total radiation dose that is acceptable for soft tissues will be greater than that acceptable for structures such as bone, spinal cord, or brainstem. An assessment of a tissue's "forgotten dose," as described by various authors [64,65], can be valuable when trying to establish a safe re-irradiation dose. Symptoms such as pain, fungating skin lesions, and bleeding are more likely to respond to low doses of re-irradiation than symptoms requiring significant reduction in the overall bulk of disease.

Unfortunately the advantage of re-irradiating (whether high dose or low dose) compared to chemotherapy alone for unresectable loco-regional recurrences is unanswered. A phase III RTOG trial that attempted to compare re-irradiation and chemotherapy to chemotherapy alone closed early because of poor accrual.

The promise of emerging technologies

There is widespread use of intensity modulated radiation therapy (IMRT) in radical treatment of HNC because of the expectation of reducing late treatment toxicities without compromise of loco-regional control. The proven benefits of IMRT to date in the radical treatment of HNC [66–68] have been in relation to parotid sparing and reduction in xerostomia. There is expectation, but not yet proof, that use of IMRT will also reduce both dental complications and osteoradionecrosis.

There is no consensus for the use of IMRT in the palliative setting. This is not only because of the issue of access, but also because of the traditional belief that palliative treatments should be quick, simple, and inexpensive. However, the dose and fractionation may still remain quick and simple, but when delivered by IMRT there is also the potential to significantly reduce acute treatment toxicities. There could also be scope for pushing the palliative radiation dose higher (for the potential benefit of a more durable remission) whilst keeping acute toxicities low, potentially improving the overall therapeutic ratio in palliative treatments. This is an area that would clearly benefit from appropriately designed prospective studies that include both TWiST and cost benefit analyses as endpoints.

Chemotherapy in palliative head and neck squamous cell carcinomas

In patients with loco-regionally or distant recurrent disease, palliative chemotherapy is often the only active treatment option. There are multiple trials that have investigated chemotherapy in this setting [39–47]. Response rates range from 15 to 40%. Toxicity from chemotherapy is, however, not insignificant with grade 3 to 4 toxicity ranging from 10 to 70%.

An adequately powered trial has never been performed to show that chemotherapy leads to a survival advantage over supportive care and no trials have shown that combination chemotherapy leads to a survival advantage over single agents [69]. Recently, however, a phase III randomized trial (EXTREME) has shown that the addition of the biologic agent, cetuximab (an EGF receptor inhibitor) resulted in an improvement in overall survival in patients with recurrent or metastatic head and neck squamous cell carcinoma [40]. Despite having a low response rate when used alone, cetuximab significantly improved the response rate of cisplatin/5-FU or carboplatin/5-FU from 20 to 36%. It also improved patients' median progression free and overall survival from 3.3 to 5.6 months and 7.4 to 10.1 months, respectively. Unfortunately this trial, along with most chemotherapy trials in this setting, lacked symptom control analysis, a quality of life component, and a cost benefit analysis. These components are particularly vital in trials of palliative treatment regimens where the traditional endpoint of overall survival is probably inadequate to assess the true value of a palliative regimen.

In general, patients with metastatic disease have a median survival around 6 months, with only 20% surviving one year [39–47]. A caveat, however, is in patients with limited distant metastasis. Five-year survival of 26.5% and 29% has been reported in selected patients who undergo resection of lung metastasis from squamous cell head and neck primaries [70,71]. Of course it is often unclear whether these tumors are truly a HNSCC metastasis rather than a new lung primary. To date attempts to generate a genetic fingerprint to separate these two clinical possibilities, and hence instigate appropriate treatment, have been largely unsuccessful [72].

The question of appropriate treatment intensity for small volume metastatic disease has become a particular clinical issue with the widespread use of staging FDG-PET-CT in HNSCC. Studies show a significant detection of previously unsuspected distant metastatic disease [73–80]. The natural history in this group of patients may be different to those described in current literature where the metastatic disease was symptomatic or of significant volume to be detected by conventional imaging. The life expectancy of patients with PET-CT detected asymptomatic small volume metastatic disease or an oligometastasis is currently unclear. It could possibly be as long as 12–18 months, in which case more aggressive treatment to both the loco-regional disease or the distant disease may be appropriate. This is another area requiring active clinical research.

Non-squamous cell carcinomas histologies

Undifferentiated nasopharyngeal cancer deserves a separate mention in the context of management of locally recurrent or distant metastatic disease.

There are data to suggest that patients with limited metastatic disease from undifferentiated nasopharyngeal cancer can have a very durable PFS with aggressive treatment [81–83]. There are also retrospective studies showing reasonably good long-term outcomes for selected patients with locally recurrent disease [84–86]. However, this may not remain the case for recurrent disease following IMRT treatment. The improved radiation dose delivery using IMRT to the whole primary gross disease seems to result in lower local failure rates [87,88], but in those who do fail locally the scope for re-irradiation will subsequently be lower.

Specific issues in palliation of head and neck squamous cell carcinomas

Upper airway obstruction (UAO) from HNSCC is sadly not uncommon. It is a symptom that is terrifying for patients and one that needs a careful holistic approach for appropriate palliative management decisions to be made. Generally, if there are no further active tumor treatment options available, the palliative treatment options for this symptom include one or all of the following: high dose dexamethasone, insertion of a tracheostomy tube, provision of medications to induce a medical coma.

The discussion regarding management options for UAO needs to occur with the patient before it becomes a medical emergency. Although a difficult topic, patients can gain major reduction in anxiety knowing that there is a clear management plan in place for that contingency, and one that they have had a major role in determining.

A major decision is whether or not to insert a tracheostomy tube in the setting of incurable untreatable disease. This may offer only short relief due to the ability of the tumor to subsequently obstruct the tracheostomy tube, or just prolong suffering for the patient. In most countries patients are able to choose the option of not having this intervention, opting for medical management only.

Another HNSCC specific complication is that of near or complete dysphagia. Again this can be a very distressing symptom that needs to be managed appropriately within the context of the patient's overall illness. When patients present with this symptom, active treatment options can alleviate or reduce this symptom. However, when there are no further active treatment options, there needs to be discussion with the patient and their family about the role of insertion of a feeding tube, either a nasogastric tube or percutaneous endoscopic gastrostomy tube. Ultimately it is the patient's choice as to whether they want this intervention or not. It is important to discuss the indications and implications of insertion of a feeding tube with patients and their families as it can be more stressful to remove an ill-considered feeding tube than to never have placed one.

Special considerations in developing countries

Head and neck cancers represent a large burden of cancers in developing countries and patients often present with advanced, incurable disease. In general, palliative radiotherapy techniques that have been described in the literature to date are simple and easily replicable in developing countries. They usually involve treatment of gross symptomatic disease only using simple parallel-opposed fields that can be shaped using simple blocks [28–38].

Two innovative treatment regimens from India have been published in an attempt to rationally allocate limited resources [31,32]. The regimens used an initial low radiation dose but then gave further radiotherapy to those who had at least partial responses and tolerated the treatment. In one scheme patients were treated with 40 Gy in 16 fractions initially and then escalated with a further 10 Gy in 4 fractions if there was evidence of complete or partial response and less than grade 3 mucosal or skin toxicity [32]. Another scheme used 20 Gy in 5 fractions initially over one week, and those patients who had at least partial response to treatment at one month had further escalation of treatment with 2 Gy per fraction daily to a biologic equivalent of 70 Gy [31]. These trials had a response rate (complete and partial) of 47% and 73%, and progression-free survival was 55.1% at one year in one study (with no reported overall survival) and a median survival of 6.7 months (in patients completing 20 Gy) in the other study; longer survival was seen in those who received escalated doses. While using initial response to radiotherapy with smaller doses is an attractive option in order to allocate resources, those patients who could potentially have radical treatment with high doses may potentially have their outcomes compromised by having treatment breaks. Further work needs to be done on clinical and prognostic markers to better select patients for lower dose or higher dose treatments from the outset.

Conclusion

Radiotherapy offers a high response rate and thus useful palliation in HNSCC, particularly for loco-regional symptoms. The best palliative radiotherapy regimen is not clear. Whilst higher radiotherapy dose regimens give higher tumor response rates, they are also more likely to produce significant treatment side effects. Our current approach is to use a low side-effect regimen (e.g. 14 Gy in 4 fractions, twice per day, repeated at monthly intervals to a total dose of 42 Gy) in the majority of patients, and to reserve higher doses (e.g. 50 Gy in 20 fractions, daily over 4 weeks) for selected patients whose life expectancy is estimated to be in the order of 12 months. Supportive care only is recommended for those patients with a very poor prognosis (less than 3 months) unless there are uncontrolled symptoms, in which case a very abbreviated regime (e.g. single 8 Gy) may be used (Figure 12.1).

References

1. Boyle P, Levin B (eds) *World Cancer Report 2008*. Lyon: International Agency for Research on Cancer, 2008.
2. World Health Organization. The global burden of disease: 2004 update. Available at: http://www.who.int/evidence/bod (accessed May 7, 2012).
3. Mehanna H, Paleri V, West C, *et al*. Head and neck cancer - Part 1: epidemiology, presentation, and prevention. *BMJ* 2010; **341**: c4684.
4. Mathers CD, Loncar D. Projections of global mortality and burden of disease from 2002 to 2030. *PLoS Med* 2006; **3**: e442.
5. Mehanna H, Jones TM, Gregoire V, *et al*. Oropharyngeal carcinoma related to human papillomavirus. *BMJ* 2010; **340**: c1439.
6. Ang KK, Harris J, Wheeler R, *et al*. Human papillomavirus and survival of patients with oropharyngeal cancer. *N Engl J Med* 2010; **363**: 24–35.
7. Rischin D, Richard JY, Fisher R, *et al*. Prognostic significance of p16INK4A and human papillomavirus in patients with oropharyngeal cancer treated on TROG 02.02 phase III trial. *J Clin Oncol* 2010; **28**: 4142–4148.
8. Pignon JP, Le Maître A, Maillard E, *et al*. Meta-analysis of chemotherapy in head and neck cancer [MACH-NC]: an update on 93 randomized trials and 17,346 patients. *Radiother Oncol* 2009; **92**: 4–14.
9. Wendt TG, Grabenbauer GG, Rodel CM, *et al*. Simultaneous Radiochemotherapy versus radiotherapy alone in advanced head and neck cancer: a randomized multicentre trial. *J Clin Oncol* 1998; **16**: 1318–1324.
10. Calais G, Alfonsi M, Bardet E, *et al*. Randomized trial of radiation therapy versus concomitant chemotherapy and radiation therapy for advanced-stage oropharynx carcinoma. *J Natl Cancer Inst* 1998; **91**: 2018–2086.
11. Aldelstein DJ, Levertu P, Saxton JP, *et al*. Mature results of a Phase III trial comparing concurrent cheoradiotherpay with radiation therapy alone in patients with stage III and IV SCC of the head and neck. *Cancer* 2000; **88**: 876–883.
12. Rischin D, Peters LJ, Fisher R, *et al*. Tirapazamine, Cisplatin and radiation versus Flurouracil, cisplatin and radiation in patients with locally advanced head and neck cancer: a randomized phase II trial of the Trans-Tasman Radiation Oncology Group (TROG 98.02). *J Clin Oncol* 2005; **23**: 79–87.
13. Albain KS, Crowley JJ, LeBlanc M, *et al*. Survival determinants in extensive-stage non-small-cell lung cancer: the South- west Oncology Group experience. *J Clin Oncol* 1991; **9**: 1618–1626.
14. Huang SH, O'Sullivan B, Waldron J, *et al*. Patterns of care in elderly head-and-neck cancer radiation oncology patients: a single-center cohort study. *Int J Radiat Oncol Biol Phys* 2011; **79**: 46–51.
15. Sesterhenn AM, Teymoortash A, Folz BJ, *et al*. Head and neck cancer in the elderly: a cohort study in 40 patients. *Acta Oncol* 2005; **44**: 59–64.
16. Sanabria A, Carvalho AL, Vartanian JG, *et al*. Comorbidity is a prognostic factor in elderly patients with head and neck cancer. *Ann Surg Oncol* 2007; **14**: 1449–1457.
17. Ledeboer QC, van der Schroeff MP, Pruyn JF, *et al*. Survival of patients with palliative head and neck cancer. *Head Neck* 2011; **33**: 1021–1026.
18. Paleri V, Wight RG, Silver CE, *et al*. Comorbidity in head and neck cancer: a critical appraisal and recommendations for practice. *Oral Oncol* 2010; **46**: 712–719.
19. Kaplan MH, Feinstein AR. The importance of classifying initial co-morbidity in evaluating the outcome of diabetes mellitus. *J Chronic Dis* 1974; **27**: 387–404.

20. Charlson ME, Pompei P, Ales KL, *et al*. A new method of classifying prognostic comorbidity in longitudinal studies: development and validation. *J Chronic Dis* 1987; **40**: 373–383.

21. Knegjens JL, Hauptmann M, Pameijer FA, *et al*. Tumor volume as prognostic factor in chemoradiation for advanced head and neck cancer. *Head Neck* 2011; **33**: 375–382.

22. Tsou YA, Hua JH, Lin MH, *et al*. Analysis of prognostic factors of chemoradiation therapy for advanced hypopharyngeal cancer—does tumor volume correlate with central necrosis and tumor pathology? *J Otorhinolaryngol Relat Spec* 2006; **68**: 206–212.

23. Mendenhall WM, Morris CG, Amdur RJ, *et al*. Parameters that predict local control after definitive radiotherapy for squamous cell carcinoma of the head and neck. *Head Neck* 2003; **25**: 535–542.

24. Doweck I, Denys D, Robbins KT. Tumor volume predicts out- come for advanced head and neck cancer treated with targeted chemoradiotherapy. *Laryngoscope* 2002; **112**: 1742–1749.

25. Chen SW, Yang SN, Liang JA, *et al*. Prognostic impact of tumor volume in patients with stage III–IVA hypo- pharyngeal cancer without bulky lymph nodes treated with definative concurrent chemoradiotherapy. *Head Neck* 2009; **31**: 709–716.

26. Jansen JF, Schöder H, Lee NY, *et al*. Tumor metabolism and perfusion in head and neck squamous cell carcinoma: pretreatment multimodality imaging with (1)H magnetic resonance spectroscopy, dynamic contrast-enhanced MRI, and [(18)F]FDG-PET. *Int J Radiat Oncol Biol Phys* 2011; **82**: 299–307.

27. Castaldi P, Rufini V, Bussu F, *et al*. Can "early" and "late"(18)F-FDG PET-CT be used as prognostic factors for the clinical outcome of patients with locally advanced head and neck cancer treated with radio-chemotherapy? *Radiother Oncol* 2012; **103**: 63–68.

28. Corry J, Peters LJ, Costa ID, *et al*. The 'QUAD SHOT' - a phase II study of palliative radiotherapy for incurable head and neck cancer. *Radiother Oncol* 2005; **77**: 137–142.

29. Porceddu SV, Rosser B, Burmeister BH, *et al*. Hypofractionated radiotherapy for the palliation of advanced head and neck cancer in patients unsuitable for curative treatment-"Hypo Trial." *Radiother Oncol* 2007; **85**: 456–462.

30. Al-Mamgani A, Tans L, Van Rooij PH, *et al*. Hypofractionated radiotherapy denoted as the "Christie scheme": an effective means of palliating patients with head and neck cancers not suitable for curative treatment. *Acta Oncol* 2009; **48**: 562–570.

31. Mohanti BK, Umapathy H, Bahadur S, *et al*. Short course palliative radiotherapy of 20 Gy in 5 fractions for advanced and incurable head and neck cancer: AIIMS study. *Radiother Oncol* 2004; **71**: 275–280.

32. Agarwal JP, Nemade B, Murthy V, *et al*. Hypofractionated, palliative radiotherapy for advanced head and neck cancer. *Radiother Oncol* 2008; **89**: 51–56.

33. Ghoshal S, Chakraborty S, Moudgil N, *et al*. Quad shot: a short but effective schedule for palliative radiation for head and neck carcinoma. *Indian J Palliat Care* 2009; **15**: 137–140.

34. Paris KJ, Spanos WJ Jr, Lindberg RD, *et al*. Phase I-II study of multiple daily fractions for palliation of advanced head and neck malignancies. *Int J Radiat Oncol Biol Phys* 1993; **25**: 657–660.

35. Stevens CM, Huang SH, Fung S, *et al*. Retrospective study of palliative radiotherapy in newly diagnosed head and neck carcinoma. *Int J Radiat Oncol Biol Phys* 2011; **81**: 958–963.

36. Chen AM, Vaughan A, Narayan S, *et al*. Palliative radiation therapy for head and neck cancer: toward an optimal fractionation scheme. *Head Neck* 2008; **30**: 1586–1591.

37. Kancherla KN, Oksuz DC, Prestwich RJ, *et al.* The role of split-course hypofractionated palliative radiotherapy in head and neck cancer. *Clin Oncol (R Coll Radiol)* 2011; **23**: 141–148.

38. Erkal HS, Mendenhall WM, Amdur RJ, *et al.* Squamous cell carcinomas metastatic to cervical lymph nodes from an unknown head and neck mucosal site treated with radiation therapy with palliative intent. *Radiother Oncol* 2001; **59**: 319–321.

39. Vermorken JB, Trigo J, Hitt R, *et al.* Open-label, uncontrolled, multicenter phase II study to evaluate the efficacy and toxicity of cetuximab as a single agent in patients with recurrent and/or metastatic squamous cell carcinoma of the head and neck who failed to respond to platinum-based therapy. *J Clin Oncol* 2007; **25**: 2171–2177.

40. Vermorken JB, Mesia R, Rivera F, *et al.* Platinum-based chemotherapy plus cetuximab in head and neck cancer. *N Engl J Med* 2008; **359**: 1116–1127.

41. Forastiere AA, Shank D, Neuberg D, *et al.* Final report of a phase II evaluation of paclitaxel in patients with advanced squamous cell carcinoma of the head and neck: an Eastern Cooperative Oncology Group trial (PA390). *Cancer* 1998; **82**: 2270–2274.

42. Gibson MK, Li Y, Murphy B, *et al.* Randomized phase III evaluation of cisplatin plus fluorouracil versus cisplatin plus paclitaxel in advanced head and neck cancer (E1395): an intergroup trial of the Eastern Cooperative Oncology Group. *J Clin Oncol* 2005; **23**: 3562–3567.

43. Forastiere AA, Metch B, Schuller DE, *et al.* Randomized comparison of cisplatin plus fluorouracil and carboplatin plus fluorouracil versus methotrexate in advanced squamous-cell carcinoma of the head and neck: a Southwest Oncology Group study. *J Clin Oncol* 1992; **10**: 1245–1251.

44. Samlowski WE, Moon J, Kuebler JP, *et al.* Evaluation of the combination of docetaxel/carboplatin in patients with metastatic or recurrent squamous cell carcinoma of the head and neck (SCCHN): a Southwest Oncology Group phase II study. *Cancer Invest* 2007; **25**: 182–188.

45. Jacobs C, Lyman G, Velez-Garcia E, *et al.* A phase III randomized study comparing cisplatin and fluorouracil as single agents and in combination for advanced squamous cell carcinoma of the head and neck. *J Clin Oncol* 1992; **10**: 257–263.

46. Clavel M, Vermorken JB, Cognetti F, *et al.* Randomized comparison of cisplatin, methotrexate, bleomycin and vincristine (CABO) versus cisplatin and 5 fluorouracil (CF) versus cisplatin (C) in recurrent or metastatic squamous cell carcinoma of the head and neck. A phase III study of the EORTC Head and Neck Cancer Cooperative Group. *Ann Oncol* 1994; **5**: 521–526.

47. Stewart JS, Cohen EE, Licitra L, *et al.* Phase III study of gefitinib compared with intravenous methotrexate for recurrent squamous cell carcinoma of the head and neck. *J Clin Oncol* 2009; **27**: 1864–1871.

48. Spanos W, Guse C, Perez C, *et al.* Phase II study of multiple daily fractions in the palliation of advanced pelvic malignancies: preliminary report of 8502. *Int J Radiat Oncol Biol Phys* 1989; **17**: 659–661.

49. Olmi P, Crispino S, Fallai C, *et al.* Locoregionally advanced carcinoma of the oropharynx: conventional radiotherapy vs. accelerated hyperfractionated radiotherapy vs. concomitant radiotherapy and chemotherapy–a multicenter randomized trial. *Int J Radiat Oncol Biol Phys* 2003; **55**: 78–92.

50. Adelstein DJ, Saxton JP, Lavertu P, *et al.* A phase III randomized trial comparing concurrent chemotherapy and radiotherapy with radiotherapy alone in resectable stage III and IV squamous cell head and neck cancer: preliminary results. *Head Neck* 1997; **19**: 567–575.

51. Minatel E, Gigante M, Franchin G, *et al*. Combined radiotherapy and bleomycin in patients with inoperable head and neck cancer with unfavourable prognostic factors and severe symptoms. *Oral Oncol* 1998; **34**: 119–122.

52. Gelber RD, Cole BF, Gelber S, Goldhirsch A. Comparing treatments using quality-adjusted survival: the Q-TWiST method. *Am Stat* 1995; **49**: 161–169.

53. Weber RS, Berkey BA, Forastiere A, *et al*. Outcome of salvage total laryngectomy following organ preservation therapy: the Radiation Therapy Oncology Group trial 91-11. *Arch Otolaryngol Head Neck Surg* 2003; **129**: 44–49.

54. Nichols AC, Kneuertz PJ, Deschler DG, *et al*. Surgical salvage of the oropharynx after failure of organ-sparing therapy. *Head Neck* 2011; **33**: 516–524.

55. van der Putten L, de Bree R, Kuik DJ, *et al*. Salvage laryngectomy: oncological and functional outcome. *Oral Oncol* 2011; **47**: 296–301.

56. Spencer SA, Harris J, Wheeler RH, *et al*. Final report of RTOG 9610, a multi-institutional trial of reirradiation and chemotherapy for unresectable recurrent squamous cell carcinoma of the head and neck. *Head Neck* 2008; **30**: 281–288.

57. Langer CJ, Harris J, Horwitz EM, *et al*. Phase II study of low-dose paclitaxel and cisplatin in combination with split-course concomitant twice-daily reirradiation in recurrent squamous cell carcinoma of the head and neck: results of Radiation Therapy Oncology Group Protocol 9911. *J Clin Oncol* 2007; **25**: 4800–4805.

58. Lee N, Chan K, Bekelman JE, *et al*. Salvage re-irradiation for recurrent head and neck cancer. *Int J Radiat Oncol Biol Phys* 2007; **68**: 731–740.

59. Dawson LA, Myers LL, Bradford CR, *et al*. Conformal re-irradiation of recurrent and new primary head-and-neck cancer. *Int J Radiat Oncol Biol Phys* 2001; **50**: 377–385.

60. Salama JK, Vokes EE, Chmura SJ, *et al*. Long-term outcome of concurrent chemotherapy and reirradiation for recurrent and second primary head-and-neck squamous cell carcinoma. *Int J Radiat Oncol Biol Phys* 2006; **64**: 382–391.

61. Watkins JM, Shirai KS, Wahlquist AE, *et al*. Toxicity and survival outcomes of hyperfractionated split-course reirradiation and daily concurrent chemotherapy in locoregionally recurrent, previously irradiated head and neck cancers. *Head Neck* 2009; **31**: 493–502.

62. Mendenhall WM, Mendenhall CM, Malyapa RS, *et al*. Re-irradiation of head and neck carcinoma. *Am J Clin Oncol* 2008; **31**: 393–398.

63. Wong SJ, Machtay M, Li Y. Locally recurrent, previously irradiated head and neck cancer: concurrent re-irradiation and chemotherapy, or chemotherapy alone? *J Clin Oncol* 2006; **24**: 2653–2658.

64. Ang KK, Price RE, Stephens LC, *et al*. The tolerance of primate spinal cord to re-irradiation. *Int J Radiat Oncol Biol Phys* 1993; **25**: 459–464.

65. Mason KA, Withers HR, Chiang CS. Late effects of radiation on the lumbar spinal cord of guinea pigs: re-treatment tolerance. *Int J Radiat Oncol Biol Phys* 1993; **26**: 643–648.

66. Nutting CM, Morden JP, Harrington KJ, *et al*. PARSPORT trial management group. Parotid-sparing intensity modulated versus conventional radiotherapy in head and neck cancer (PARSPORT): a phase 3 multicentre randomised controlled trial. *Lancet Oncol* 2011; **12**: 127–136.

67. Pow EH, Kwong DL, McMillan AS, *et al*. Xerostomia and quality of life after intensity-modulated radiotherapy vs conventional radiotherapy for early-stage nasopharyngeal carcinoma: initial report on a randomized controlled clinical trial. *Int J Radiat Oncol Biol Phys* 2006; **66**: 981–991.

68. Kam MK, Leung SF, Zee B, *et al*. Prospective randomized study of intensity-modulated radiotherapy on salivary gland function in early-stage nasopharyngeal carcinoma patients. *J Clin Oncol* 2007; **25**: 4873–4879.

69. Colevas AD. Chemotherapy options for patients with metastatic or recurrent squamous cell carcinoma of the head and neck. *J Clin Oncol* 2006; **24**: 2644–2652.

70. Shiono S, Kawamura M, Sato T, *et al*. Pulmonary Metastasectomy for Pulmonary Metastases of Head and Neck Squamous Cell Carcinomas. *Ann Thorac Surg* 2009; **88**: 856–861.

71. Finley RK, Verazin GT, Driscoll DL, *et al*. Results of surgical resection of pulmonary metastases of squamous cell carcinoma of the head and neck. *Am J Surg* 1992; **164**: 594–598.

72. Lal A, Panos R, Marjanovic M, *et al*. A gene expression profile test to resolve squamous cell carcinomas of head & neck from squamous cell carcinomas of the lung. Proc AACR 2012 Abstract 1724.

73. Ng SH, Chan SC, Yen TC, *et al*. Staging of untreated nasopharyngeal carcinoma with PET/CT: comparison with conventional imaging work-up. *Eur J Nucl Med Mol Imaging* 2009; **36**: 12–22.

74. Chua ML, Ong SC, Wee JT, *et al*. Comparison of 4 modalities for distant metastasis staging in endemic nasopharyngeal carcinoma. *Head Neck* 2009; **31**: 346–354.

75. Goerres GW, Schmid DT, Grätz KW, *et al*. Impact of whole body positron emission tomography on initial staging and therapy in patients with squamous cell carcinoma of the oral cavity. *Oral Oncol* 2003; **39**: 547–551.

76. Connell CA, Corry J, Milner AD, *et al*. Clinical impact of, and prognostic stratification by, F-18 FDG PET/CT in head and neck mucosal squamous cell carcinoma. *Head Neck* 2007; **29**: 986–995.

77. Lonneux M, Hamoir M, Reychler H, *et al*. Positron emission tomography with [18F] fluorodeoxyglucose improves staging and patient management in patients with head and neck squamous cell carcinoma: a multicenter prospective study. *J Clin Oncol* 2010; **28**: 1190–1195.

78. Sigg MB, Steinert H, Grätz K, *et al*. Staging of head and neck tumors: [18F]fluorodeoxy-glucose positron emission tomography compared with physical examination and conventional imaging modalities. *J Oral Maxillofac Surg* 2003; **61**: 1022–1029.

79. Schwartz DL, Rajendran J, Yueh B, *et al*. Staging of head and neck squamous cell cancer with extended-field FDG-PET. *Arch Otolaryngol Head Neck Surg* 2003; **129**: 1173–1178.

80. Senft A, de Bree R, Hoekstra OS, *et al*. Screening for distant metastases in head and neck cancer patients by chest CT or whole body FDG-PET: a prospective multicenter trial. *Radiother Oncol* 2008; **87**: 221–229.

81. Hui EP, Leung SF, Au JS, *et al*. Lung metastasis alone in nasopharyngeal carcinoma: a relatively favourable prognostic group- A study by the Hong Kong Nasopharyngeal Carcinoma Study Group. *Cancer* 2004; **101**: 300–306.

82. Fandi A, Bachouchi M, Azli N, *et al*. Long-term disease-free survivors in metastatic undifferentiated carcinoma of nasopharyngeal type. *J Clin Oncol* 2000; **18**: 1324–1330.

83. Cheng LC, Sham JS, Chiu CS, *et al*. Surgical resection of pulmonary metastases from nasopharyngeal carcinoma. *Aust N Z J Surg* 1996; **66**: 71–73.

84. Wang CC. Re-irradiation of recurrent nasopharyngeal carcinoma-treatment techniques and results. *Int J Radiat Oncol Biol Phys* 1987; **13**: 953–956.

85. Lee AW, Law SC, Foo W, *et al.* Retrospective analysis of patients with nasopharyngeal carcinoma treated during 1976-1985: survival after local recurrence. *Int J Radiat Oncol Biol Phys* 1993; **26**: 773–782.

86. Wei WI. Salvage surgery for recurrent primary nasopharyngeal carcinoma. *Crit Rev Oncol Hematol* 2000; **33**: 91–98.

87. Lee N, Xia P, Quivey JM, *et al.* Intensity-modulated radiotherapy in the treatment of nasopharyngeal carcinoma: an update of the UCSF experience. *Int J Radiat Oncol Biol Phys* 2002; **53**: 12–22.

88. Ng WT, Lee MC, Hung WM, *et al.* Clinical outcomes and patterns of failure after intensity-modulated radiotherapy for nasopharyngeal carcinoma. *Int J Radiat Oncol Biol Phys* 2011; **79**: 420–428.

CHAPTER 13

The role of palliative radiotherapy in breast cancer

Ian H. Kunkler
Department of Clinical Oncology, Western General Hospital, Edinburgh, UK

Introduction

Palliative radiotherapy (PRT) plays an important role in the management of breast cancer, the most common malignancy in women in developed countries and the second leading cause of death among females [1]. While mortality rates from breast cancer have been falling in the UK and North America since the 1990s as a result of screening and better treatment, nearly a third of patients with breast cancer will relapse despite initial treatment [2]. Local recurrence rates following mastectomy alone may be as high as 45% for T3 or T4 or node positive patients [3]. Bedwinek noted that 62% of patients with uncontrolled disease experience one or more distressing symptoms (pain, ulceration, arm edema, bleeding, or brachial plexopathy) for the duration of their life (see Box 13.1) [4]. Axillary relapse after primary surgery, adjuvant radiotherapy, and systemic therapy for early breast cancer may occur in about 10% of cases [5]. Less than 10% of American breast cancer patients present with locally advanced breast cancer (LABC) and less than 2% with inflammatory breast cancer [6]. The proportion of LABC is higher in younger women and among racial ethnic minorities [7].The rate of LABC in American women aged 30–39 is 15% in Caucasians, 18% in African Americans, and 19% in women of Hispanic descent [7]. For stage IIIA and IIIB disease, 5-year survival is 52% and 48% respectively.

Box 13.1 Symptoms commonly associated with locally advanced or recurrent breast cancers

- Pain
- Ulceration
- Arm edema

- Bleeding
- Infection
- Brachial plexopathy

Radiation Oncology in Palliative Cancer Care, First Edition. Edited by Stephen Lutz, Edward Chow, and Peter Hoskin.
© 2013 John Wiley & Sons, Ltd. Published 2013 by John Wiley & Sons, Ltd.

With the age related rise in incidence of the disease, the burden of loco-regional recurrence will rise in the elderly where issues of comorbidities complicate disease management and issues of dose fractionation for palliative radiotherapy need to be carefully considered. The psychologic distress induced by visible local recurrence, odorous or bleeding tumors on the chest wall, breast, or in axillary nodes is very substantial. Palliative radiotherapy has anti-secretory, anti-inflammatory, and analgesic effects [8].

Palliative radiotherapy (PRT) is but one component in the multi-disciplinary management of breast cancer, and close liaison is needed between the surgeon, oncologist, family doctor, specialist breast care nurses, and palliative care specialists to plan treatment flexibly around the changing needs of the patient. The need for PRT has been diminished by the advent of more effective systemic therapies, better quality surgery, and improved options for tumor debulking or mastectomy and reconstruction for locally advanced disease. In particular, the introduction of anthracycline and taxane based neoadjuvant chemotherapy followed by mastectomy and post-operative radiotherapy has improved outcomes with loco-regional control rates in excess of 80% for inflammatory breast cancer [9]. In advanced disease, neoadjuvant systemic therapy shows equivalent overall survival to post-operative chemotherapy and better operability rates from pre-operative downsizing and potential for breast conserving surgery [10].

It should also be appreciated that there is a wide spectrum of clinical manifestations and prognoses of loco-regional recurrence ranging from aggressive inflammatory breast cancer to more indolent solitary recurrences in the mastectomy scar. Most patients with loco-regional recurrence will eventually develop distant metastases (81–93%), with a median survival of 12–53 months [4,11,12]. In general, patients with regional nodal relapse have a poorer prognosis than with chest wall or breast recurrences [13]. Therefore, no "one size fits all approach" can be appropriate.

The technical requirements of radiotherapy planning and dose fractionation need to be individualized, taking into account the site and extent of disease to be irradiated, constraints of previous radiotherapy, radiation technology available, the presence and extent of metastatic disease, and the general condition and wishes of the patient.

Every effort should be made to plan and deliver palliative radiotherapy within 1–2 weeks of intention to treat to minimize persistent cancer-related symptomatology and associated psychologic distress. A rapid response clinic such as that described by Holt and Yau in Australia for palliative radiotherapy including breast cancer increased the likelihood of patients being treated within 24 hours of assessment [14].

Given the clinical heterogeneity, this chapter reviews a variety of typical clinical scenarios to illustrate the different roles that PRT may play (Figure 13.1). These circumstances include de novo locally advanced breast cancer (LABC), isolated chest wall recurrence, cancer-induced brachial plexopathy,

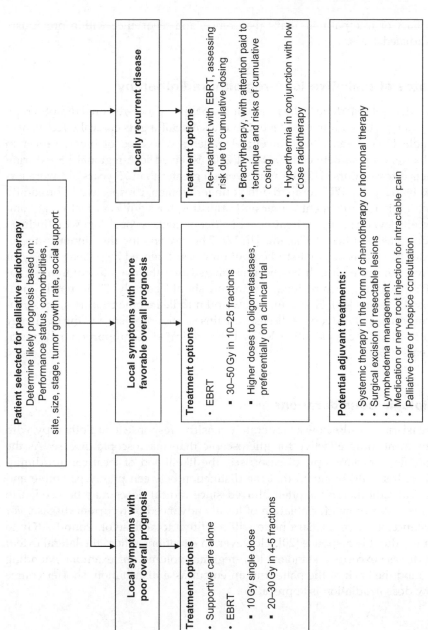

Figure 13.1 Algorithm for use of palliative radiotherapy for patients with locally advanced or recurrent breast cancer.

axillary or internal mammary recurrence, and recurrence within previously irradiated areas.

Rates of palliative loco-regional radiotherapy

The data set that defines the rationale for palliative loco-regional radiotherapy is incomplete, with limited level 1 evidence detailing its clinical effectiveness (Table 13.1). Twenty-two percent of patients who died of breast cancer in Alberta, Canada between 2000 and 2004 received loco-regional PRT during their disease course [15]. Of note, women greater than 75 years old were less likely to receive PRT compared to younger women, irrespective of proximity to a radiation treatment center and adjusting for significant factors at community level. The under-treatment of older patients is consistent with findings from other studies in Canada [16,17]. The reasons for this under-usage in older patients is not well-studied but may be influenced by patient, family, or physician preference. It has been estimated that the overall requirement for PRT (including loco-regional treatment) should be only 2% in newly diagnosed patients [18]. However, in low and middle income countries, presentation with locally advanced disease remains a major problem and the frequency with which local palliative RT will be indicated is proportionately much greater [19].

Biologic considerations

Breast cancer cells show a moderately sensitive response to radiotherapy, with treatment more effective for microscopic than macroscopic disease. As the volume of macroscopic disease rises, the likelihood of local control diminishes. It should be noted that the distinction between purely palliative and radical radiotherapy is often blurred since radical doses may be needed to achieve symptomatic palliation of locally advanced or recurrent disease. For instance, a 2–3 cm axillary node will require a total dose of around 70 Gy to gain a durable response [20]. However, in situations where the lateral extent of disease exceeds a standard loco-regional volume, for example extending around the back of the patient in an en cuirasse distribution, shorter course low dose irradiation is appropriate.

Definitions, clinical features, and multi-disciplinary approach

Locally advanced or locally recurrent breast cancer spans a broad and heterogeneous spectrum of clinical manifestations and behaviors. Locally advanced disease, or stage III breast cancer, is defined by the TNM classification system as a primary tumor larger than 5 cm in diameter with chest wall or skin

Table 13.1 Studies suggesting lack of association between loco-regional treatment and survival in patients with metastatic breast cancer at diagnosis.

Study (year)	Study period	Patients (n)	Patients treated with surgery n (%)	RT information	Systemic therapy information	Survival with versus without surgery/p-value	MVA of association between loco-regional treatment and survival: adjusted HR (95% CI)	Analyzed variables in MVA (significant variables in bold)
Hazard et al. (2008) [61]	Lynn Sage Comprehensive Breast Center, (IL, USA) 1995–2005	111	47 (42)	RT: 60 (55%) No RT: 48 (45%) Use of RT higher in the surgery group (67 vs 29%; p < 0.001)	AC CT: 18 (16%) AC-T CT: 45 (41%) HD CT with autologous bone marrow support: 8 (7%) Other combination CT: 6 (5%) Trastuzumab: 7 (6%) HT: 34 (39%)	3-year OS: 43 vs 37%	0.80 (0.40–.52) with surgery; P = 0.52	Hormone receptor status, age, RT, site of metastasis, number of metastatic sites. **Significant:** NR
Leung et al. (2010) [62]	Virginia Commonwealth University (VA, USA) 1990–2000	157	52 (33)	RT: 58 (36%) No RT: 99 (63%)	CT: 84 (54%) No CT: 73 (46%) HT: 80 (51%) No HT: 77 (49%)	Surgery: Medial OS: 25 vs 13 months; P = 0.06 RT: Medial OS: 17 vs 17 months; P = 0.2	ns	**CT**, RT, HT, age

MVA, multivariate analysis

involvement. Strictly speaking, stage T3 cancers are therefore only locally advanced when accompanied by fixed axillary nodes (N2) or spread to the supraclavicular or internal mammary nodes. Inflammatory breast cancer (stage T4d) is included in the category of LABC, and it may be difficult to distinguish from neglected breast cancers which more commonly present in low resource countries that have limited facilities for screening and treatment.

Clinical scenarios

Locally advanced disease

Locally advanced breast cancer may occur by virtue of its position in the breast (e.g. in or close to the inframammary fold), due to neglect, or because of biologically aggressive disease such as inflammatory breast cancer (T4d) [10]. Conventionally, locally advanced breast cancer is treated with neoadjuvant systemic therapy [21] with the goal of achieving a complete pathologic response at subsequent surgery. The systemic regimens used in the adjuvant setting are also appropriate in the neoadjuvant setting.

For patients not fit enough for neoadjuvant chemotherapy and not candidates for cytoreductive hormonal therapy, high dose palliative radiotherapy can achieve partial and occasionally complete and durable responses. Much of the data on primary radiotherapy alone are from older literature [21,22]. Non-randomized studies showed that radiotherapy alone can achieve response rates of 60–80% for LABC [23,24], though responses were only maintained until death in 27–35% of cases. A trend toward increased local control rates approaching 75% may be achieved with higher total doses, though doses beyond 60 Gy are associated with side-effect risks including fibrosis, necrosis, lymphedema, and brachial plexopathy [25–27].

Flap recurrence after mastectomy

Isolated loco-regional recurrence on the chest wall occurs in about 10–15% of patients following radical or modified radical mastectomy [4]. Chest wall recurrence carries a much worse prognosis than in-breast recurrence after breast conserving therapy, with an overall survival and disease free survival at 5 years of 36% and 13%, respectively [4]. About 80% of patients with loco-regional recurrence will subsequently develop distant metastases.

Flap recurrence after mastectomy is of three distinct types: solitary spot recurrence, multiple spot recurrence, and field change. It is usually possible to control spot recurrences by local excision and post-operative radiotherapy. If there are positive margins then conventional chest wall irradiation is given to 50 Gy in 20 to 25 fractions for tumors less than 1 cm and at least 60 Gy for larger lesions [28]. Treatment is given with tangential fields using 6–8 MV photons and bolus over the whole of the chest wall to ensure full dose to the skin. Treating less than the entire chest wall reduces local control from 55–75% to 6–35% [29]. Patients with a solitary site of recurrence and negative lymph

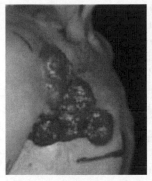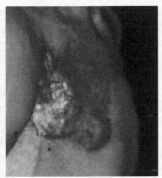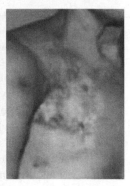

Figure 13.2 Clinical case: pain, lymphedema, bleeding, and ulceration before, 2 months, and 3 years after radiotherapy (see Plate 13.1). Reproduced from van Oorschot *et al.* [8], with permission from Karger.

nodes may achieve as high as a 78% rate of local control, with many of those who fail suffering further recurrences in adjacent, non-irradiated sites [30]. Figure 13.2 shows that even widespread local recurrences can achieve a complete or near-complete response.

For multiple spot recurrences the same radiotherapy is given, but no attempt is made surgically to excise the recurrences given that surgery will not likely add to local control in this setting [28]. For patients with three tumor nodules less than 3 cm in maximum diameter and a disease free interval of at least 12 months, the addition of tamoxifen improves disease free survival [31]. The special circumstance of field change flap recurrence is associated with aggressive primary tumors and a poor prognosis [32]. This clinical presentation should first be managed with cytoreductive chemotherapy followed by chest wall radiotherapy.

Recurrence within a previously irradiated area
Patients who have undergone adjuvant radiotherapy may suffer a local recurrence within the breast, on the chest wall, or in the draining lymphatic regions. Local recurrence in the breast is the most common site of recurrence [33], with subsequent management options including surgical excision, mastectomy and reconstruction, systemic therapy, or re-irradiation. Such cases should be discussed with a multi-disciplinary team so that the risks and benefits are carefully assessed. Chemotherapy is often of limited effect in areas treated by previous surgery and radical radiotherapy. Where recurrences are inoperable, re-irradiation alone or in combination with chemotherapy or hyperthermia are potential options.

The role of re-irradiation for chest wall recurrences is uncertain, and there is little guidance on the role of palliative radiotherapy in this setting. There are legitimate concerns that a second course of radiotherapy to radical doses may induce significant toxicity to skin, subcutaneous tissues and ribs, and it should therefore be considered with caution. Radiotherapy techniques for this situation vary and may include brachytherapy, intraoperative radiotherapy, or external beam irradiation. Small series of patients re-treated with radical courses of external beam therapy to combined total doses of over 100 Gy do suggest the potential for reasonable local control with limited acute side effects [34,35]. Brachytherapy has been used in this setting, though the data documenting its effectiveness and safety are limited, and its application requires a clinician who is experienced in its use [36,37].

Within the author's institution, lower doses of irradiation such as 20 Gy in 5 daily fractions are often used to limited areas of recurrence with 6–9 MeV electrons of appropriate energy using build up to maximize skin dose. Tumor shrinkage or healing of ulceration can often be achieved without any significant toxicity.

Hyperthermia with or without additional radiotherapy or systemic therapy

The results of re-irradiation alone for recurrences in previously irradiated areas are relatively poor, so alternative approaches such as hyperthermia have been investigated to improve local control. Tissue heating can be an effective cell killing agent, and it may have radiosensitizing properties due to its specific effects on hypoxic and therefore radiotherapy-resistant tumor cells [38]. An example of a complete clinical response following radiotherapy plus hyperthermia is shown in Figure 13.3.

There is limited level 1 evidence about the role of hyperthermia in locally recurrent breast cancer, and sample sizes from individual trials are too small to make meaningful conclusions. Pooled data from 5 randomized trials [39] identified 317 lesions randomized in 307 patients, with 213 lesions on the chest wall (69%) and 79 (26%) in breast tissue. A complete response was achieved in 41% of those randomized to RT alone and in 59% of those who received radiotherapy plus hyperthermia (p < 0.001).

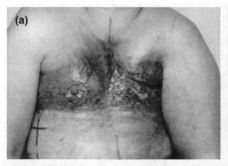 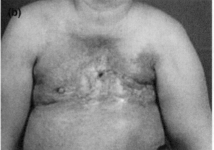

Figure 13.3 Complete response to combination of radiotherapy and hyperthermia to treat bilateral chest wall recurrent before cancer (a) before treatment, (b) after treatment (see Plate 13.2). Courtesy of Dr. G. van Tienhoven, Academic Medical Centre, Amsterdam.

Some of the patients randomized to receive hyperthermia could not complete the treatment due to discomfort associated with the heating procedure. Non-randomized data suggest up to a 73% rate of local control following radiotherapy plus hyperthermia, with a median duration of control of 32 months and a subcutaneous fibrosis rate of 14% [40]. Hyperthermia given in conjunction with chemotherapy and radiotherapy is known as thermochemoradiotherapy. Phase I and II trials have shown this approach to be well-tolerated and associated with modest response rates [40–42]. However, studies have demonstrated that response rates are lower for more bulky or extensive disease [43].

Axillary recurrence and brachial plexopathy
The optimal management of axillary recurrence is uncertain [44]. In general, palliative radiotherapy is reserved for symptomatic and inoperable axillary disease. Axillary dissection is the treatment of choice in this setting because it yields a higher local control rate than radiotherapy, alone [44,45]. Patients who are not suitable for surgery may undergo chemotherapy to diminish the bulk of the recurrent tumor before starting radiotherapy [5]. Brachial plexopathy due to axillary recurrence is particularly distressing for patients since the pain and dysesthesia can be difficult to control. Involvement of palliative care and pain control specialists is important to optimize symptom control.

Supraclavicular node metastases
Supraclavicular lymph node metastases are classified as stage IV, even if not associated with distant metastases at other anatomic sites. In the absence of metastatic disease elsewhere, supraclavicular relapse should be treated by radical dose fractionation schedules. Though the data regarding response rates with this radical approach are scant, a series of patients with supraclavicular nodal relapse achieved a complete subjective response rate of 71% after salvage radiotherapy [46]. Overall median survival was 11.5 months, with 5 patients (23%) surviving 2 years.

Symptom control

Bleeding
Bleeding is a feature of locally advanced or recurrent disease that normally takes the form of continuous oozing from friable tumor. Bleeding is distressing to the patient and family, and substantial blood loss can lead to anemia-related fatigue. Palliative radiotherapy should be started within a few days using an initial large dose of 10 Gy to stem the bleeding. This may be sufficient alone but an additional 8–20 Gy in 2–5 fractions may be given to consolidate hemostasis. Non-adherent dressings should be applied to the affected area to avoid precipitating bleeding when the dressing is removed.

Ulceration, discharge, and infection

Chronic discharge from the breast, chest wall, or axilla due to ulcerative disease can be accompanied by infection with anaerobic bacteria that cause a foul odor. This malodor commonly leads to anxiety, depression, low morale, and social isolation. Palliative radiotherapy with 20–30 Gy in 5–10 fractions using electrons of appropriate energy or photons usually reduces the discharge and can lead to complete healing of ulcerated areas within a month after completion of the course. Treatment of infection with antibiotics and a charcoal-impregnated dressing can substantially reduce odor and improve morale and quality of life.

Palliative loco-regional radiotherapy for oligometastatic disease

There has recently been increasing interest in the role of loco-regional treatment for oligometastatic disease. While the benefit of this approach remains controversial, some studies do suggest that surgery or radiotherapy to the primary tumor site can improve survival in some patients presenting with stage IV disease [47–49]. One French study revealed that patients who had synchronous metastases at the time of initial disease presentation had a statistically significantly increased 3-year survival rate with loco-regional radiotherapy than without radiotherapy [47]. Table 13.2 summarizes studies showing an association or lack of association between loco-regional radiotherapy with or without surgery with outcome in oligometastatic disease. Randomized trials are needed to better define the role of loco-regional radiotherapy with or without surgery in this setting, with studies active in India and Turkey [50,51].

Radiotherapy dosing schedules

Standard dose fractionation

There is a wide range of dose fractionation schedules used for the loco-regional palliation of breast cancer. Box 13.2 shows some of the schedules in use in the UK. As stated earlier, radical doses are commonly used in fitter patients to achieve loco-regional control. Shorter courses are commonly 20–30 Gy in 5–10 fractions. The variation in dose fractionation schedules in large part reflects the absence of randomized trials to define the best approach, thereby leaving many physicians to follow schedules based upon their own experience and local trends.

Alternative fractionation

Both hyper and hypofractionated dose schedules have been used for palliation. There does not seem to be any specific advantage of using a hyperfractionated dose schedule in LABC. A randomized trial of 200 patients [52] with stage III non-inflammatory breast cancer randomized to hyperfractionated RT

Table 13.2 Studies suggesting association between loco-regional radiotherapy and survival in oligometastatic breast cancer (modified from [49]).

Author (year)	Institution and period of study	Patients (no)	Patients treated with surgery n (%)	RT	Systemic therapy	Survival with versus without surgery/p-value	MVA of association between loco-regional treatment and survival: adjusted HR (95% CI)	Significant variables in MVA
Bafford et al. (2009) [64]	Brigham and Women's Hospital) MA, USA 1998–2005	147	64 (41)	Use of RT higher in surgery group (38 vs 16%; p < 0.01)	CT: 123 (84%) HT: 86 (59%) Trastuzumab: 40 (27%)	Median OS: 42 vs 28 months; P = 0.09	0.47 with surgery; P = 0.003	ER status, HER2/neu status, CNS metastasis
Le Scodan et al. (2009) [48]	Centre Rene Huguenin (Paris, France) 1980–2004	581	71 (12)	RT (and surgery): 320 (55%) No RT: 261 (45%)	CT: 92 (16%) HT: 168 (29%) Both: 307 (53%) None: 14 (2%) Comparable use of CT in RT and no RT group	Radiotherapy: 3-year OS: 43 vs 27%; p < 0.001	0.70 (0.58–0.85) with radiotherapy; p < 0.001	Age, metastatic sites, involvement of multiple sites, HT
Ruiterkamp et al. (2009) [65]	The Netherlands Comprehensive Cancer Centre (Amsterdam, the Netherlands) 1993–2004	728	288 (40)	Use of RT higher in surgery group (34 vs 10%; p < 0.001)	Use of systemic therapy higher in surgery group (89 vs 79%; p < 0.001)	5-year OS: 25 vs 13%; p < 0.001	0.62 (0.51–0.76) with surgery	Age, number of metastatic sites, systemic treatment

MVA, multivariate analysis

Box 13.2 Dose fractionation schedules for loco-regional palliative radiotherapy for breast cancer in UK cancer centers

20 Gy in 5 daily fractions over 1 week
500 cGy weekly in 4–5 treatments for elderly patients (Tobias, 1986 [63])
30 Gy in 10 fractions over 2 weeks
30 Gy in 6 fractions weekly
36 Gy in 6 fractions weekly
39 Gy in 13 fractions over 2 weeks
40 Gy in 12 fractions alternate days over 4 weeks
45 Gy in 12 fractions @ 3 fractions per week
45 Gy in 15 fractions over 3 weeks
45–50 Gy in 20–25 fractions over 4–5 weeks with boost of 10–15 Gy to tumor mass on breast/chest wall

---

to 72 Gy in 1.2 Gy twice daily fractions versus a once daily schedule to 60 Gy in 30 fractions and found no statistically significant difference between the two arms with respect to loco-regional recurrence, acute toxicity, or late complications, though there was a slightly higher rate of moist desquamation in the hyperfractionated arm.

Hypofractionated radiotherapy is typically delivered in daily doses of 3–8 Gy per fraction [53]. Equivalent local control rates are achievable with once weekly hypofractionated loco-regional schedules for older patients who have non-metastatic breast cancer [54,55]. A series from Institut Curie in Paris showed that hypofractionated treatment to the breast with 32.5 Gy in weekly fractions of 6.5 Gy provided equivalent local control and cause specific survival as a more conventional fractionation scheme [56].

Radiotherapy technique and the promise of newer technology

Traditionally, short course palliative radiotherapy to 20–30 Gy has been based on simple radiotherapy techniques with single or parallel opposed fields with generous fields to ensure tumor coverage of the breast, chest, axilla, or supraclavicular nodes. However, where radical doses are required for the control of loco-regional recurrence, CT-based 3D planning is recommended to achieve good field matching and a more homogeneous dose distribution.

For locally advanced disease, there is no consensus as to whether the regional nodes including the internal mammary nodes should be routinely treated [57]. If the internal mammary nodes are irradiated, there is an increased risk of cardiac toxicity. The use of a matched electron field over the medial part of the chest wall field to reduce dose to the heart may result in an area of under-dosage where the risk of recurrence is higher [58]. Until the results of the EORTC 22922-10925 IMC trial are known, it seems advisable not to treat the internal mammary chain nodes unless they are radiologically involved.

To treat the breast or chest wall and the supraclavicular fossa, a megavoltage (6–10 MV) single isocentric technique is recommended with half beam blocks to match the tangential fields with the nodal field. Bolus is applied to ensure full skin dose if there is macroscopic disease or a positive excision margin after mastectomy. A posterior axillary boost may be needed if the depth of the supraclavicular and axillary nodes differs significantly. CT-based treatment planning is advised to contour the nodal volumes. For local recurrence within previously irradiated fields, electron beam field with appropriate thickness of degrader ensures full skin dose to limited areas are effective [58].

It is uncertain whether more conformal techniques such as IMRT, image-guided radiation therapy (IGRT), or stereotactic body radiation therapy (SBRT) for LABC can improve local control or reduce long-term toxicity to lung, ribs, brachial plexus, or heart. One report from Chatterjee *et al.* [59] describes the use of helical tomotherapy to spare the brachial plexus in treating the supraclavicular field with a sequential or simultaneous integrated boost as practical and safe, and further advancements are due to come (Figure 13.4).

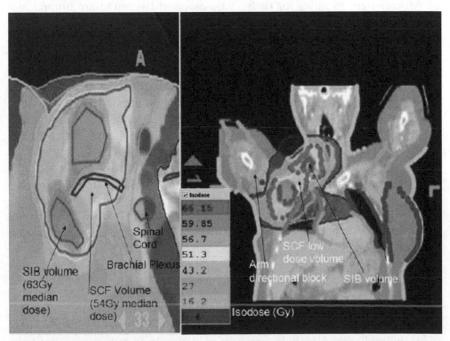

Figure 13.4 Simultaneous integrated boost technique using helical tomotherapy to spare the brachial plexus outside the "boost" volume (see Plate 13.3). Reproduced from Chatterjee *et al.* [59], with permission from Elsevier.

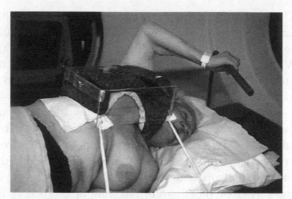

Figure 13.5 Breast jig for palliative treatment of locally advanced disease. Reproduced from Kunkler [60], with kind permission from Elsevier.

Special considerations in developing countries

In low resource countries, particularly in Africa and Asia, it is difficult to estimate accurately the burden of LABC since there are few tumor registries. Mortality-incidence ratios have been used as a reasonable proxy for the burden of LABC. These ratios are highest in the less well-developed regions of Africa where facilities for early diagnosis and treatment are limited and lowest in western developed countries. Rates of LABC between 25–50% have been reported from impoverished populations in Singapore, Egypt, North Africa, India, and Sub-Saharan Africa. Within China, an example of a rapidly developing country, the incidence of LABC in Shanghai has fallen from 25% before 1990 to <10% in 2007, although the incidence of breast cancer has risen from 17 per 100,000 to 40 per 100,000 over the same period [60].

Where there is no access to linear accelerator technology, palliative radiotherapy with cobalt-60 using parallel opposed fields to the breast/chest wall is recommended. A breast jig may help ensure the glancing fields are parallel (Figure 13.5). Where the peripheral lymphatics need to be treated, for example in locally advanced disease with axillary nodal involvement, an "en bloc" technique can be used encompassing the chest/breast, axilla, and supraclavicular nodes in a pair of large tangential fields with skin bolus. The ipsilateral arm is positioned behind the head and the body rotated slightly to the opposite side [60].

Follow up

The most appropriate follow-up schedule following PRT includes a first visit one month after the completion of therapy with the timing of subsequent visits individualized to help provide palliative care but also to limit the burdens associated with frequent appointments, especially for older and frailer patients.

Conclusion

Breast cancer remains the most common malignancy in women in developed countries as well as the second leading cause of death among females in those locales. Palliative radiotherapy plays an important role for women with this disease, both in developed countries and in developing countries where the incidence of neglected and therefore locally advanced breast cancer is much higher. Local symptoms from advanced or recurrent disease can be physically and emotionally debilitating, requiring coordinated palliative care from several different types of specialist. The continued improvement of systemic therapy for patients with this disease will undoubtedly necessitate further study of, and improvements in, the management of symptomatic local disease by radiotherapy.

References

1. Cancer Research UK. Breast Cancer – UK Mortality Statistics. Available at: http://info.cancerresearchuk.org/cancerstats/types/breast/mortality/ (accessed June 17, 2012).
2. Glück S. The prevention and management of distant metastases in women with breast cancer. *Cancer Invest* 2007; **25**: 6–13.
3. Lee MC, Jagsi R. Postmastectomy radiation therapy: indications and controversies. *Surg Clin North Am* 2007; **87**: 511–526.
4. Bedwinek JM, Lee J, Fineberg B, *et al.* Prognostic indicators in patients with isolated local-regional recurrence of breast cancer. *Cancer* 1981; **47**: 2232–2235.
5. McKinna F, Gothard L, Ashley S, *et al.* Lymphatic relapse in women with early breast cancer: a difficult management problem. *Eur J Cancer* 1999; **35**: 1065–1069.
6. Chang S, Parker SL, Pham T, *et al.* Inflammatory breast carcinoma incidence and survival: the surveillance, epidemiology, and end results program of the National Cancer Institute, 1975–1992. *Cancer* 1998; **82**: 2366–2372.
7. Newman LA. Epidemiology of locally advanced breast cancer. *Semin Radiat Oncol* 2009; **19**: 195–203.
8. van Oorschot B, Beckmann G, Schulze W, *et al.* Radiotherapeutic options for symptom control in breast cancer. *Breast Care* 2011; **6**: 14–19.
9. Liao Z, Strom EA, Buzdar AU, *et al.* Locoregional irradiation for inflammatory breast cancer: effectiveness of dose escalation in decreasing recurrence. *Int J Radiat Oncol Biol Phys* 2000; **47**: 1191–2000.
10. Rodger A, Leonard RC, Dixon JM. ABC of breast disease. Locally advanced breast cancer. *BMJ* 1994; **309**: 1431–1433.
11. Aberizk WJ, Silver B, Henderson IC, *et al.* The use of radiotherapy for treatment of isolated locoregional recurrence of breast carcinoma after mastectomy. *Cancer* 1986; **58**: 1214–1218.
12. van der Zee J, van der Holt B, Rietveld PJ, *et al.* Reirradiation combined with hyperthermia in recurrent breast cancer results in worthwhile local palliation. *Br J Cancer* 1999; **79**: 483–490.
13. Buccholz TA, Haffty BG. *Breast Cancer: Locally Advanced and Recurrent Disease, Postmastectomy Radiation and Systemic Therapies in: Perez and Brady's Principles and Practice of*

Radiation Oncology, 5th edn. Wolters Kluwer/Lippincott: Williams & Wilkins, 2008, p. 1311.

14. Holt TR, Yau VK. Innovative program for palliative radiotherapy in Australia. *J Med Imaging Radiat Oncol* 2010; **54**: 76–81.

15. Danielson B, Winget M, Gao Z, *et al.* Palliative radiotherapy for women with breast cancer. *Clin Oncol* 2008; **20**: 506–512.

16. Huang J, Zhou S, Groome P, *et al.* Factors affecting the use of palliative radiotherapy in Ontario. *J Clin Oncol* 2001; **19**: 137–144.

17. Johnston GM, Boyd CJ, Joseph P, *et al.* Variation in delivery of palliative radiotherapy in persons dying of cancer in Nova Scotia, 1994–1998. *J Clin Oncol* 2001; **19**: 3323–3332.

18. Jacob S, Wong K, Delaney GP, *et al.* Estimation of an optimal utilisation rate for palliative radiotherapy in newly diagnosed cancer patients. *Clin Oncol* 2010; **22**: 56–64.

19. Anderson BO, Cazap E, El Saghir NS. Optimisation of breast cancer management in low-resource and middle-resource countries: executive summary of the Breast Health Global Initiative consensus, 2010. *Lancet Oncol* 2011; **12**: 387–398.

20. Montague ED. Radiation management of advanced breast cancer. *Int J Radiat Oncol Biol Phys* 1978; **4**: 305–307.

21. Specht J, Gralow JR. Neoadjuvant chemotherapy for locally advanced breast cancer. *Semin Radiat Oncol* 2009; **19**: 222–228.

22. Rodger A, Jack WJ, Hardman PD, *et al.* Locally advanced breast cancer: report of phase II study and subsequent phase III trial. *Br J Cancer* 1992; **65**: 761–765.

23. Griscom NT, Wang CC. Radiation therapy of inoperable breast carcinoma. *Radiology* 1962; **79**: 18–32.

24. Langlands AO, Kerr GR, Shaw S. The management of locally advanced breast cancer by X-ray therapy. *Clin Oncol* 1976; **2**: 365–371.

25. Spanos WJ Jr, Montague ED, Fletcher GH. Late complications of radiation only for advanced breast cancer. *Int J Radiat Oncol Biol Phys* 1980; **6**: 1473–1476.

26. Sheldon T, Hayes DF, Cady B, *et al.* Primary radiation therapy for locally advanced breast cancer. *Cancer* 1987; **60**: 1219–1225.

27. Price A, Kerr GR, Rodger A. Primary radiotherapy for T4 breast cancer. *Clin Oncol* 1992; **4**: 217–221.

28. Parker RG. Palliative use of ionizing radiations. *Acta Oncol* 1996; **35**: 981–987.

29. Halverson KJ, Perez CA, Kuske RR, *et al.* Isolated local-regional recurrence of breast cancer following mastectomy: radiotherapeutic management. *Int J Radiat Oncol Biol Phys* 1990; **19**: 851–858.

30. Chen KK, Montague ED, Oswald MJ. Results of irradiation in the treatment of locoregional breast cancer recurrence. *Cancer* 1985; **56**: 1269–1273.

31. Borner M, Bacchi M, Goldhirsch A, *et al.* First isolated locoregional recurrence following mastectomy for breast cancer: results of a phase III multicenter study comparing systemic treatment with observation after excision and radiation. Swiss Group for Clinical Cancer Research. *J Clin Oncol* 1994; **12**: 2071–2077.

32. Blacklay PF, Campbell FC, Hinton CP. Patterns of flap recurrence following mastectomy. *Br J Surg* 1985; **72**: 719–720.

33. Barton MB, Hudson HM, Delaney G, *et al.* Patterns of retreatment by radiotherapy. *Clin Oncol* 2011; **23**: 10–18.

34. Würschmidt F, Dahle J, Petersen C, *et al.* Reirradiation of recurrent breast cancer with and without concurrent chemotherapy. *Radiat Oncol* 2008; **3**: 1–9.

35. Harkenrider MM, Wilson MR, Dragun AE. Reirradiation as a component of the multi-disciplinary management of locally recurrent breast cancer. *Clin Breast Cancer* 2011; **11**: 171–176.

36. Harms W, Krempien R, Hensley FW, *et al*. Results of chest wall reirradiation using pulsed-dose-rate (PDR) brachytherapy molds for breast cancer local recurrences. *Int J Radiat Oncol Biol Phys* 2001; **49**: 205–210.

37. Delanian S, Housset M, Brunel P, *et al*. Iridium 192 plesiocurietherapy using silicone elastomer plates for extensive locally recurrent breast cancer following chest wall irradiation. *Int J Radiat Oncol Biol Phys* 1992; **22**: 1099–1104.

38. Field SB. In vivo aspects of hyperthermic oncology. In: Field SB, Hand JW (eds) *An Introduction to the Practical Aspects of Clinical Hyperthermia*. London: Taylor and Francis, 1990, pp. 55–58.

39. Vernon CC, Hand JW, Field SB, *et al*. Radiotherapy with or without hyperthermia in the treatment of superficial localized breast cancer: results from five randomized controlled trials. International Collaborative Hyperthermia Group. *Int J Radiat Oncol Biol Phys* 1996; **35**: 731–744.

40. Kouloulias VE, Dardoufas CE, Kouvaris JR, *et al*. Liposomal doxorubicin in conjunction with reirradiation and local hyperthermia treatment in recurrent breast cancer: a phase I/II trial. *Clin Cancer Res* 2002; **8**: 374–382.

41. Feyerabend T, Wiedemann GJ, Jäger B, *et al*. Local hyperthermia, radiation, and chemotherapy in recurrent breast cancer is feasible and effective except for inflammatory disease. *Int J Radiat Oncol Biol Phys* 2001; **49**: 1317–1325.

42. Bornstein BA, Zouranjian PS, Hansen JL, *et al*. Local hyperthermia, radiation therapy, and chemotherapy in patients with local-regional recurrence of breast carcinoma. *Int J Radiat Oncol Biol Phys* 1993; **25**: 79–85.

43. Kapp DS. Efficacy of adjuvant hyperthermia in the treatment of superficial recurrent breast cancer: confirmation and future directions. *Int J Radiat Oncol Biol Phys* 1996; **35**: 1117–1121.

44. Newman LA, Hunt KK, Buchholz T, *et al*. Presentation, management and outcome of axillary recurrence from breast cancer. *Am J Surg* 2000; **180**: 252–256.

45. Fisher B, Montague E, Redmond C, *et al*. Comparison of radical mastectomy with alternative treatments for primary breast cancer. A first report of results from a prospective randomized clinical trial. *Cancer* 1977; **39**: 2827–2839.

46. Ampil FL, Caldito G, Li BD, *et al*. Supraclavicular nodal relapse of breast cancer: prevalence, palliation and prognosis. *Eur J Gynaecol Oncol* 2003; **24**: 233–235.

47. Khan SA, Stewart AK, Morrow M. Does aggressive local therapy improve survival in metastatic breast cancer? *Surgery* 2002; **132**: 620–626.

48. Le Scodan R, Stevens D, Brain E, *et al*. Breast cancer with synchronous metastases: survival impact of exclusive locoregional radiotherapy. *J Clin Oncol* 2009; **27**: 1375–1381.

49. Nguyen DH, Truong PT. A debate on locoregional treatment of the primary tumor in patients presenting with stage IV breast cancer. *Expert Rev Anticancer Ther* 2011; **11**: 1913–1922.

50. Badwe R, Hawaldar RW, Khare A, *et al*. Role of local-regional treatment in metastatic breast at presentation: a randomised trial. Presented at 2008 Breast Cancer Symposium, Washington DC, USA 5–7 September, 2008.

51. Soran A, Ozbas S, Kelsey SF, *et al*. Randomized trial comparing locoregional resection of primary tumor with no surgery in Stage IV Breast cancer at the Presentation (Protocol

MF07-01): a Study of Turkish federation of the National Societies for Breast Diseases. *Breast J* 2009; **15**: 399–403.

52. Buchholz TA, Strom EA, Oswald MJ, *et al*. Fifteen-year results of a randomized prospective trial of hyperfractionated chest wall irradiation versus once daily chest wall irradiation after chemotherapy and mastectomy for patients with locally advanced non inflammatory breast cancer. *Int J Radiat Oncol Biol Phys* 2006; **65**: 1155–1160.

53. Lutz ST, Chow EL, Hartsell WF, *et al*. A review of hypofractionated palliative radiotherapy. *Cancer* 2007; **109**: 1462–1470.

54. Maher M, Campana F, Mosseri V, *et al*. Breast cancer in elderly women: a retrospective analysis of combined treatment with tamoxifen and once-weekly irradiation. *Int J Radiat Oncol Biol Phys* 1995; **31**: 783–789.

55. Ortholan C, Hannoun-Levi JM, Ferrero JM, *et al*. Long-term results of adjuvant hypofractionated radiotherapy for breast cancer in elderly patients. *Int J Radiat Oncol Biol Phys* 2005; **61**: 154–162.

56. Kirova YM, Campana F, Savignoni A, *et al*. Breast-conserving treatment in the elderly: long-term results of adjuvant hypofractionated and normofractionated radiotherapy. *Int J Radiat Oncol Biol Phys* 2009; **75**: 76–81.

57. Moran MS, Haffty BG. Radiation techniques and toxicities for locally advanced breast cancer. *Semin Radiat Oncol* 2009; **19**: 244–255.

58. Laramore GE, Griffin TW, Parker RG, *et al*. The use of electron beams in treating local recurrence of breast cancer in previously irradiated fields. *Cancer* 1978; **41**: 991–995.

59. Chatterjee S, Lee D, Kent N, *et al*. Managing supraclavicular disease from breast cancer with brachial plexus-sparing techniques using helical tomotherapy. *Clin Oncol* 2011; **23**: 101–107.

60. Kunkler IH. Cancer of the Brest. In: Bomford CK, Kunkler IH and Sheriff S. (eds) *Walter and Miller's Textbook of Radiotherapy Fifth Edition*. Churchill Livingston (1993), p. 389.

61. Hazard H, Gorla S, Scholtens D, *et al*. Surgical resection of the primary tumor, chest wall control, and survival in women with metastatic breast cancer. *Cancer* 2008; **113**: 2011–2019.

62. Leung A, Vu H, Nguyen K, *et al*. Effects of surgical excision on survival of patients with stage IV breast cancer. *J Surg Res* 2010; **161**: 83–88.

63. Tobias J. Radiotherapy and breast conservation. *Br J Radiol* 1986; **59**: 653–666.

64. Bafford A, Burstein H, Barkley C, *et al*. Breast surgery in stage IV breast cancer: impact of staging and patient selection on overall survival. *Breast Cancer Res Treat* 2009; **115**: 7–12.

65. Ruiterkamp J, Ernst M, van de Poll-Franse L, *et al*. Surgical resection of the primary tumour is associated with improved survival in patients with distant metastatic breast cancer at diagnosis. *Eur J Surg Oncol* 2009; **35**: 1146–1151.

CHAPTER 14

Palliative radiotherapy in advanced lung cancer

George Rodrigues[1], Benjamin Movsas[2]
[1]Department of Radiation Oncology, London Health Sciences Centre and University of Western Ontario, London, ON, Canada
[2]Department of Radiation Oncology, Henry Ford Health System, Detroit, MI, USA

Introduction

Lung cancer is an entity related with high incidence of disease burden requiring palliative interventions (Box 14.1). This can commonly be due to metastatic disease (e.g. brain and bone metastases), seen in approximately 40% of incident cases. However, the local disease burden within the lung and mediastinum can often require palliative management in order to optimize patient health-related quality-of-life and to minimize clinically significant symptom burden. In the context of stage IV lung cancer, palliative treatment is often directed towards symptom control as well as the prevention/delay of anticipated symptoms. Survival prolongation with treatment interventions such as palliative radiotherapy (RT) and chemotherapy is modest with a 5-year survival of 5–10% for patients diagnosed with *de novo* stage IV lung cancer.

The utilization of palliative radiotherapy directed to thoracic lung tumors has been a mainstay of radiation oncology practice for decades. The primary goal of this type of therapy has been the palliation of symptoms related to tumor effects on various anatomic structures located in or around the thorax. Frequently observed symptoms can usually be referenced back to anatomically related sites affected by primary and regionally metastatic lung cancer tumors. These sites include the respiratory system (e.g. lung, bronchus, and trachea), vascular system (e.g. superior vena cava, pulmonary vessels), as well as other organs/tissues including the rib and esophagus. Specific symptoms and scenarios that may require palliation include cough, shortness of breath, hemoptysis, bronchial/tracheal obstruction, esophageal obstruction, superior vena cava obstruction, and brachial plexopathy.

Radiation Oncology in Palliative Cancer Care, First Edition. Edited by Stephen Lutz, Edward Chow, and Peter Hoskin.
© 2013 John Wiley & Sons, Ltd. Published 2013 by John Wiley & Sons, Ltd.

Box 14.1 Symptoms commonly associated with advanced lung cancer

- Shortness of breath
- Cough
- Hemoptysis
- Chest pain
- Superior vena cava syndrome
- Dysphagia
- Brachial plexopathy
- Post-obstructive pneumonia

Prospective clinical trials assessing a variety of patient-related endpoints have investigated various palliative interventions in this patient population. These interventions include surgical (e.g. stenting and pleurodesis), radiotherapeutic (external beam and brachytherapy), and chemotherapeutic options given either as stand-alone interventions or commonly as integrated sequential interventions to optimize palliative management. In the context of the utility of radiotherapy in the palliation of lung cancer, the majority of randomized controlled trials and meta-analyses or systematic reviews have focused on the questions of external beam radiation therapy (EBRT) dose fractionation and the use of endobronchial brachytherapy in the initial or salvage palliative management (either alone or in conjunction with other treatment modalities) of lung cancer. In addition, the use of concurrent chemotherapy with palliative radiotherapy has been the subject of various investigations. Practice guidelines and consensus statements have been previously prepared to provide guidance to practitioners and patients with regard to treatment options [1–8].

The primary aim of clinical trials assessing palliative thoracic radiotherapy is the improvement in clinical symptomatology related to local and/or regional tumor burden. Clinical trials have used an assortment of patient-reported outcomes to assess symptoms and health-related quality-of-life. Among health-related quality-of-life instruments, the European Organisation for Research and Treatment of Cancer (EORTC QLQ-C30/LC-13) and the Functional Assessment of Cancer Therapy (FACT-L) are the two most commonly used questionnaires with strong development and validation methodologies. Various symptom scores were reported as separate individual scores and usually not as a combined aggregate score. The issue of a common endpoint symptom definition has not been resolved in the medical literature. The reason for difficulty in a common definition is the heterogeneity of symptom complexes observed in this patient population. Symptoms such as cough, dyspnea, and chest pain are common, while hemoptysis, dysphagia, and hoarseness are less regularly observed. Fatigue and anorexia or weight loss are also very common; however, whether they can respond to thoracic RT is highly debatable. Establishing a broad consensus, to define a clinically relevant endpoint to cover this complexity may prove to be difficult.

Limited information exists on the utility and efficacy of advanced radiotherapy technologies such as image guided radiation therapy (IGRT) and intensity modulated radiation therapy (IMRT) in the optimization of the therapeutic ratio between tumor effects (survival and symptom control) and treatment toxicities such as esophagitis, tumor pain flare, fatigue, and other radiotherapy side effects. However, investigations into treatment selection from the resource setting [9], patient [10], and economic [11] viewpoints do exist in the medical literature. These investigations will be discussed in this chapter and are instructive to the clinician in informing evidence-based decision-making.

Radiotherapy treatment

Overview
The majority of palliative thoracic radiotherapy is delivered using an external beam radiation therapy approach due to its widespread availability compared to high-dose rate brachytherapy. Various dose-fractionation schedules are available for the efficient palliation of thoracic symptomology (see below). Common fractionation schedules utilized include: 16–17 Gy in 2 fractions, 20 Gy in 5 fractions, 30 Gy in 10 fractions, and 39–45 Gy in 12–15 fractions. Palliative thoracic radiotherapy has been shown in multiple prospective clinical trials to improve clinical symptom burden in approximately 60% of patients. Acute side effects of thoracic radiotherapy commonly include: fatigue, skin reaction, esophagitis, shortness of breath, and chest pain. Due to the nature of advanced lung cancer, late effects of radiotherapy are not usually encountered; however, esophageal stricture, pneumonitis, and lung fibrosis have been known to occur.

Despite the general effectiveness of palliative thoracic radiotherapy in the management of local disease burden and symptoms, several important limitations to this treatment modality do exist. Although the simulation and planning of palliative radiotherapy is more straightforward than comparative radical situations, there can be a delay between the decision to treat and treatment start. Additionally, a significant delay between treatment initiation and symptom alleviation of several weeks can occur. Another important limitation of palliative thoracic radiotherapy is in relation to the management of pleural disease, large volume disease, or multi-focal metastatic disease. In situations where directed local therapy may not be effective, other treatment modalities, such as palliative systemic chemotherapy and surgical modalities (pleurodesis and stenting) may be preferred options.

External beam dose fractionation
Fourteen randomized controlled trials have been concluded and published addressing the question of optimal thoracic external beam radiation therapy dose-fractionation [12–24]. A variety of fractionations have been tested ranging

Table 14.1 Common dose fractionation schemes used for palliative thoracic radiotherapy.

Dose fractionation classification	Examples
Short Fractionation	10 Gy in 1 fraction
	16–17 Gy in 2 fractions (weekly)
	20 Gy in 5 fractions
Standard Dose Fractionation	30 Gy in 10 fractions
High-Dose Fractionation	39–45 Gy in 12–15 fractions
	50–60 Gy in 25–30 fractions

from a single fraction of 10 Gy to high-dose schema like 50–60 Gy in 25–30 fractions given 2 Gy/day. Fractionation schedules commonly employed in these trials and in clinical practice include 16–17 Gy in 2 fractions, 20 Gy in 5 fractions (4 Gy/day), or 30–45 Gy in 10–15 fractions (3 Gy/day) (Table 14.1). These dose-fractionation clinical trials have recently been the subject of various knowledge translation documents including an updated Cochrane review [6], a meta-analysis [25], an American Society for Radiation Oncology (ASTRO) practice guideline [1], and an international consensus statement [2].

Considerable clinical trial heterogeneity in various factors such as performance status, patient age, dose-fractionations utilized, and clinical trial endpoints can be observed in these clinical trials. Despite these limitations in the literature, several important conclusions can be deduced from this collective clinical trial experience. Shorter fractionation schedules (e.g. 10 Gy in 1 fraction, 17 Gy in 2 fractions, and 20 Gy in 5 fractions) are highly effective and efficient at providing symptomatic relief with low treatment-related toxicity. Due to the small fraction number, this approach is highly advantageous for patients with poor performance status, limited transportation, or for patients who require palliative radiotherapy integrated between ongoing chemotherapy cycles. Higher dose fractionation schedules (e.g. 30 Gy in 10 fractions or higher) are associated with a modest 5% improvement in one-year survival (primarily in good performance status patients) but at the cost of more treatment-related toxicity, such as radiation esophagitis. The downside of protracted schedules of treatment can include the fact that patients will spend more time in treatment, which may be difficult for frail patients or patients that need to travel for therapy. Additionally, there may be more associated direct costs to the patient and insurance or government payers. Despite the available evidence in the literature, the ideal high-dose fractionation schedule to optimize the therapeutic ratio between patient outcome, symptom control, and treatment toxicity is still currently unclear. Essentially, dose fractionation selection should be based on the complete evaluation of the patient based on patient, tumor, treatment, and social factors combined with the medical evidence (Figure 14.1).

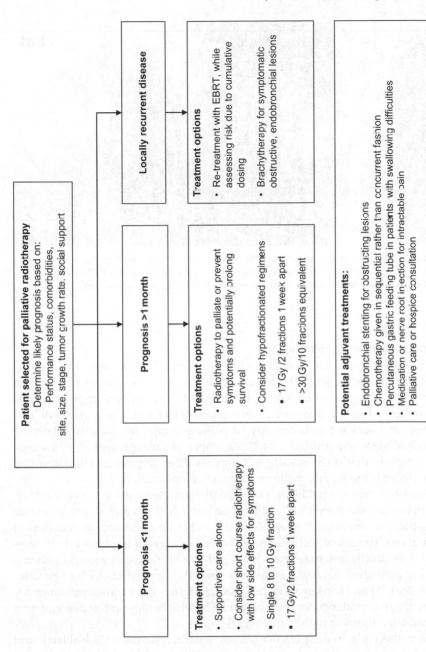

Patient selected for palliative radiotherapy
Determine likely prognosis based on:
Performance status, comorbidities,
site, size, stage, tumor growth rate, social support

Prognosis <1 month

Treatment options
- Supportive care alone
- Consider short course radiotherapy with low side effects for symptoms
  - Single 8 to 10 Gy fraction
  - 17 Gy/2 fractions 1 week apart

Prognosis >1 month

Treatment options
- Radiotherapy to palliate or prevent symptoms and potentially prolong survival
- Consider hypofractionated regimens
  - 17 Gy /2 fractions 1 week apart
  - >30 Gy/10 fractions equivalent

Locally recurrent disease

Treatment options
- Re-treatment with EBRT, while assessing risk due to cumulative dosing
- Brachytherapy for symptomatic obstructive, endobronchial lesions

Potential adjuvant treatments:
- Endobronchial stenting for obstructing lesions
- Chemotherapy given in sequential rather than concurrent fashion
- Percutaneous gastric feeding tube in patients with swallowing difficulties
- Medication or nerve root injection for intractable pain
- Palliative care or hospice consultation

Figure 14.1 Algorithm for use of palliative radiotherapy for patients with lung cancer.

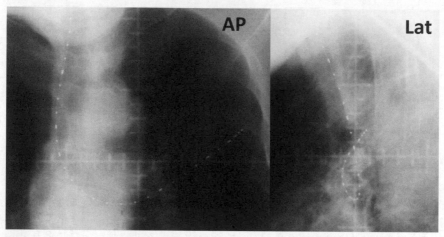

Figure 14.2 Anterior-posterior and lateral fluoroscopic projection of endobronchial brachytherapy catheter (with radiopaque guidewire). Adapted from photos by Tdrovak, available under a creative commons attribution-share alike 3.0 unported licence.

Endobronchial brachytherapy

Six randomized clinical trials have been performed on the use of endobronchial brachytherapy [26–32]. This treatment involves the placement of a catheter within the bronchial lumen to ultimately introduce a high-dose rate radioactive source near to the endobronchial obstruction. The goal is to deliver intense and focused radiotherapy to palliate symptoms directly related to bronchial obstruction (Figure 14.2). An important pre-requisite for this type of therapy is that there is sufficient lumen caliber to pass an endobronchial tube through the length of the endobronchial obstruction.

Similar to the external beam radiation therapy literature, a variety of dose-fractionations have been utilized with no published research strongly recommending one fractionation regime over another. In addition, various clinical indications, treatment techniques, and other integrated treatment modalities contribute to the heterogeneous nature of this literature. A recent Cochrane review published in 2008, as well as recently completed ASTRO practice guidelines [1] and consensus statements [2], all provide a consistent summary regarding the evidence for endobronchial brachytherapy in the management of palliative thoracic malignancies [33].

From this collective experience of completed randomized clinical trials and associated summary documents, several findings apply to the indications and utilization of endobronchial brachytherapy. In the context of an initial presentation of thoracic cancer requiring palliative radiation, there is no randomized evidence to recommend endobronchial brachytherapy either alone or in combination with other palliative treatments. However, given a scenario where evidence of a central endobronchial obstruction exists prior to definitive radiotherapy, initial endobronchial radiation followed by external beam radiation is a reasonable option given the observation of improved re-expansion rates in one prospective randomized controlled trial [29]. In the context of a patient with a documented recurrent endobronchial obstruction after palliative external beam radiation therapy, the use of endobronchial brachytherapy is a reasonable option given the lack of evidence existing to the contrary.

Concurrent chemotherapy integrated with palliative thoracic radiotherapy

The use of traditional forms of intravenous chemotherapy and the integration of newer forms of oral targeted therapy (e.g. EGFR tyrosine kinase inhibitors) are a mainstay of the treatment of patients with metastatic or recurrent lung cancer. Successive rounds of randomized controlled trials assessing important clinically relevant endpoints such as overall survival, progression-free survival, health-related quality of life, and symptom control have established these therapies as useful. In the context of palliative radiotherapy, some literature does exist regarding the a priori integration of drug treatment during the conduct of palliative radiation (i.e. concurrent chemoradiation versus sequential therapy with radiation given before, in between, or after completion of various chemotherapy cycles).

Very limited information has been published regarding the planned integration of drug therapy with palliative radiation therapy fractions [1]. This information generally is in the form of phase I and phase II clinical trials, which have assessed various drugs such as carboplatin/premetrexed, carboplatin/etoposide, cisplatin/vinorelbine, gemcitibine, and docetaxel. A single phase III clinical trial assessed continuous infusion 5-FU versus no chemotherapy in conjunction with palliative radiation therapy with 20 Gy in 5 fractions [34]. This 200 patient trial failed to find any differences in patient outcome including survival and palliation of symptoms. However, a significant increase in treatment toxicity was observed; therefore, this combination treatment was not recommended for routine clinical use. Therefore, the current available clinical trial evidence does not support the routine use of concurrent integrated chemotherapy with palliative thoracic radiotherapy. However, the use of palliative radiotherapy given in between chemotherapy cycles for specific palliative symptoms is advisable. Given the recent activity in newer targeted agents, several phase I–III clinical trials are currently underway assessing the possible synergistic effects of drug treatment and palliative radiotherapy in optimizing patient outcomes both in terms of patient survival as well as symptom and health-related quality-of-life endpoints.

The impact of emerging technologies

The past decade has seen a proliferation of technological advancements that have improved our ability to provide highly conformal treatment (e.g. IMRT)

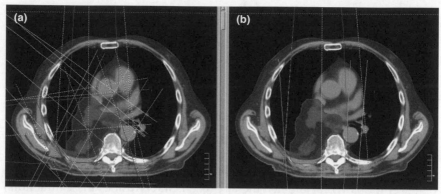

Figure 14.3 Beam arrangement for (a) 4-field 3D conformal palliative radiation treatment to 45 Gy in 15 fractions vs (b) 2-field parallel opposed pair palliative radiation treatment to 30 Gy in 10 fractions (see Plate 14.1). Figure courtesy of Drs. Stewart Gaede and Brian Yaremko (Division of Radiation Oncology, London Health Sciences Centre, UK).

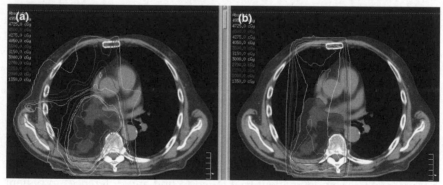

Figure 14.4 Axial dosimetry for (a) 4-field 3D conformal palliative radiation treatment to 45 Gy in 15 fractions vs (b) 2-field parallel opposed pair palliative radiation treatment to 30 Gy in 10 fractions (see Plate 14.2). Figure courtesy of Drs. Stewart Gaede and Brian Yaremko (Division of Radiation Oncology, London Health Sciences Centre, UK).

in a highly accurate manner (e.g. IGRT). Using these technologies, dose-escalated radiation therapy can be achieved in order to improve the tumor effect whilst maintaining or improving the related toxicity of treatment (Figures 14.3 and 14.4). Combined with advancements in patient immobilization, stereotactic radiation therapy has also been recently utilized in extracranial scenarios to treat localized lung cancers as well as oligometastatic lung metastases.

From an efficiency perspective, the use of advanced treatments such as IMRT and IGRT are useful tools to provide highly conformal, highly accurate, or precise therapy with potentially short treatment times (depending on the clinical scenario). As an example of the possible utility of these techniques,

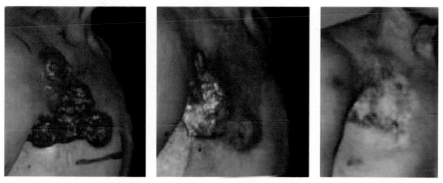

Plate 13.1 (Figure 13.2) Clinical case: pain, lymphedema, bleeding, and ulceration before, 2 months, and 3 years after radiotherapy. Reproduced from van Oorschot *et al.* [8], with permission from Karger.

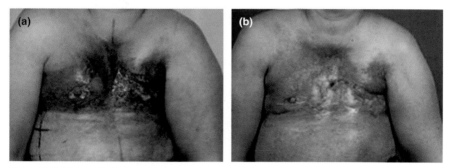

Plate 13.2 (Figure 13.3) Complete response to combination of radiotherapy and hyperthermia to treat bilateral chest wall recurrent before cancer (a) before treatment, (b) after treatment. Courtesy of Dr. G. van Tienhoven, Academic Medical Centre, Amsterdam.

Radiation Oncology in Palliative Cancer Care, First Edition. Edited by Stephen Lutz, Edward Chow, and Peter Hoskin.
© 2013 John Wiley & Sons, Ltd. Published 2013 by John Wiley & Sons, Ltd.

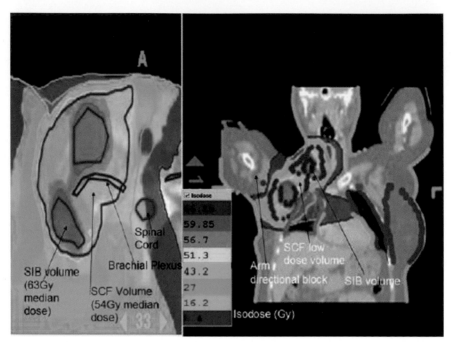

Plate 13.3 (Figure 13.4) Simultaneous integrated boost technique using helical tomotherapy to spare the brachial plexus outside the "boost" volume. Reproduced from Chatterjee *et al.* [59], with permission from Elsevier.

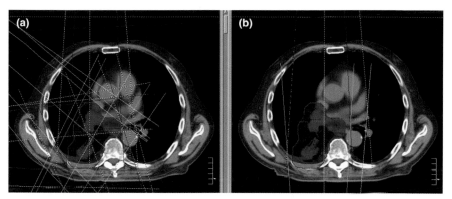

Plate 14.1 (Figure 14.3) Beam arrangement for (a) 4-field 3D conformal palliative radiation treatment to 45 Gy in 15 fractions vs (b) 2-field parallel opposed pair palliative radiation treatment to 30 Gy in 10 fractions. Figure courtesy of Drs. Stewart Gaede and Brian Yaremko (Division of Radiation Oncology, London Health Sciences Centre, UK).

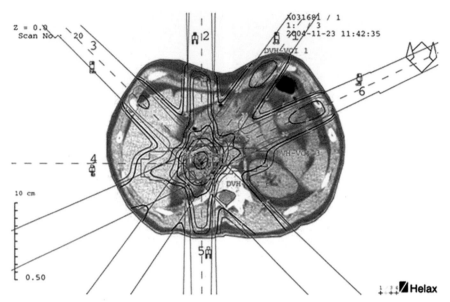

Plate 24.1 (Figure 24.3) Stereotactic body radiotherapy used to treat a small asymptomatic right adrenal metastasis using a 6 static field photon beam technique. Reproduced from Holy *et al.* [14], with permission from Urban und Vogel.

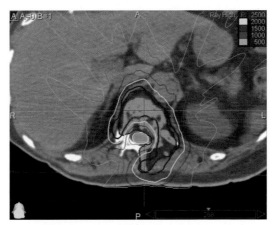

Plate 28.1 (Figure 28.1) Stereotactic body radiotherapy for re-irradiation of breast cancer spinal metastasis at T12 which had prior external beam radiotherapy to 37.5 Gy in 15 fractions; a dose of 25 Gy in 5 fractions was prescribed to 78%, while limiting the spinal cord maximum point dose to 10 Gy in 5 fractions; the beams were manipulated by the computer such that the radiation dose was steered away from the spinal cord; the patient obtained prompt pain relief after the treatment (pain decreased from 6 to 1 on an 11-point scale).

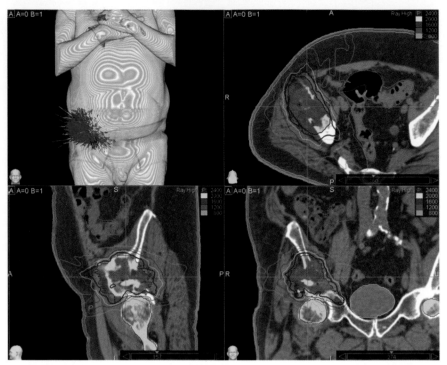

Plate 28.2 (Figure 28.2) CyberKnife-based stereotactic body radiotherapy for the treatment of a single large painful right iliac bone metastasis from renal cell carcinoma; a dose of 24 Gy in 3 fractions was prescribed to 70%; OARs included the right femoral head and the small bowels.

investigations into arc-based radiation therapy (e.g. tomotherapy or volumetric arc-based radiotherapy) to optimize treatment in the palliative setting are available in the literature. These publications do provide some guidance for general palliative patient populations that may benefit from the use of advanced radiation technologies such as IMRT and IGRT [35–38].

These populations/clinical scenarios that will likely benefit most from advanced technology include:

• tumors near (and/or wrapping around) critical structures in the setting of dose-escalation where traditional techniques will overdose critical structures

• large tumors where meeting dose-volume constraints are difficult or impossible with standard 2D/3D conformal approaches.

• scenarios in which a microscopic area is to be treated with an integrated macroscopic boost. Traditional shrinking field techniques can be used; however, simultaneous in-field boost radiotherapy delivered with arc-based techniques (IMRT as well) can provide highly efficient therapy by utilizing intralesional hypofractionation. This approach has been successfully employed in the treatment of oligometastatic brain metastases.

• complex re-irradiation scenarios may also benefit from advanced IMRT and IGRT techniques to maximize delivered dose to the target and concurrently minimize critical structure dose.

• treatment of oligometastasis of the lung with stereotactic body radiation therapy (SBRT) [39].

Important circumstances

Patient selection

Despite the common use of treatment maneuvers (including radiotherapy) for the palliation of thoracic symptoms with locally advanced cancer, little original research exists to assist the clinician in identifying patients that would be best managed by a radical versus palliative approach. Various consensus documents and practice guidelines have previously attempted to provide guidance on this topic [4,5,40,41]. These summary documents have identified various patient features such as performance status, treatment tolerability, radiotherapy volume, pulmonary function, presence of metastatic disease, presence of malignant pleural effusion, patient age, disease stage, and weight loss as important considerations when making radiotherapeutic dose-fractionation decisions. However, no widely accepted schema for patient selection criteria is available.

In the context of an asymptomatic patient, the Medical Research Council Lung Cancer Working Party reported on a phase III clinical trial in 2002 randomizing between immediate versus delayed thoracic radiotherapy for locally advanced lung cancer with minimal baseline symptoms [42]. Radiotherapy utilized in this trial included 10 Gy/1 fraction or 17 Gy in 2 fractions over 1 week. Patients were generally ECOG performance status 0–1 with only 12% of patients having metastatic disease at baseline. No differences in survival or health-related quality of life were observed between the immediate arm (90% radiotherapy utilization) and delayed arm (42% radiotherapy utilization). This study therefore suggests that patients who do not wish to have a radical course of upfront therapy may consider an observation strategy with delayed intervention upon progressive symptoms or patient preference.

Patient preferences

Additionally, patients themselves routinely have strong opinions regarding the conduct of their treatment course. Tang *et al.* evaluated a decision-making aid to assist patients with the decision of radiotherapy treatment fraction length in the treatment of metastatic lung cancer [10]. This aid listed the various advantages and disadvantages of two palliative fractionation schedules (17 Gy/2 fractions vs 39 Gy/13 fractions) in terms of various patient specific and economic endpoints. Interestingly, the majority (55%) of patients selected the longer fractionation schedule mainly because of information suggesting better local control and survival. Shorter fractionation schedules were selected by 45% of patients primarily because of shorter treatment time, greater convenience, lower cost, and better symptom control. This investigation suggests that patient decision-making regarding palliative radiotherapy can be based on multiple complex factors.

Economic considerations

Randomized controlled trials and other summary forms of evidence can provide insight into the efficacy and effectiveness of medical interventions (such as palliative radiotherapy) on defined patient populations. However, the health economic impacts of various treatments can also be assessed by demonstration of the resource cost (usually described in currency) to provide a desired clinical effect (e.g. years of life saved). Very limited information currently exists in the medical literature regarding the health economic impacts regarding palliative radiotherapy.

One important economic analysis has been published on the topic of palliative thoracic dose-fractionation. A cost-utility analysis based on a Dutch randomized clinical trial randomizing patients between 16 Gy/2 fractions vs 30 Gy/10 fractions was published in 2006 [11]. Using both survival and utility (health-related quality-of-life) information from the trial, the authors demonstrated that the incremental cost-utility ratio for longer fractionated therapy was $40,900/QALY (quality-adjusted life year) and that this therapy could be justified on economic grounds. The authors recommended that while the use of 1–2 fraction regimens was appropriate in many situations, patients with a good performance status should be considered for higher dose regimens based on the observed survival differences. There can be significant limitations of extrapolating economic information from one jurisdiction to another;

at the same time, it is important to note that these conclusions are consistent with the recently published ASTRO practice guideline [1] and international consensus statements [2].

Special considerations in developing countries

Resource constrained practice

Macbeth *et al.* have recently published International Atomic Energy Agency (IAEA) guidelines for lung cancer management in limited resource settings [9]. A variety of fractionation schedules for palliative thoracic radiotherapy were recommended based on clinical characteristics such as performance status, stage, and symptoms. Recommended dose regimens included: 10 Gy/1fraction, 16–17 Gy/2 fractions, 20 Gy/5 fractions, 30 Gy/10 fractions, and 39 Gy/13 fractions. In particular, patients with poor performance status can be treated with either 10 Gy/1 fraction or 16–17 Gy in 2 fractions as these fractionation schedules have been tested against other fractionation schedules (such as 30 Gy/10 fractions) demonstrating equivalent symptom control. Higher dose (≥30 Gy) treatment can be used for patients with good performance status, as these patients are more likely to tolerate and benefit from the additional dose.

Conclusion

The medical literature suggests that patients with good performance status may benefit from higher-dose/fractionation external beam radiation therapy palliation (30 Gy/10-fraction equivalent or greater) because of the observed modest observed survival benefit. No defined role for endobronchial brachytherapy for the routine initial palliative treatment of chest disease has been demonstrated; however, endobronchial brachytherapy remains an option for the palliation of endobronchial lesions causing obstructive symptomatology in the EBRT failure scenario or in locally advanced non-metastatic cancer patients with endobronchial disease who require lung re-expansion before or in conjunction with radical RT. The integration of concurrent chemotherapy with palliative intent/fractionated RT is not currently supported by the medical literature. However, integration of palliative chemotherapy and RT in a non-concurrent fashion is important for the optimal palliation of lung cancer patients with thoracic symptoms.

Recent (and ongoing) improvements in pre-treatment lung cancer imaging, targeted systemic agents, and radiation planning/delivery technologies (e.g. IMRT, IGRT, and SBRT) will require continued prospective evaluation to optimize patient clinical and health-related quality of life outcome in this patient population. Important knowledge translation documents and other decision-making investigations exist in the medical literature to guide the clinician to optimize clinical care for this challenging patient population.

References

1. Rodrigues G, Videtic GMM, Sur R, *et al*. Palliative thoracic radiotherapy in lung cancer: an American Society for Radiation Oncology evidence-based clinical practice guideline. *Pract Radiat Oncol* 2011; **1**: 60–71.
2. Rodrigues G, Macbeth F, Burmeister B, *et al*. Consensus statement on palliative lung radiotherapy: Third International Consensus Workshop on Palliative Radiotherapy and Symptom Control. *Clin Lung Cancer* 2011; doi: 10.1016/j.cllc.2011.04.004
3. Scottish Intercollegiate Guidelines Network: Management of patients with lung cancer: a national clinical guideline. Available at: http://www.sign.ac.uk/pdf/sign80.pdf (accessed July 13, 2010).
4. No authors listed. Clinical practice guidelines for the treatment of unresectable non-small-cell lung cancer. Adopted on May 16, 1997 by the American Society of Clinical Oncology. *J Clin Oncol* 1997; **15**:2996–3018.
5. Graham MV, Byhardt RW, Sause WT, *et al*. Non-aggressive, non-surgical treatment of inoperable non-small cell lung cancer (NSCLC). American College of Radiology. ACR Appropriateness Criteria. *Radiology* 2000; **215**(Suppl): 1347–1362.
6. Lester JF, Macbeth FR, Toy E, *et al*. Palliative radiotherapy regimens for non-small cell lung cancer. *Cochrane Database Syst Rev* 2006; (4): CD002143.
7. National Comprehensive Cancer Network: Treatment guidelines – NCCN Clinical Practice Guidelines in Oncology Non-Small Cell Lung Cancer V.2, 2010. Available at: http://www.nccn.org/professionals/physician_gls/PDF/nscl.pdf (accessed July 13, 2010).
8. Okawara G, Mackay JA, Evans WK, *et al*. Lung Cancer Disease Site Group of Cancer Care Ontario's Program in Evidence-based Care. Management of unresected stage III non-small cell lung cancer: a systematic review. *J Thorac Oncol* 2006; **1**: 377–393.
9. Macbeth FR, Abratt RP, Cho KH, *et al*. International Atomic Energy Agency. Lung cancer management in limited resource settings: guidelines for appropriate good care. *Radiother Oncol* 2007; **82**: 123–131.
10. Tang JI, Shakespeare TP, Lu JJ, *et al*. Patients' preference for radiotherapy fractionation schedule in the palliation of symptomatic unresectable lung cancer. *J Med Imaging Radiat Oncol* 2008; **52**: 497–502.
11. van den Hout WB, Kramer GW, Noordijk EM, Leer JW. Cost-utility analysis of short-versus long-course palliative radiotherapy in patients with non-small cell lung cancer. *J Natl Cancer Inst* 2006; **98**: 1786–1794.
12. Simpson JR, Francis ME, Perez-Tamayo R, *et al*. Palliative radiotherapy for inoperable carcinoma of the lung: final report of an RTOG multi-institutional trial. *Int J Radiat Oncol Biol Phys* 1985; **11**: 751–758.
13. Teo P, Tai TH, Choy D, *et al*. A randomized study on palliative radiation therapy for inoperable non small cell carcinoma of the lung. *Int J Radiat Oncol Biol Phys* 1988; **14**: 867–871.
14. Medical Research Council Lung Cancer Working Party. Inoperable non-small-cell lung cancer (NSCLC): a Medical Research Council randomised trial of palliative radiotherapy with two fractions or ten fractions. *Br J Cancer* 1991; **63**: 265–270.
15. Medical Research Council Lung Cancer Working Party. A Medical Research Council (MRC) randomised trial of palliative radiotherapy with two fractions or a single fraction in patients with inoperable non-small cell lung cancer (NSCLC) and poor performance status. *Br J Cancer* 1992; **65**: 934–941.

16. Medical Research Council Lung Cancer Working Party. Randomized trial of palliative two-fraction versus more intensive thirteen fraction radiotherapy for patients with inoperable nonsmall cell lung cancer and good performance status. *Clin Oncol* 1996; **8**: 167–175.

17. Rees GJ, Devrell CE, Barley VL, *et al.* Palliative radiotherapy for lung cancer; two versus five fractions. *Clin Oncol* 1997; **9**: 90–95.

18. Reinfuss M, Glinski B, Kowalska T, *et al.* Radiotherapy in stage III, unresectable, asymptomatic non-small cell lung cancer. Final results of a prospective randomized study of 240 patients. *Cancer Radiother* 1999; **3**: 475–479.

19. Nestle U, Nieder N, Walter K, *et al.* A palliative accelerated irradiation regimen for advanced non-small cell lung cancer vs conventionally fractionated 60 Gy: results of a randomized equivalence study. *Int J Radiat Oncol Biol Phys* 2000; **48**: 95–103.

20. Bezjak A, Dixon P, Brundage M, *et al.* Randomized phase III trial of single versus fractionated thoracic radation in the palliation of patients with lung cancer (NCIC CTG SC.15). *Int J Radiat Oncol Biol Phys* 2002; **54**: 719–728.

21. Sundstrom S, Bremnes R, Aasebo U, *et al.* Hypofractionated palliative radiotherapy (17 Gy per 2 fractions) in advanced non-small cell lung carcinoma is comparable to standard fractionation for symptom control and survival: a national phase III trial. *J Clin Oncol* 2004; **22**: 801–810.

22. Erridge SC, Gaze MN, Price A, *et al.* Symptom control and quality of life in people with lung cancer: a randomised trial of two palliative radiotherapy fractionation schedules. *Clin Oncol* 2005; **17**: 61–67.

23. Kramer GW, Wanders SL, Noordijk EM, *et al.* Results of the Dutch National study of the palliative effect of irradiation using two different treatment schemes for non-small cell lung cancer. *J Clin Oncol* 2005; **23**: 2962–2970.

24. Senkus-Konefka E, Dziadziuszko R, Bednaruk-Mlynski E, *et al.* A prospective randomised study to compare two palliative radiotherapy schedules for non-small cell lung cancer (NSCLC). *Br J Cancer* 2005; **92**: 1038–1045.

25. Fairchild A, Harris K, Barnes E, *et al.* Palliative thoracic radiotherapy for lung cancer: a systematic review. *J Clin Oncol* 2008; **26**: 4001–4011.

26. Mallick I, Sharma SC, Behera D, *et al.* Optimization of dose and fractionation of endobronchial brachytherapy with or without external radiation in palliative management of non-small cell lung cancer: a prospective randomized study. *J Cancer Res Ther* 2006; **2**: 119–125.

27. Sur R, Ahmed SN, Donde B, *et al.* Brachytherapy boost vs teletherapy boost in palliation of symptomatic, locally advanced nonsmall cell lung cancer: preliminary analysis of a randomized, prospective study. *J Brachyther Int* 2001; **17**: 309–315.

28. Sur R, Donde B, Mohuiddin M, *et al.* Randomized prospective study on the role of high dose rate intraluminal brachytherapy (HDRILBT) in palliation of symptoms in advanced non-small cell lung cancer (NSCLC) treated with radiation alone [abstract]. *Int J Radiat Oncol Biol Phys* 2004; **60**: S205.

29. Langendijk H, de Jong J, Tjwa M, *et al.* External irradiation versus external irradiation plus endobronchial brachytherapy in inoperable non-small cell lung cancer: a prospective randomized study. *Radiother Oncol* 2001; **58**: 257–268.

30. Chella A, Ambrogi MC, Ribechini A, *et al.* Combined Nd-YAG laser/HDR brachytherapy versus Nd-YAG laser only in malignant central airway involvement: a prospective randomized study. *Lung Cancer* 2000; **27**: 169–175.

31. Stout R, Barber P, Burt P, *et al.* Clinical and quality of life outcomes in the first United Kingdom randomized trial of endobronchial brachytherapy (intraluminal radiotherapy)

vs external beam radiotherapy in the palliative treatment of inoperable non-small cell lung cancer. *Radiother Oncol* 2000; **56**: 323–327.

32. Huber RM, Fischer R, Hautmann H, *et al*. Palliative endobronchial brachytherapy for central lung tumors. A prospective, randomized comparison of two fractionation schedules. *Chest* 1995; **107**: 463–470.

33. Cardona AF, Reveiz L, Ospina EG, *et al*. Palliative endobronchial brachytherapy for non-small cell lung cancer. *Cochrane Database Syst Rev* 2008; (2): CD004284.

34. Ball D, Smith J, Bishop J, *et al*. A phase III study of radiotherapy with and without continuous-infusion fluorouracil as palliation for non-small cell lung cancer. *Br J Cancer* 1997; **75**: 690–697.

35. Bauman G, Yartsev S, Rodrigues G, *et al*. A prospective evaluation of helical tomotherapy. *Int J Radiat Oncol Biol Phys* 2007; **68**: 632–641.

36. MacPherson M, Montgomery L, Fox G, *et al*. On-line rapid palliation using helical tomotherapy: a prospective feasibility study. *Radiother Oncol* 2008; **87**: 116–118.

37. Rodrigues G, Yartsev S, Coad T, *et al*. Novel application of helical tomotherapy in whole skull palliative radiotherapy. *Med Dosim* 2008; **33**: 282–285.

38. Rodrigues G, Yartsev S, Yaremko B, *et al*. Phase I trial of simultaneous in-field boost with helical tomotherapy for patients with one to three brain metastases. *Int J Radiat Oncol Biol Phys* 2011; **8**: 1128–1133.

39. Rusthoven KE, Kavanagh BD, Burri SH, *et al*. Multi-institutional phase I/II trial of stereotactic body radiation therapy for lung metastases. *J Clin Oncol* 2009; **27**: 1579–1584.

40. Timothy AR, Girling DJ, Saunders MI, *et al*. Second Workshop on Palliative Radiotherapy and Symptom Control. Radiotherapy for inoperable lung cancer. *Clin Oncol (R Coll Radiol)* 2001; **13**: 86–87.

41. Brundage MD, Bezjak A, Dixon P, *et al*. The role of palliative thoracic radiotherapy in non-small cell lung cancer. *Can J Oncol* 1996; **6**(Suppl 1): 25–32.

42. Falk SJ, Girling DJ, White RJ, *et al*. Immediate versus delayed palliative thoracic radiotherapy in patients with unresectable locally advanced non-small cell lung cancer and minimal thoracic symptoms: randomized controlled trial. *BMJ* 2002; **325**: 465.

CHAPTER 15

Palliative radiotherapy for gastrointestinal and colorectal cancer

Robert Glynne-Jones, Mark Harrison
Mount Vernon Centre for Cancer Treatment, Mount Vernon Hospital, Northwood, London, UK

Introduction

The aims of palliative radiation therapy (RT) are to alleviate symptoms, restore function, diminish suffering, and improve quality of life. Palliative RT has been shown to be an effective and simple method of providing relatively rapid relief in both locally advanced and metastatic cancer [1,2] for symptoms of pain, bleeding, ulceration, compression, or obstruction. It is accepted that the majority of patients will have a limited life span, and the duration of symptom relief may be short. Box 15.1 lists the indications for use of palliative radiotherapy.

More than 50 years of experience means that safe doses of radiation can be delivered quickly in one or a few daily fractions. Although larger fraction sizes may lead to increased late effects, this toxicity will take months or years to develop and is unlikely to prove problematic in a population with a short life span. Current palliative radiotherapy regimens for colorectal and gastrointestinal cancer commonly deliver doses ranging from 8 Gy as a single fraction, 20–25 Gy in 5 fractions, 30 Gy in 10 fractions, to 27–30 Gy in 6 fractions over 3 weeks (Figure 15.1). We often have insufficient information to choose the optimal regimen. Very few studies have used validated endpoints for symptom relief or have included formal measures of quality of life. Hence, it is probably best to tailor radiation fraction regimens and duration of treatment to the individual and their estimated survival time, although, due to their close patient contact, oncologists tend to be overly optimistic and unrealistic.

This chapter reviews the role of palliative radiation therapy in gastrointestinal and colorectal cancer as well as the selection of patients who are appropriate for radiotherapy. Patients with advanced gastrointestinal and colorectal

Radiation Oncology in Palliative Cancer Care, First Edition. Edited by Stephen Lutz, Edward Chow, and Peter Hoskin.
© 2013 John Wiley & Sons, Ltd. Published 2013 by John Wiley & Sons, Ltd.

Box 15.1 Symptoms commonly associated with gastrointestinal cancers

- Pain
- Bleeding
- Dysphagia
- Nausea/vomiting
- Malnutrition
- Deydration
- Small or large bowel obstruction
- Fungating or ulcerative mass

---

cancers suffer from a range of symptoms which include bleeding, pain, and obstruction, but there are a number of challenges somewhat distinct from other malignancies. Though the management of bone, cerebral, and painful metastases parallels other cancers, a significant amount of palliative treatment is aimed at preserving luminal patency. Dysphagia is a uniquely distressing symptom since immediate consequences are obvious and, for those with some luminal patency, there is an obvious discomfort evident to the patient and their carers. We describe the various clinical scenarios amenable to palliation by radiotherapy, as well as the commonly used doses, fractionation schemes, and techniques. More conformal techniques such as stereotactic ablative radiotherapy (SART), CyberKnife, and brachytherapy are also described. Finally we recommend specific studies to accumulate evidence for decision-making and define the optimal way to utilize radiotherapy for palliation of colorectal cancer.

Treatment of dysphagia

Esophageal cancer generally presents at a late stage, with severe dysphagia. An inability to swallow solid foods progresses to difficulty in swallowing even liquids. In general, radical treatments for cure are only possible in the minority of patients, with the remainder requiring optimal palliation. Early intervention to prevent obstruction is important, and palliative radiotherapy has an important role to play in this scenario. Other options for management of dysphagia include stenting, laser ablation, and possibly chemotherapy, though radiotherapy has been shown to offer the best dysphagia-free survival [3].

Endoscopic dilatation can be useful in the short term, but requires serial endoscopy, with a consequent risk of perforation. Laser ablation using the Nd:YAG laser can be used if the tumor is exophytic and projects into the esophagus, but it is less effective for circumferential tumors, where perforation is a risk, especially in stenosing lesions where the direction of the lumen is not obvious [4]. Argon plasma coagulation is an alternative and addresses tumor that is more superficial, with a lower risk of perforation.

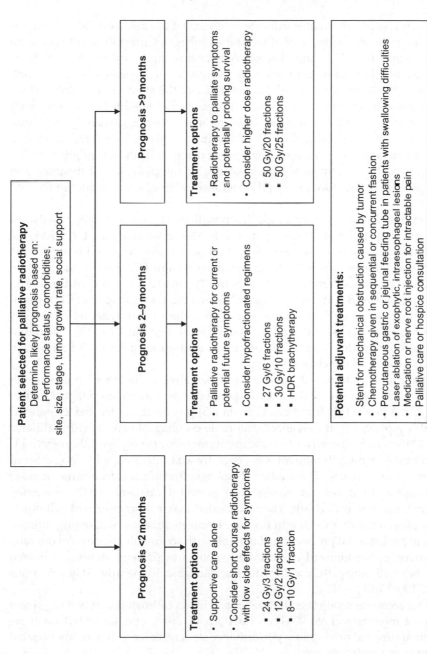

Patient selected for palliative radiotherapy
Determine likely prognosis based on:
Performance status, comorbidities,
site, size, stage, tumor growth rate, social support

Prognosis <2 months

Treatment options
- Supportive care alone
- Consider short course radiotherapy
  with low side effects for symptoms
  - 24 Gy/3 fractions
  - 12 Gy/2 fractions
  - 8–10 Gy/1 fraction

Prognosis 2–9 months

Treatment options
- Palliative radiotherapy for current or
  potential future symptoms
- Consider hypofractionated regimens
  - 27 Gy/6 fractions
  - 30 Gy/10 fractions
  - HDR brachytherapy

Prognosis >9 months

Treatment options
- Radiotherapy to palliate symptoms
  and potentially prolong survival
- Consider higher dose radiotherapy
  - 50 Gy/20 fractions
  - 50 Gy/25 fractions

Potential adjuvant treatments:
- Stent for mechanical obstruction caused by tumor
- Chemotherapy given in sequential or concurrent fashion
- Percutaneous gastric or jejunal feeding tube in patients with swallowing difficulties
- Laser ablation of exophytic, intraesophageal lesions
- Medication or nerve root injection for intractable pain
- Palliative care or hospice consultation

Figure 15.1 Algorithm for use of palliative radiotherapy for patients with esophageal cancer.

Early complication rates from stent placement are low, and 95% of patients enjoy significant improvement in their dysphagia. Currently, stent migration occurs in only 5–10%, and obstructive episodes require intervention in 3–5% of patients. However, the stent may eventually be bypassed by continuing tumor growth through or around the lattice of the stent in up to 36%, which may limit the effectiveness of the technique [4,5]. One-third of patients with dysphagia at the time of death have received previous stenting [6]. Randomized controlled trials [3,7–9] and a meta-analysis [10] have compared brachytherapy, laser ablation therapy, and argon beam coagulation (APC) therapy with self-expanding metal stents for the palliation of dysphagia in esophageal cancer. One study [11] examined external beam radiation therapy (EBRT).

Several different radiotherapy fractionation schema have improved dysphagia in up to 70% of treated patients. In Mount Vernon, our standard is the delivery of 27 Gy in 6 fractions over 3 weeks usually delivered with parallel opposed fields but occasionally to a planned volume [12]. Symptom palliation may persist for several months or years. The median survival of this group of patients was 8.2 months (range 0.2–54 months). Dysphagia was improved by radiotherapy in 77% of cases, the median duration of relief was 24 weeks (range 0–208 weeks) and was maintained until death in 40% [13]. The radiotherapy can be delivered with concurrent continuous infusion 5-fluorouracil or oral capecitabine chemotherapy.

Some studies reported the benefit of palliative radiation with concurrent 5-FU chemotherapy (CRT) for dysphagia in advanced esophageal cancer [14,15]. A phase I/II trial from Canada [15] prospectively treated 22 patients with dysphagia from advanced incurable esophageal cancer with palliative RT (30 Gy/10 fractions) and a concurrent single course of chemotherapy (5-FU and mitomycin-C). Treatment was generally well-tolerated, and 68% achieved a complete response. The median dysphagia-free interval from time of onset of improvement was 11 weeks, and overall 11 patients (50%) remained dysphagia-free until death. They concluded that a short course of radiotherapy plus chemotherapy might produce complete relief of swallowing difficulties in a substantial proportion of patients with acceptable toxicity. An ongoing Norwegian randomized clinical study compares primary stenting followed by brachytherapy 8 Gy × 3, with standard brachytherapy 8 Gy × 3 alone (NCT00653107).

Our recommendation is that patients with an estimated survival of greater than 2 months receive 27 Gy/6 fractions of EBRT and those with a more limited survival or very low performance status receive a shorter fractionated regime or brachytherapy.

Gastric cancer

Radiation therapy is effective in up to 75% of patients in palliating symptoms of gastric outlet or biliary obstruction, pain, and bleeding [16]. Exophytic tumors tend to respond better than a linitis plastica. Diffuse histology may not respond as well as other histologies. In the situation where the patient is losing 1–2 units of blood a week without suffering cardiovascular instability, most will respond to a short course of EBRT [17]. Regimens vary but may comprise anything from 8 Gy in a single dose or 20 Gy in 5 fractions over 5 days (probably the most common). Others suggest at least 30 Gy in 10 fractions or even higher doses are required [18].

If patients have a good performance status, CRT may improve response. In one study of advanced gastric cancer, 37 patients were treated with palliative RT (median dose 35 Gy), the majority of whom received CRT [19]. The symptoms of bleeding, dysphagia/obstruction, and pain were relieved in 70% (14/20), 81% (13/16), and 86% (6/7) respectively, with an overall symptom control rate of almost 70%, compared to 25–54% control rate for palliative RT alone [20]. Patients receiving CRT also had a trend towards better overall survival than RT alone (median 6.7 vs 2.4 months, $P = 0.08$) [21]. The same unit suggests patients with potentially resectable gastric cancer treated with pre-operative CRT, but progressing with peritoneal disease and not suitable for surgery, have outcomes similar to that with chemotherapy alone. In these circumstances, CRT provides both symptom relief and durable local control for most patients, though the omission of radiotherapy may not diminish the results and might decrease side-effect risks.

Palliation of biliary obstruction

Patients in whom standard treatments for relief of biliary obstruction have failed may be considered for palliative radiotherapy. EBRT directed at the porta hepatis/common bile ducts can relieve biliary obstruction. There are a small number of case reports that look at EBRT as a single agent for relief of jaundice. For those patients in whom a biliary stent is inserted there is significant experience – predominantly in the management of cholangiocarcinoma – that a combination of EBRT and intraluminal brachytherapy provides good short-term palliation but does not significantly alter the long-term prognosis.

Nodes at origin of the superior mesenteric artery

The extrinsic compression of the third part of the duodenum as it passes through the aorto-mesenteric angle, anterolateral to the aorta, is known as the superior mesenteric artery syndrome (SMAS). This syndrome, also known as Wilkie syndrome, is a rare mechanical cause of upper intestinal obstruction, with a reported incidence of between 0.2% and 0.78%. Nodes enlarge at the root of the superior mesenteric artery and paralyze small bowel motility. Chronic symptoms include intermittent gastric pain, fullness, and occasional episodes of post-prandial vomiting, whilst acute symptoms include intractable vomiting, oral intolerance, epigastric distension, and abdominal pain.

Stomach and small bowel studies show that contrast proceeds through the small bowel, albeit slowly, and there is no mechanical obstruction. Drugs which stimulate propulsion such as metoclopramide are ineffective, and the patient describes symptoms of bloating after eating and vomiting if more than small volumes are eaten. CT scans usually highlight macroscopically involved lymph nodes at the root of the SMA. Pallative radiotherapy using up to 30 Gy is effective in giving prompt symptom relief.

High dose rate brachytherapy

High dose rate intraluminal brachytherapy (HDR-ILBT) has the advantage of high conformality – i.e. a rapid fall-off of radiation dose, which allows the delivery of a high dose to the tumor to provide symptom control, while sparing normal surrounding structures such as the adjacent normal rectal mucosa, bladder, and small bowel [22]. Brachytherapy is quick to administer, simple, and acceptable to the patients with poor performance status, limited mobility, and the elderly.

This technique has been used at Mount Vernon Cancer Centre for the last 10 years [23] for short-term palliation for advanced symptomatic rectal tumors, particularly in patients with a poor performance status and the very elderly and frail.

It is possible to place clips at the superior inferior extent of the tumor although these can only be relied upon to be maintained for 10–12 days. When the tumor is not circumferential, it is possible to use segmental shielding with an applicator which shields 25% or 50% of the rectal circumference. Treatment prescription is defined at 1 cm from the source access. Fractionated courses of 6 Gy up to 36 Gy for radical treatments or 10–12 Gy in 1–2 fractions can be delivered. In a group of 25 assessable patients treated at the Mount Vernon Cancer Centre, 14 have achieved complete clinical response. Median survival for the entire group was 6 months (range 1–54 months) and for patients treated with radical intent, 25 months (range 1.5–54) [24].

However, there are limited data available evaluating the advantages of HDR-ILBT with EBRT as compared to EBRT alone. HDR-ILBT for advanced or inoperable tumors of the rectum has been used both in the palliative setting and to dose escalate after chemoradiation for curative treatment [25]. It also offers an effective conservative approach to the treatment of early stage rectal adenocarcinoma in appropriately selected (most often elderly unfit for radical surgery) patients.

Locally advanced/recurrent rectal cancer

Rectal cancer may be considered unsuitable for surgery or radical radio-therapy / CRT by virtue of the extensive local infiltration requiring unacceptable extensive resection, poor performance status, extreme age, severe comorbidity, or in the setting of locally recurrent or metastatic disease. Locally advanced and unresectable rectal cancer may present with bleeding, pain on defecation or pain in the distribution of the sciatic nerve, a copious mucous discharge, infections, and rarely, obstruction. EBRT has been considered an effective palliative treatment. Studies of palliative RT for rectal cancer have shown statistically significant improvements in pain control for patients suffering from locally advanced disease [26–28].

Studies reported in the 1960s–1980s showed that relief of pain and/or bleeding was achieved in approximately 75% of patients with doses as low as 20 Gy in 10 fractions over 2 weeks or various doses of 40–60 Gy in 1.8–2.5 Gy per fraction [29–31]. However, median duration of symptom relief is often short at 3–9 months. Later reports showed similar or improved results for symptom palliation: control of pain in 78–93% of patients, control of bleeding in 68–100%, and control of mass in 35–88% [32,33].

Several different radiotherapy fractionation schema have produced acceptable rates of symptom control in this setting. The delivery of 30 Gy in 6 fractions over 3 weeks with concurrent continuous infusion 5-fluorouracil chemotherapy for locally advanced or unresectable colorectal cancer provided good pain control and acceptable toxicity and prevented the need for eventual colostomy placement in two-thirds of treated patients [33]. Expected acute side effects include nausea, vomiting, diarrhea, proctitis, tenesmus, urinary frequency and dysuria, erythema, and moist desquamation of the perineum in low rectal cancers.

The published literature is sparse on the benefits of brachytherapy for advanced inoperable rectal cancer [35,36]. However, there are limited data available evaluating the advantages of HDR-ILBT with EBRT as compared to EBRT/CRT [37]. HDR-ILBT has been used palliatively [23]. One experience of 79 patients treated 2001–2007 with HDR-ILBT in our own departments using a single line source 2-cm diameter rectal applicator has also shown encouraging tumor and symptom response rates and acceptable toxicity [23].

Isolated local recurrence after pre-operative radiotherapy and total mesorectal excision (TME) surgery is infrequent, rarely isolated, and has almost invariably been associated with a fatal outcome [34]. Recurrent rectal cancer in the pelvis carries a poor prognosis with a median survival of under a year without treatment. Most experience progressive symptoms of bleeding, tenesmus, mucous discharge, and severe neuropathic pain, all of which can significantly impact the quality of life. Currently in the UK, the widespread use of pre-operative radiotherapy either short course or long course with chemoradiation has ensured that isolated local pelvic recurrence is a rarity.

If local recurrence occurs and radiotherapy has not previously been administered, radiotherapy or chemoradiation [35] can produce good palliation of symptoms if the patient is reasonably fit with a good performance status, but long-term local control is seldom achieved. For frail and elderly patients a short course may be preferable.

The duration of effective palliation is usually short with further progression of symptoms within 3–6 months after irradiation [36]; complete responses are rarely achieved even with high radical doses in the region of 60 Gy [38]. Rectal mucous discharge is often an extremely difficult symptom to palliate with radiotherapy but occasionally may be relieved by octreotide.

Re-irradiation

After previous neoadjuvant radiotherapy, chemotherapy is often ineffective with only very temporary symptom relief. Further re-irradiation in these circumstances remains a controversial issue [39,40], and doses are usually limited to 36–45 Gy applied with small safety margins due to the normal tissue constraints from prior radiotherapy. Some single center experience suggests this practice may be safe in the short term, although long-term evidence is sparse [38,41], and there is a potential risk of treatment-related side effects [42]. The present authors would not usually recommend doses in excess of 36 Gy in combination with 5-FU based chemotherapy, and they should only be considered in circumstances where concerns regarding small bowel toxicity were small.

Anal cancer

Local recurrence in anal cancer is also complicated by pain, bleeding, and discharge. Recurrent disease within the pelvis is similar to the situation experienced by patients with recurrent rectal cancer, i.e. pelvic pain extending into the buttocks and often in a sciatic distribution; if the recurrence is predominantly pre-sacral there will be irritation of the lumbar sacral plexus. Bi-lateral ureteric obstruction is often encountered. Re-irradiation is often surprisingly effective, but again the benefit is usually not durable.

The promise of highly conformal therapy

There are a number of systems that allow a stereotactic approach. Current literature on their value is limited though treatment systems such as the CyberKnife (Accurray) show interesting results in a number of situations including locally advanced carcinoma of the pancreas.

Special considerations in developing countries

Patients in developing countries may present with advanced disease because of limited access to health care or poor socioeconomic conditions that limit the ability of the patient to pay for screening or oncology care. Additionally, some diagnoses with relatively poor prognoses such as gastric cancer or primary hepatocellular cancer are more prevalent in developing countries. Finally, developing countries may have limitations in diagnostic capabilities, surgical sophistication, chemotherapy availability, and/or up-to-date radiotherapy equipment. As such, some of the most useful radiotherapy approaches may need to be modified to match the available resources.

Conclusion

The optimal palliative radiotherapy fractionation regimen has not been adequately defined. Retrospective audits and population studies cannot capture all the data to identify the optimal choice of fractionation regimens. In some countries this is driven partially by reimbursement issues. Randomized studies have not specifically addressed this issue. In retrospective studies, the patient's performance status and perceived life expectancy appear to be the most common reasons for selecting single fractions. More clinical research in palliative care is also needed to guide selection of an optimal palliative radiation schedule for the treatment of patients with many of the common symptoms from gastrointestinal cancer. There is little evidence to support the common prejudice that better and longer palliation is achieved with higher doses delivered in multiple smaller fractions, and future studies will require clinically relevant validated endpoints to capture symptom relief and quality of life. Increasing options in terms of chemotherapy and biological agents which improve survival make these decisions more difficult. Research will enable us to provide guidelines to support radiation oncologists in evaluating suitability and recommending the most appropriate palliative treatments. Patients also need to be part of the decision-making with tailored information in an acceptable format, aimed at supporting those undergoing palliative treatment.

References

1. Konski A, Feigenberg S, Chow E. Palliative radiation therapy. *Semin Oncol* 2005; **32**: 156–164.
2. Dolinsky C, Metz JM. Palliative radiation therapy in oncology. *Anesthesiol Clin* 2006; **24**: 113–128, viii–ix.
3. Tytgat GN, Bartelink H, Bernards R, *et al*. Cancer of the esophagus and gastric cardia: recent advances. *Dis Esophagus* 2004; **17**: 10–26.
4. Adam A, Ellul J, Watkinson AF, *et al*. Palliation of inoperable esophageal carcinoma: a prospective randomised trial of laser therapy and stent placement. *Radiology* 1997; **202**: 344–348.
5. O'Sullivan GJ, Grundy A. Palliation of malignant dysphagia with expanding metallic stents. *J Vasc Interv Radiol* 1999; **10**: 346–351.
6. Bone Pain Trial Working Party. 8 Gy in single fraction radiotherapy for the treatment of metastatic skeletal pain: randomised comparison with a multifraction schedule over 12 months of patient follow-up. *Radiother Oncol* 1999; **52**: 111–121.
7. Dallal HJ, Smith GD, Grieve DC, *et al*. A randomized trial of thermal ablative therapy versus expandable metal stents in the palliative treatment of patients with esophageal carcinoma. *Gastrointest Endosc* 2001; **54**: 549–557.

8. Homs MY, Steyerberg EW, Eijkenboom WM, *et al*. Palliative treatment of esophageal cancer with dysphagia: more favourable outcome from single-dose internal brachytherapy than from the placement of a self-expanding stent; a multicenter randomised study. *Ned Tijdschr Geneeskd* 2005; **149**: 2800–2806.

9. Bergquist H, Wenger U, Johnsson E, *et al*. Stent insertion or endoluminal brachytherapy as palliation of patients with advanced cancer of the esophagus and gastroesophageal junction. Results of a randomized, controlled clinical trial. *Dis Esophagus* 2005; **18**: 131–139.

10. Sgourakis G, Gockel I, Radtke A, *et al*. The use of self-expanding stents in esophageal and gastroesophageal junction cancer palliation: a meta-analysis and meta-regression analysis of outcomes. *Dig Dis Sci* 2010; **55**: 3018–3030.

11. Shenfine J, McNamee P, Steen N, *et al*. A pragmatic randomised controlled trial of the cost-effectiveness of palliative therapies for patients with inoperable oesophageal cancer. *Health Technol Assess* 2005; **9**: 1–121.

12. Chong I, Ah-See M, Harrison M. Evaluation of the efficacy and tolerability of a high dose palliative radiotherapy regimen in oesophageal carcinoma. *Radiother Oncol* 2006; **81**(Suppl 1): 149–150.

13. Leslie MD, Dische S, Saunders M, *et al*. The role of radiotherapy in carcinoma of the thoracic oesophagus: an audit of the Mount Vernon experience 1980–1989. *Clin Oncol (R Coll Radiol)* 1992; **4**: 114–118.

14. Coia LR, Soffen EM, Schultheiss TE, *et al*. Swallowing function in patients with esophageal cancer treated with concurrent radiation and chemotherapy. *Cancer* 1993; **71**: 281–286.

15. Hayter CR, Huff-Winters C, Paszat L, *et al*. A prospective trial of short-course radiotherapy plus chemotherapy for palliation of dysphagia from advanced esophageal cancer. *Radiother Oncol* 2000; **56**: 329–333.

16. Perez C, Brady LW, Halperin EC. *Principles and Practice of Radiation Oncology*, 4th edn. Philadelphia: Lippincott Williams & Wilkins, 2004.

17. Mackay S, Hayes T, Yeo A. Management of gastric cancer. *Aust Fam Physician* 2006; **35**: 208–211.

18. Lee JA, Lim do H, Park W, *et al*. Radiation therapy for gastric cancer bleeding. *Tumori* 2009; **95**: 726–730.

19. Kim MM, Rana V, Janjan NA, *et al*. Clinical benefit of palliative radiation therapy in advanced gastric cancer. *Acta Oncol* 2008; **47**: 421–427.

20. Tey J, Back MF, Shakespeare TP, *et al*. The role of palliative radiation therapy in symptomatic locally advanced gastric cancer. *Int J Radiat Oncol Biol Phys* 2007; **67**: 385–388.

21. Vuong T, Belliveau PJ, Michel RP, *et al*. Conformal preoperative endorectal brachytherapy treatment for locally advanced rectal cancer: early results of a phase i/ii study. *Dis Colon Rectum* 2002; **45**: 1486–1493.

22. Corner C, Bryant L, Chapman C, *et al*. High-dose-rate afterloading intraluminal brachytherapy for advanced inoperable rectal carcinoma. *Brachytherapy* 2010; **9**: 66–70.

23. Hoskin PJ, de Canha SM, Bownes P, *et al*. High dose rate afterloading intraluminal brachytherapy for advanced inoperable rectal carcinoma. *Radiother Oncol* 2004; **73**: 195–198.

24. Jakobsen A, Mortensen JP, Bisgaard C, *et al*. Preoperative chemoradiation of locally advanced T3 rectal cancer combined with an endorectal boost. *Int J Radiat Oncol Biol Phys* 2006; **64**: 461–465.

25. Wong R, Thomas G, Cummings B, *et al*. The role of radiotherapy in the management of pelvic recurrence of rectal cancer. *Can J Oncol* 1996; **6**(Suppl 1): 39–47.

26. Wong R, Thomas G, Cummings B, *et al.* In search of a dose-response relationship with radiotherapy in the management of recurrent rectal carcinoma in the pelvis: a systematic review. *Int J Radiat Oncol Biol Phys* 1998; **40**: 437–446.
27. Ito Y, Ohtsu A, Ishikura S, *et al.* Efficacy of chemoradiotherapy on pain relief in patients with intrapelvic recurrence of rectal cancer. *Jpn J Clin Oncol* 2003; **33**: 180–185.
28. Gunderson LL, Cohen AM, Welch CW. Residual, inoperable, or recurrent colorectal cancer: surgical radiotherapy interaction. *Am J Surg* 1980; **139**: 518–525.
29. Rominger CJ, Gunderson LL, Gelber RD, Conner N. Radiation therapy alone or in combination with chemotherapy in the treatment of residual or inoperable carcinoma of the rectum and rectosigmoid or pelvic recurrence following colorectal surgery. Radiation Therapy Oncology Group study (76-16). *Am J Clin Oncol* 1985; **8**: 118–127.
30. Gunderson LL, Martenson JA. Irradiation of adenocarcinomas of the gastrointestinal tract. *Front Radiat Ther Oncol* 1988; **22**: 127–148.
31. Willett CG, Gunderson LL. Palliative treatment of rectal cancer: is radiotherapy alone a good option? *J Gastrointest Surg* 2004; **8**: 277–279.
32. Bae SH, Park W, Choi DH, *et al.* Palliative radiotherapy in patients with a symptomatic pelvic mass of metastatic colorectal cancer. *Radiat Oncol* 2011; **6**: 52.
33. Janjan NA, Breslin T, Lenzi R, *et al.* Avoidance of colostomy placement in advanced colorectal cancer with twice weekly hypofractionated radiation plus continuous infusion 5-fluorouracil. *J Pain Symptom Manage* 2000; **20**: 266–272.
34. Arnott SJ. The value of combined 5-fluorouracil and x-ray therapy in the palliation of locally recurrent inoperable rectal carcinoma. *Clin Radiol* 1975; **26**: 177–182.
35. James RD, Johnson RJ, Eddleston B, *et al.* Prognostic factors in locally recurrent rectal carcinoma treated by radiotherapy. *Br J Surg* 1983; **70**: 469–472.
36. Wong CS, Cummings BJ, Brierley JD, *et al.* Treatment of locally recurrent rectal carcinoma – results and prognostic factors. *Int J Radiat Oncol Biol Phys* 1998; **40**: 427–435.
37. Mohiuddin M, Lingareddy V, Rakinic J, Marks G. Reirradiation for rectal cancer and surgical resection after ultra-high doses. *Int J Radiat Oncol Biol Phys* 1993; **27**: 1159–1163.
38. Mohiuddin M, Marks G, Marks J. Long-term results of reirradiation for patients with recurrent rectal carcinoma. *Cancer* 2002; **95**: 1144–1150.
39. Glimelius B, Gronberg H, Jarhult J, *et al.* A systematic overview of radiation therapy effects in rectal cancer. *Acta Oncol* 2003; **42**: 476–492.
40. Lingareddy V, Ahmad NR, Mohiuddin M. Palliative reirradiation for recurrent rectal cancer. *Int J Radiat Oncol Biol Phys* 1997; **38**: 785–790.
41. Gunderson LL, Nelson H, Martenson JA, *et al.* Intraoperative electron and external beam irradiation with or without 5-fluorouracil and maximum surgical resection for previously unirradiated, locally recurrent colorectal cancer. *Dis Colon Rectum* 1996; **39**: 1379–1395.
42. Haddock MG, Gunderson LL, Nelson H, *et al.* Intraoperative irradiation for locally recurrent colorectal cancer in previously irradiated patients. *Int J Radiat Oncol Biol Phys* 2001; **49**: 1267–1274.

CHAPTER 16

Genitourinary malignancies

Gillian M. Duchesne

Peter MacCallum Cancer Centre, University of Melbourne and Monash University, Melbourne, Victoria, Australia

Introduction

Urologic cancers encompass a disparate group of malignancies which have in common their association with the genitourinary tract, excluding gynecologic malignancy in the female, but including the male genital tumors of prostate, penis, and testis (Box 16.1). The origins of many are from the urothelium, transitional cell in particular, and others include glandular adenocarcinoma (the most common type of carcinoma of the prostate), squamous carcinoma, germ cell tumors, and other rare entities such as lymphoma or sarcoma. Where tumor origin, site, or histopathology differ significantly in terms of their palliative management, the details will be discussed in other chapters.

Incidence and etiology

The incidence and rates of diagnosis of the various genitourinary tumors vary significantly from country to country, mainly because of lifestyle influences on etiology, the average life expectancy of the populations, and the relationship to public health factors in particular areas.

Urothelial cancers, including those arising in the ureter, the urinary bladder, and the proximal urethra, are most commonly transitional cell (TCC) in origin, with adenocarcinoma and squamous carcinomas representing only a few percent of the total, except where schistosomiasis as the causative agent is endemic. Many urothelial cancers are caused by smoking or ingestion of other carcinogenic toxins, and their incidence mirrors that of lung cancer. Two distinct clinical patterns are seen, with the majority of TCC being low grade, non-invasive, and managed successfully by local means. The minority of tumors are high grade, invasive, and have lethal potential, with mortality rates over 50% for those extending beyond the local organ.

Radiation Oncology in Palliative Cancer Care, First Edition. Edited by Stephen Lutz, Edward Chow, and Peter Hoskin.
© 2013 John Wiley & Sons, Ltd. Published 2013 by John Wiley & Sons, Ltd.

Box 16.1 Symptoms commonly associated with genitourinary cancers

- Bleeding
- Pain
- Urinary tract infection
- Urinary frequency
- Dysuria
- Hematuria
- Pyelonephritis
- Urinary retention or obstruction
- Bowel obstruction
- Lower extremity edema

In the western world the incidence of prostate cancer has been said to have reached epidemic proportions, with attendant concerns that much over-diagnosis of insignificant cancer takes place, leading to inappropriate treatments and unnecessary toxicity. Nonetheless, prostate cancer still kills, with a mortality-to-incidence ratio of 17% [1] , and those patients who go on to die of their disease carry a significant burden of locally advanced, locally recurrent, and/or metastatic disease and related symptomatology in the community, particularly because of their potential longevity. Prostate cancer incidence is also increasing in traditionally low-risk populations such as the Indian and Chinese societies: for example, a recent publication on incidence and mortality changes in Singapore Chinese men suggests that standardized incidence rates are increasing by over 5% a year [2]. These results may in part arise from increased detection and diagnosis, but they may also reflect a true increase in incidence. In communities where early detection is not commonly practiced, presentation with metastatic disease, requiring palliation, may be the norm.

Testis cancer remains a rare disease, with its etiologic factors generally still to be pinned down, but it is the supreme model of chemo-curable malignancy, and the role of palliative radiotherapy is limited and will not be further discussed. Palliative management of the other rare cancers should be based on first principles in the absence of substantive evidence to support a standard of care.

Renal cancer is increasing in incidence in the western world for reasons which are not clear, with an increase of up to 15% predicted in Victoria, Australia between 2010 and 2013, and similar findings reported elsewhere [3]. The largest increase in observed incidence is in the younger population, prompting the need for a better understanding of etiologic factors that could translate into preventative measures.

Clinical behavior

Palliation of advanced genitourinary cancer, as for all advanced malignancy, should be considered in terms of management of the loco-regional disease if this is troublesome, and management of the sites of disease dissemination and the systemic effects of malignancy (Figure 16.1). Given that management of metastatic disease is discussed in detail elsewhere in this publication, specific reference has not been made in this chapter.

Bladder cancer

Incurable bladder cancer frequently causes significant local pelvic symptoms from soft tissue disease including bladder frequency, dysuria, pain, hematuria, and bowel obstruction. Renal function may be impaired secondary to primary or nodal disease. Nodal enlargement may cause lower abdominal, genital, and leg edema. Local bony spread may lead to bone pain and fracture.

Systemic features are common and may include weight loss, cachexia, and malaise, as well as symptoms related to site-specific metastatic spread. Hypercalcemia of malignancy is not common. It is rare to see oligometastatic disease in bladder cancer, and palliation is generally based around systemic chemotherapy or simple radiation approaches to reduce troublesome local symptoms.

Prostate cancer

Patients with incurable prostate cancer may live for some years with asymptomatic recurrence, or they may develop symptoms from local disease, or soft tissue or bony metastasis. Locally recurrent prostate cancer after prior definitive radiation therapy is becoming rare as a consequence of the successful use of accurate high-dose curative radiation techniques, but when it occurs it can cause significant difficulties with bladder emptying, bleeding from the tumor bed, pain, bowel obstruction, ureteric and urethral obstruction, and edema.

Specific measures for managing bony metastasis from prostate cancer that may not be applicable for other tumor types will be discussed, including denosumab and radium-223.

Renal cancer

The recent increases in kidney cancer incidence are predominantly because of increasing numbers of cases with stage I disease, readily curable with surgical resection. Nonetheless, it remains relatively common to see advanced and unresectable primary cancers presenting with hematuria from erosion of the renal vessels, back and abdominal pain from local infiltration, or site-specific symptoms from metastases.

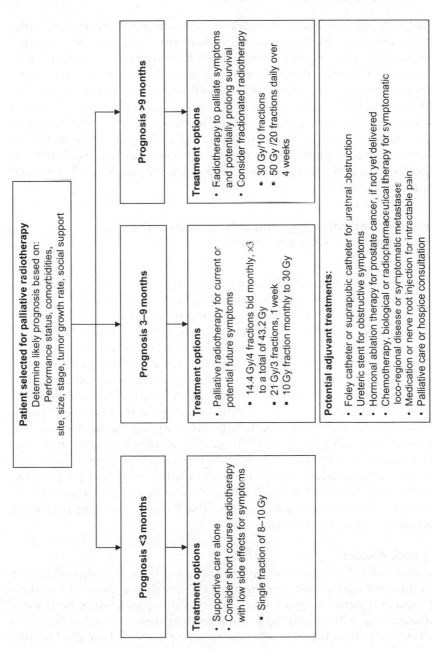

Patient selected for palliative radiotherapy
Determine likely prognosis based on:
Performance status, comorbidities,
site, size, stage, tumor growth rate, social support

Prognosis <3 months

Treatment options
- Supportive care alone
- Consider short course radiotherapy with low side effects for symptoms
  - Single fraction of 8–10 Gy

Prognosis 3–9 months

Treatment options
- Palliative radiotherapy for current or potential future symptoms
  - 14.4 Gy/4 fractions bid monthly, ×3 to a total of 43.2 Gy
  - 21 Gy/3 fractions, 1 week
  - 10 Gy fraction monthly to 30 Gy

Potential adjuvant treatments:
- Foley catheter or suprapubic catheter for urethral obstruction
- Ureteric stent for obstructive symptoms
- Hormonal ablation therapy for prostate cancer, if not yet delivered
- Chemotherapy, biological or radiopharmaceutical therapy for symptomatic loco-regional disease or symptomatic metastases
- Medication or nerve root injection for intractable pain
- Palliative care or hospice consultation

Prognosis >9 months

Treatment options
- Radiotherapy to palliate symptoms and potentially prolong survival
- Consider fractionated radiotherapy
  - 30 Gy/10 fractions
  - 50 Gy /20 fractions daily over 4 weeks

Figure 16.1 Algorithm for use of palliative radiotherapy for patients with genitourinary cancers.

Metastatic disease has a very variable course in renal cancer, with some patients living in near-symbiosis with disseminated disease for prolonged periods, and others rapidly developing fulminant disease. Some patients present with metastatic disease in anatomic sites which are rare in other types of malignancy, such as thyroid or paranasal sinuses. Others develop single sites of metastatic disease which may remain solitary for many years, if not life-long. There are strong systemic influences at work, demonstrated by the abscopal effect of successfully treating bulky primary or metastatic disease resulting in regression of disease at distant sites (e.g. [4]). Malignant hypercalcemia and other metabolic problems are common in advanced disease.

Palliative radiotherapy and other approaches for management of primary disease

Bladder cancer

The only published trial of palliative radiotherapy in primary bladder cancer [5] was completed some years ago and hence used relatively simple radiation therapy techniques, such as parallel opposed megavoltage fields, to palliate locally advanced disease. Patients were randomized between two fractionation schedules of 21 Gy in 3 fractions and 35 Gy in 10 fractions; and, although no significant advantage was found for either schedule, the results provide a benchmark of palliative efficacy against which the value of newer techniques or agents may be measured. At 3 months, 82% of patients overall showed improvement in urinary frequency, with improvement rates of 88% for hematuria and 72% for dysuria. Median time to symptom progression after response was 6 months and median survival was 7.5 months indicating that even simple approaches can provide worthwhile palliative responses. Anecdotal evidence also suggests that single fractions of radiation therapy (8 Gy), or the use of short-course schedules such as 4 fractions of 4 Gy over 2 days, are useful particularly for hematuria, with commendable limited commitment of patient time and use of scarce resources.

Prostate cancer

The first step in managing locally advanced, incurable prostate cancer is to introduce androgen deprivation therapy (ADT), with or without a local surgical maneuver such as trans-urethral resection to relieve severe obstructive symptoms. As with other stages of disease, response rates following these interventions are in excess of 80% and may be maintained for good lengths of time. Management of local disease which has become castrate-resistant is a different matter, and low-dose palliative radiation may be inadequate to control the symptoms and tumor bulk. Hindson et al. [6] demonstrated that use of high dose palliative radiotherapy to 60 Gy in this group resulted in complete symptom response in only a minority of patients (3/35, all whose hematuria was controlled), but worthwhile partial responses in a further 50%

of patients. Others have employed more hypofractionated schedules such as 45–60 Gy in 18 to 24 fractions, appropriate in the palliative setting, with good effect [7].

The desire to avoid having to manage progressive local disease led to the trial reported by Warde *et al.* [8], which examined the effect of adding radiotherapy to ADT to pre-empt the need for a later local intervention. Not only was local control achieved in the majority of patients, but overall survival at 7 years was higher in the combined modality group. While this trial included patients without systemic disease at presentation, they were all high risk, a group not uncommonly managed with palliative intent (depending on other circumstances). The benefits of adding radiation therapy to ADT should be discussed with this group of patients.

Recurrent primary disease following external beam radiation or brachytherapy is a challenge to palliate, and the patient should be managed in a multi-disciplinary setting with the urologist because of the potential need for urethral or ureteric stenting, transurethral prostate resection, or control of bleeding. Very rarely is this circumstance regarded as potentially curable disease, and salvage cysto-prostatectomy is not generally applicable, although appropriate case selection in expert centers may yield acceptable oncologic results with limited toxicity [9].

The roles of other modalities such as high intensity focused ultrasound (HIFU), hyperthermia, and cryotherapy remain to be established in this setting. HIFU for example has been reported to improve symptoms and produce prostate specific antigen (PSA) responses in patients who have local failure after attempted curative radiation therapy, but may be associated with debilitating toxicities such as fistula formation [10] and bladder outlet obstruction. The results of re-irradiation to control symptomatic recurrence are also disappointing, because effective doses may be associated with significant local toxicity, although salvage low dose rate [11] or high dose rate [12] brachytherapy may be useful. Management of these cases has to be very individualized, with the patient fully informed of the risks of toxicity to bowel, urinary, and sexual function. Careful consideration needs to be given as to whether salvage therapy is intended with curative or solely palliative intent – if the latter, then the least toxic approach is to be preferred. Overall, it is generally more appropriate to consider instigation of systemic therapy with androgen deprivation strategies to manage local radio-recurrence. If local recurrence occurs in the setting of developing castrate-resistant disease, low dose palliative external radiation doses may provide some reduction in tumor volume and relief of urinary or bowel obstruction, or bleeding arising from soft tissue metastases.

Renal cancer

Renal cancer has conventionally been regarded as relatively radio-resistant, requiring higher doses and fractionated courses for effective disease control. Early trials looking at the potential benefits of post-operative radiotherapy to treat the tumor bed with simple techniques demonstrated an adverse therapeutic ratio because the sensitivity of organs such as the liver in the upper abdomen meant that side effects generally outweighed the benefits. Radiotherapy has therefore generally only played a minor role in either curative or palliative settings, with the mainstays of treatment being surgery and systemic agents such as immune response modulators, and drugs targeting VEGF and PI3K-mTOR molecular pathways (see [13] for Review), which can provide useful albeit expensive palliation.

Other approaches

There is now a large literature supporting the use of palliative surgical nephrectomy to remove the primary renal cancer and to enhance the efficacy of systemic therapies in combating metastatic disease, quite apart from palliating local symptoms such as bleeding [14]. Other techniques such as percutaneous radiofrequency or cryotherapy ablation [15] of lesions may be useful where surgery is not contemplated or where nephron-sparing approaches are required, though they tend to be more effective for smaller rather than larger lesions, limiting their applicability. Stereotactic ablative radiotherapy has also been used in this setting with some success.

Specific management of metastatic disease in urologic malignancies

In general, the management of metastases in all urologic cancer types follows the same principles as detailed in other chapters in this resource. There are, however, particularly features of metastatic prostate cancer and renal cancer that deserve specific mention.

Prostate cancer

No other malignancy produces such a consistent sclerotic response to metastatic bone disease than prostate cancer. This osteoblastic component has made it particularly attractive to target the metastatic cells with drugs that specifically interact with bone formation, although the high rates of bone turnover are associated with a significant lytic component, too. The radionuclide strontium-89 is handled similarly to calcium and is taken up into areas of bone turnover, giving a high localized radiation dose through the emission of beta particles [16]. Other isotopes include rhenium-188 (also a beta emitter) [17] and samarium-153, which is targeted to bone through chelation to ethylene diamine tetramethylene phosphonate (EDTMP) and is both a beta and gamma emitter [18]. All the radionuclides produce relief of bone pain in up to 80% of prostate cancer patients [19]. Generalized or multiple sites of bone pain are well-managed by these agents. It is perhaps unfortunate that the current practice of using docetaxel chemotherapy in refractory disease induces some reluctance to use these agents early because of the potential reduction in bone marrow reserve.

The publication of the preliminary results of a randomized phase II trial of radium-223 in prostate cancer [20] is a landmark event because of its demonstration of a clinically important prolongation of survival despite the study having predominantly palliative endpoints. The study was conducted in patients with castrate-resistant metastatic prostate cancer bone disease causing pain requiring radiotherapy, and patients were randomized between four intravenous injections of the isotope every 4 weeks or placebo. The primary endpoint of reduction in bony alkaline phosphatase showed a significant benefit to radium-223, with a non-significant reduction in skeletal-related events. Median overall survival, a secondary endpoint, was 65.3 weeks for radium-223 and 46.4 weeks for placebo, although the difference was not statistically significant. Time to PSA progression was significantly increased from 8 weeks to 26 weeks. The survival gain is markedly greater than is usually seen in clinical trials assessing the activity and benefit of new systemic agents for advanced disease, and the drug is well-tolerated. The place of this new agent in palliation is still in evolution, and reports of its potential efficacy continue [21].

Denosumab [22] is another novel systemic agent that is now available for the management of metastatic bone disease in castrate-resistant prostate cancer. It is a fully humanized monoclonal antibody to the RANK ligand, a molecule produced by osteoclasts which mediates bone resorption. Despite the dominance of sclerotic metastasis in prostate cancer, it is the underlying lytic component which is targeted by the drug. Administered subcutaneously once monthly, it is well-tolerated and reduces skeletal-related events (defined as pathologic fracture, the need for radiation therapy for bone pain, surgery for skeletal complications or spinal cord compression), with resulting improvements in quality of life, although it does not prolong survival.

Finally, while bony metastasis dominates the clinical picture in metastatic prostate cancer, relatively modest doses of palliative external beam radiation therapy (EBRT) (such as 20 Gy in 10 fractions) can be useful to palliate local symptoms from soft tissue metastasis.

Renal cancer

Despite the controversy over the radioresponsiveness of renal cancer, especially with small fraction sizes, worthwhile palliative responses to radiation therapy can be achieved in the metastatic setting using radiation doses which are similar to those known to be effective in other malignancies, such as 30 Gy in 10 fractions [23]. Debate continues as to the relative efficacies of single fractions (such as 8 Gy) and higher dose fractionated courses for relief of bone pain. Patient numbers for renal cancer in the randomized bone pain trials have been too low to be able to draw definitive conclusions, because of their relative scarcity compared with breast and prostate cancer patients.

The frequency with which solitary metastasis or oligometastases occur with renal cancer has led to the development of interest in using stereotactic radiosurgery or radiotherapy to deliver tumoricidal doses to metastatic disease with quasi-curative intent. Delivery of doses capable of sterilization of the target metastases rather than merely damping disease down may change the treatment philosophy of treating metastatic disease from palliation to long-term control or even cure. The considerations around the use of stereotactic techniques apply equally to the metastatic setting and for palliation and control of the primary disease. In particular, optimization of fractionation schedules to achieve the therapeutic aim in a cost-effective fashion is critical.

The promise of highly conformal therapy

With the development of stereotactic technology, the role of radiotherapy in treating inoperable primary renal cancers is being re-evaluated using hypo-fractionated schedules, which have not been feasible to date with standard external beam techniques because of the tolerance limits of adjacent normal structures. Several programs are in development, with early indications that effective palliation can be achieved using extreme hypo-fractionation schedules such as 39 Gy in 3 fractions [24] without prejudicing the integrity of the surrounding normal tissues.

As an example, one of the largest series was reported by Gilson *et al.* [25]. This publication described a cohort of 92 patients who had a total of 204 local and metastatic renal cell carcinoma lesions treated with stereotactic techniques, using a median dose of 40 Gy (12–60 Gy) and a median of 5 fractions (2 to 10 fractions). For metastatic lesions, early local control with a median follow-up just under a year was 87%. Perhaps more significant clinically was the local control rate of treated primary renal cell carcinoma lesions of 94% at 17 months mean follow-up. Other series [26] report hypofractionated dose schedules such as 32 Gy in 4 fractions, 45 Gy in 3 fractions, or 48 Gy in 6 fractions, or up to 30 Gy in a single fraction for stereotactic radiosurgery. The series from these expert institutions report very acceptable toxicity profiles, with no cases of grade 4 or grade 5 toxicities being noted. On this basis the therapeutic ratio of tumor control versus the morbidity of a palliative procedure appears highly acceptable.

The aim of these treatment approaches is somewhat different from the conventional interpretation of palliative treatments given to patients with limited prognoses. As such, the protection of normal tissues from the risk of late effects is paramount, and these techniques may prove to be pivotal in the provision of good quality of life and long survival.

One of the difficulties that faces us in disseminating this type of treatment more broadly is defining what the most appropriate and effective fractionation schedules should be, given the relatively extreme hypo-fractionation employed. Small variations in fraction size or total dose may significantly change the chances of local control or the development of toxicity. Many departments also face practical constraints for patient access, because of the complexity of the planning and treatment processes, the stringent quality assurance processes required, and the pressures of heavy caseloads requiring treatment, which might preclude using complex treatments for palliative patients.

Special considerations in developing countries

Not only is the incidence of certain diagnoses such as squamous cell carcinoma of the bladder more prevalent in countries where schistosomiasis prevails, so too is there variability in diagnostic and treatment capabilities of genitourinary cancers between different countries. Optimal palliation of all genitourinary cancers requires the availability of multi-disciplinary involvement, chemotherapy, adequate radiotherapy equipment, and radiopharmaceuticals, any of which may be in short supply in developing countries.

Conclusion

Genitourinary malignancies are a common and diverse group of cancers that require multi-disciplinary management of both local and metastatic manifestations of incurable disease. Radiotherapy effectively palliates many of the symptoms caused by this set of diseases, though the data sets that describe the proper fractionation schemes for several clinical scenarios are incomplete. The circumstances of treatment may differ greatly between developed and developing countries, with marked disparities in the availability of useful and technologically developed treatments.

References

1. Thursfield V, Farrugia H. Cancer in Victoria: statistics and trends 2010. 2011. Melbourne, Cancer Council Victoria.
2. Chia SE, Tan CS, Lim GH, *et al*. Incidence, mortality and five-year relative survival ratio of prostate cancer among Chinese residents in Singapore from 1968 to 2002 by metastatic staging. *Ann Acad Med Singapore* 2010; **39**: 466–471.
3. Nepple KG, Yang L, Grubb RL III, Strope SA. Population based analysis of the increasing incidence of kidney cancer in the United States: evaluation of age specific trends from 1975 to 2006. *J Urol* 2012; **187**: 32–38.
4. Sadler GM, Duchesne GM. Regression of lung metastases after local treatment of bone metastasis of renal adenocarcinoma. *Br J Urol* 1994; **73**: 714–715.
5. Duchesne GM, Bolger JJ, Griffiths GO, *et al*. A randomized trial of hypofractionated schedules of palliative radiotherapy in the management of bladder carcinoma: results of medical research council trial BA09. *Int J Radiat Oncol Biol Phys* 2000; **47**: 379–388.
6. Hindson B, Turner S, Do V. Palliative radiation therapy for localized prostate symptoms in hormone refractory prostate cancer. *Australas Radiol* 2007; **51**: 584–588.
7. Gogna NK, Baxi S, Hickey B, *et al*. Split-course, high-dose palliative pelvic radiotherapy for locally progressive hormone-refractory prostate cancer. *Int J Radiat Oncol Biol Phys* 2012; **83**: e205–e211.
8. Warde P, Mason M, Ding K, *et al*. Combined androgen deprivation therapy and radiation therapy for locally advanced prostate cancer: a randomised, phase 3 trial. *Lancet* 2011; **378**: 2104–2111.

9. Corcoran NM, Godoy G, Studd RC, *et al*. Salvage prostatectomy post-definitive radiation therapy: the Vancouver experience. *Can Urol Assoc J* 2012; **24**: 1–6.

10. Ahmed HU, Cathcart P, Chalasani V, *et al*. Whole-gland salvage high-intensity focused ultrasound therapy for localized prostate cancer recurrence after external beam radiation therapy. *Cancer* 2011; doi: 10.1002/cncr.26631.

11. Burri RJ, Stone NN, Unger P, Stock RG. Long-term outcome and toxicity of salvage brachytherapy for local failure after initial radiotherapy for prostate cancer. *Int J Radiat Oncol Biol Phys* 2010; **77**: 1338–1344.

12. Nguyen PL, Devlin PM, Beard CJ, *et al*. High-dose-rate brachytherapy for prostate cancer in a previously radiated patient with polyethylene glycol hydrogel spacing to reduce rectal dose: case report and review of the literature. *Brachytherapy* 2012; [Epub ahead of print]

13. Suarez C, Morales R, Munoz E, *et al*. Molecular basis for the treatment of renal cell carcinoma. *Clin Transl Oncol* 2010; **12**: 15–21.

14. Russo P, O'Brien MF. Surgical intervention in patients with metastatic renal cancer: metastasectomy and cytoreductive nephrectomy. *Urol Clin North Am* 2008; **35**: 679–686.

15. Venkatesan AM, Wood BJ, Gervais DA. Percutaneous ablation in the kidney. *Radiology* 2011; **261**: 375–391.

16. Robinson RG, Blake GM, Preston DF, *et al*. Strontium-89: treatment results and kinetics in patients with painful metastatic prostate and breast cancer in bone. *Radiographics* 1989; **9**: 271–281.

17. Liepe K, Kropp J, Runge R, Kotzerke J. Therapeutic efficiency of rhenium-188-HEDP in human prostate cancer skeletal metastases. *Br J Cancer* 2003; **89**: 625–629.

18. Resche I, Chatal JF, Pecking A, *et al*. A dose-controlled study of 153Sm-ethylene-diaminetetramethylenephosphonate (EDTMP) in the treatment of patients with painful bone metastases. *Eur J Cancer* 1997; **33**: 1583–1591.

19. Finlay IG, Mason MD, Shelley M. Radioisotopes for the palliation of metastatic bone cancer: a systematic review. *Lancet Oncol* 2005; **6**: 392–400.

20. Nilsson S, Franzen L, Parker C, *et al*. Bone-targeted radium-223 in symptomatic, hormone-refractory prostate cancer: a randomised, multicentre, placebo-controlled phase II study. *Lancet Oncol* 2007; **8**: 587–594.

21. Sartor A, Heinrich D, Helle S, *et al*. Radium-223 chloride impact on skeletal-related events in patients with castration-resistant prostate cancer (CRPC) with bone metastases: a phase III randomized trial (ALSYMPCA). *J Clin Oncol* 2012; **30**(Suppl 5; abstr 9).

22. Iranikhah M, Wilborn TW, Wensel TM, Ferrell JB. Denosumab for the prevention of skeletal-related events in patients with bone metastasis from solid tumor. *Pharmaco-therapy* 2012; **32**: 274–284.

23. Lee J, Hodgson D, Chow E, *et al*. A phase II trial of palliative radiotherapy for metastatic renal cell carcinoma. *Cancer* 2005; **104**: 1894–1900.

24. Kaplan I, Redrosa I, Martin C, *et al*. Results of a Phase I dose escalation study of stereotactic radiosurgery for primary renal tumours. *Int J Radiat Oncol Biol Phys* 2010; **78**(3S): S191.

25. Gilson B, Lederman G, Qian G, *et al*. Hypofractionated stereotactic extra-cranial radiosurgery (HFSR) for primary and metastatic renal cell carcinoma. *Int J Radiat Oncol Biol Phys* 2006; **66**(3S): S349.

26. Svedman C, Sandstrom P, Pisa P, *et al*. A prospective Phase II trial of using extracranial stereotactic radiotherapy in primary and metastatic renal cell carcinoma. *Acta Oncol* 2006; **45**: 870–875.

CHAPTER 17

Palliative radiotherapy in locally advanced and locally recurrent gynecologic cancer

Firuza Patel
Department of Radiotherapy and Oncology, Post Graduate Institute of Medical
Education and Research, Chandigarh, India

Introduction

Gynecologic cancers are a diverse group of malignancies with incidence and stage at presentation varying in different regions of the world. Uterine corpus and ovarian cancers are common in the developed world, while cancer of the cervix is more common in developing countries. In the United States it is estimated that in 2012 there will be 88,750 women who will suffer from gynecologic malignancies, resulting in 29,520 deaths. Uterine corpus is the most common site of origin, accounting for 53% of all gynecologic cancers, and they are followed in incidence by ovarian cancer and carcinoma of the cervix. However, deaths from ovarian cancer will be the highest of the three due to its propensity for late stage at presentation [1].

Patients with locally advanced or recurrent gynecologic malignances constitute a heterogeneous population with varied treatment options. In carcinoma of the cervix, stage IIB to IVA is defined as locally advanced disease. However, a majority of patients with Stage II and III disease are treated by radical radiotherapy with combination chemotherapy and can achieve a 5-year survival of 30–50% depending on primary tumor size and lymph node involvement. Given that patients with even relatively advanced disease may be treated with curative intent, the delivery of palliative intent only treatment is appropriate for a small subsection of the affected population. Hence, patients selected for palliative radiotherapy are:
- those with poor performance status or extreme old age who cannot tolerate a protracted treatment schedule
- those with very advanced loco-regional disease who would require radiation fields or total dose that would be poorly tolerated

Radiation Oncology in Palliative Cancer Care, First Edition. Edited by Stephen Lutz,
Edward Chow, and Peter Hoskin.
© 2013 John Wiley & Sons, Ltd. Published 2013 by John Wiley & Sons, Ltd.

- patients with distant metastatic spread, or
- patients with recurrent disease following previous treatment.

Patterns of loco-regional failures for gynecologic cancers

In cervical cancer, primary tumor stage and lymph node involvement are the most important prognostic factors for patients with non-metastatic disease. Approximately 35% of women with cervical cancer will suffer recurrence of their disease. A recurrence rate of 10–20% is reported following primary treatment for Stage IB and IIA tumors with no lymph node involvement, whereas 70% of patients with nodal metastasis and/or more advanced tumors will relapse [2]. As the bulk of pelvic tumor increases, so do the chances of having residual or recurrent disease in the pelvis following completion of therapy. Patients treated only with external beam radiation therapy (EBRT) and no brachytherapy are also more likely to fail locally. The omission of brachytherapy may result from patient wishes, lack of its availability in a specific geographic locale, or because of a belief on the part of the practitioner that its contributions may be negligible in controlling pelvic sidewall disease for patients with FIGO stage III tumors.

After definitive radical radiotherapy most regional recurrences occur within the first 2 years. The residual or recurrent disease may occur in-field, suggesting a deficiency in the dose, or there may be a marginal failure, suggesting a deficiency in target volume coverage. Another problem faced by geographic locales that do not have adequately trained manpower is that cancer patients are subjected to inadequate surgery in the form of a simple hysterectomy which only temporarily relieves the patients' symptoms. They then seek medical advice only when the symptoms recur, by which time the disease is often far advanced and suitable only for palliation.

Though endometrial carcinoma generally presents at an early stage, in developing countries it is not uncommon for patients to present with advanced disease. Women with a lack of cancer awareness may incorrectly attribute post-menopausal or irregular vaginal bleeding to normal circumstances of menopause, thereby leading those women to put off seeking medical advice. Undiscovered endometrial tumors may grow to a significant size before causing additional symptoms due to obstruction or direct bone invasion, leading these women to present with incurable disease.

Carcinoma of the vulva is a rare tumor and tends to spread locally before it metastasizes to distant organs. Its prognosis depends on stage of disease, lymph node involvement, and depth of invasion of the primary tumor. While tumor growth is often indolent, it is not uncommon for patients to present initially with a large local growth on the vulva with fixed or fungating inguinal nodes. Chances of local recurrence are high even after surgery, especially if the surgeon cannot achieve negative margins around the primary disease or complete dissection of involved inguinal lymph node regions.

Management

In the era of multi-modality treatment, a majority of cancer patients will require radiation at some point during the course of their disease. Yet, nearly 50% of all radiation delivered will be with a palliative intent. Radiation is one of the most valuable palliative tools available as it has a major role in symptom management. Palliative radiotherapy for an advanced loco-regional or recurrent gynecologic malignancy is a very small part of the total holistic management of a patient with advanced gynecologic malignancy. Optimum palliative care can only be provided by a team that may include a gynecologic oncologist, a radiation oncologist, an interventional radiologist, a palliative care physician, nurse, and a social worker to address the various problems faced by these patients.

Various symptoms with which a patient with advanced gynecologic malignancy may present are listed in Box 17.1. It is important to understand that radiation is a localized form of treatment and hence can only be used to relieve some of these symptoms. Palliative radiation can be employed for achieving hemostasis for patients with bleeding growths from the cervix or vagina. It is also useful for palliating fungating lymph nodes or cutaneous ulcers, either of which may respond after only a short course of radiation. Additional indications for palliative EBRT include relief from obstruction and pressure effects due to large pelvic masses as well as pain management due to direct extension or metastatic spread of tumor to pelvic bones (Figure 17.1).

Vaginal bleeding or discharge is the most common presenting symptom of advanced or recurrent gynecologic malignancy. Patients may initially ignore bleeding if it is minimal and potentially attributable to menses. However, direct invasion of blood vessels by tumor may come to cause massive bleeding. Initial management of pathologic vaginal bleeding requires a proper gynecologic examination and considerations of placement of tight vaginal

---

Box 17.1 Symptoms commonly associated with advanced gynecologic cancers

- Vaginal bleeding
- Foul smelling vaginal discharge
- Pain
- Fungation and ulceration
- Lower extremity edema
- Deep venous thrombosis (DVT)
- Urinary or bowel fistulas
- Dyspnea from pleural or pulmonary involvement
- Bowel obstruction
- Ascites

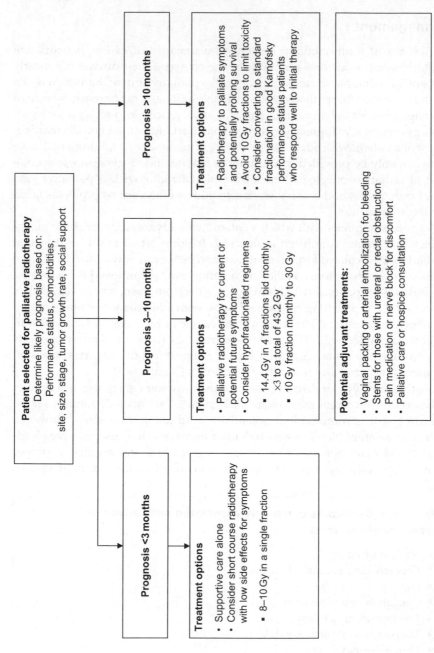

Figure 17.1 Algorithm for use of palliative radiotherapy for patients with gynecologic cancer.

packing with hemodynamic support. The packing should be left in place for 24–48 hours, though persistent bleeding may require urgent initiation of either EBRT or brachytherapy. Alternatively, an interventional radiologist may attempt to occlude the vessels that are supplying the anatomic sites of uncontrolled bleeding.

External radiation can be delivered using a cobalt machine or linear accelerator, and sophisticated equipment is not required as patients are treated to the whole pelvis using parallel opposed anterior and posterior fields or four-field box techniques. The upper border is generally placed at the L4-L5 interspace while the lower border is positioned either at the lower end of the obturator foramen or at least 2 cm below the most distal vaginal extension of the growth. When using a four-field technique, the anterior border of the lateral field is located anterior to the symphysis pubis while the posterior border should cover the entire sacrum to include disease which may be located in the sacral hollows. Alternatively, if available, virtual simulation using CT may be used to define simple palliative fields.

The optimal palliative dose and fractionation scheme cannot be established from the available literature. A systematic review only showed eight studies applicable to this circumstance, with all of them observational retrospective studies except for the results reported by the Radiation Therapy and Oncology (RTOG) group [3]. Treatment responses in all of these studies may be misleading as patients may not have finished treatment either because they had a good response following only part of the intended course or because they suffered deterioration due to progressive disease that did not allow them to continue the intended course. Treatment-related toxicities have been incompletely reported in these studies, and evaluation is made more difficult by the fact that symptoms of tumor progression (i.e. fistula formation) may mimic radiation side effects.

The results of some of the published studies are summarized in Table 17.1. Boulware *et al.* [4] reported the M.D. Anderson experience with advanced gynecologic malignancies that were treated between 1954 and 1975. They used a fraction size of 10 Gy to the whole pelvis which was then repeated after 3–4 week intervals for a maximum of 3 fractions. Out of 86 patients, the second fraction was received by 55 patients, and only 20 completed the third fraction. Vaginal bleeding was controlled in 45%, 85%, and 100%, while pelvic pain was palliated in 45%, 59%, and 63% of patients receiving 1, 2, or 3 fractions respectively. Of the 20 patients who were able to receive all 3 fractions, 50% had complete clinical tumor regression. The authors commented that the evaluation of long-term toxicity was limited due to the short survival of the treated patients. They noted 23 complications, describing 8 "minimal" reactions, 11 instances of fistula formation, and 4 more serious bowel injuries.

Hodson and Krepart [5] used a similar fractionation of 10 Gy repeated monthly to a total dose of 30 Gy for 27 patients with advanced gynecologic malignancies. Their results showed that the palliative response obtained was good with a consistent cessation of vaginal bleeding and relief of pelvic pain.

Table 17.1 Overview of selected studies, radiation schedule, symptom and tumor response.

Author & year of publication	Radiation dose (Gy) per fraction/No. of fractions	No. of patients	>50% improvement in symptoms			> 50% tumor response	Complications
			Bleeding No. (%)	Pain No. (%)	Obstruction No. (%)	No. (%)	
Boulware et al. 1979 [4]	10 Gy/1	86	39/86 (45)	14/31 (45)	4/17 (24)	16/86 (19)	23/86
	10 Gy/2	55	47/55 (85)	13/22 (59)	12/16 (75)	33/55 (60)	15 also had uncontrolled pelvic tumor
	10 Gy/3	20	20/20 (100)	5/8 (63)	3/4 (75)	17/20 (85)	
Hodson & Krepart 1983 [5]	10 Gy/3	27	22/22 (100)	4/4 (100)	1/1 (100)	17/19 (89)	3/19 chronic morbidity
Halle et al. 1986 [6]	10 Gy/1-3	42	27/30 (90)	4/9 (44)		15/28 (54)	5/42 (12%) 2 also had uncontrolled pelvic tumor
Spanos et al. 1989 [8]	3.7 Gy/4 in 2 days, 3 such cycles	136	71/73 (97)	44/65 (68)	14/16 (88)	41/136 (30) 40/92 (43) for patients receiving all 3 fractions	10/87 (12%) Gr-3 late morbidity
Mishra et al. 2005 [9]	10 Gy/1	100	(31)	(3)		24/70 (34)	10 patients had Grade 3–4 late morbidity
	10 Gy/2	61		(41)		28/45 (62)	
	10 Gy/3	33	(100)	(17)		25/33 (75)	

Although this therapy was planned for palliation and the median survival was 7 months, there was one long-term survivor at 35 months.

Halle *et al.* [6] reported on 42 patients with advanced gynecologic cancers between 1980 and 1986. They used a similar treatment schedule of 10 Gy repeated at regular intervals. Twenty-five patients received a single fraction, 15 received 2 fractions, and 2 patients received 2 fractions of 10 Gy and a third fraction of 7 Gy. Of the 30 patients who presented with bleeding, 18 (60%) had complete resolution of the problem and 9 (30%) had partial relief. However, only 8 (27%) remained permanently free from bleeding. Similarly 4 of 9 (44%) patients had partial or complete pain relief, but only one patient remained totally pain free until death. Five patients (12%) suffered serious complications, and in two of these patients uncontrolled pelvic tumor was documented as being a contributing factor. Four of the complications occurred 10 months or more after completion of treatment. Therefore, the authors concluded that only patients with a life expectancy of less than one year should be treated with 10 Gy per fraction protocol, as these patients will not live long enough to either get complications or recurrence of their symptoms.

On the basis of these trials the Radiation Therapy and Oncology Group initiated a Phase I/II study (RTOG 7905) using three fractions of 10 Gy each at monthly intervals given concurrently with the hypoxic cell radiosensitizer misonidazole at a dose of 4 gm/m^2, administered 4–6 hours prior to radiation [7]. The patient group consisted of those with locally advanced pelvic malignancies, including 20 with primary gynecologic cancer, 24 with colorectal cancer, and 2 with prostate malignancies. For the 37 patients who completed all 3 fractions, the overall response was 41% with a 16% complete response. The overall grade 3 to 4 gastrointestinal complication rate was 45%, with an 80% complication rate for those who had a complete tumor response. The severity of the complications also showed a progressive increase in incidence with longer survival. Due to this high toxicity, the subsequent RTOG studies omitted misonidazole and decreased the dose per fraction.

In the Phase II RTOG 8502 study, 4 fractions were planned over 2 days at a rate of 3.7 Gy per fraction given twice per day for a total of 1480 cGy per course. This course was repeated at 3–6 weeks interval for a total of 3 courses and a total potential dose of 4440 cGy [8]. This protocol was equally effective in palliation rates as the previous RTOG study with a 43% response rate for patients completing all three courses. However, this protocol reported a 12% incidence of late complications, which was markedly decreased when compared to the 45% incidence in the previous RTOG 7905 protocol. This study was continued as a Phase III trial which compared a 2 week rest to a 4 week rest without any obvious difference in response rates detected between the different intervals.

Mishra *et al.* [9] in a series of 100 patients also used 10 Gy per fraction to a maximum of 3 fractions. They reported a tumor response of 75% in patients who received all 3 fractions.

Therefore, a summary of the literature suggests that the most commonly described fractionation scheme for these patients is 10 Gy repeated at one month intervals to a total of 30 Gy as clinical circumstances dictate and tolerance of the dosing allows. Patients who receive all 3 fractions have superior outcomes compared to those who do not, though those with the longest survival often face a recurrence of their local symptoms and an increased incidence of severe toxicity. It is therefore prudent to consider a lower dose-per-fraction for patients who may survive 10 to 12 months, or longer.

Several single institution trials have also used palliative radiation for patients with symptomatic refractory ovarian cancers failing chemotherapy regimens who present with bleeding and pain. Adelson *et al.* [10] reported that the safest and most efficient dose may be one or two fractions of 10 Gy given at 4-weekly intervals. May *et al.* [11] investigated the use of different dose schedules varying from 1.8 to 3 Gy per day for up to 2 weeks versus a single 10 Gy fraction.

Most published studies on palliative radiotherapy have focused on pain and bleeding. Soft tissue masses causing lymphatic or bowel obstruction have been less commonly addressed. There are no randomized trials for gynecologic malignancies, but trials using different fractionation schemes have been performed for other primary sites such as urinary bladder and can be extrapolated to gynecologic patients. An international randomized clinical trial of bladder cancer compared 35 Gy in 10 fractions to 21 Gy in 3 fractions. There was no difference in overall symptomatic improvement (50% vs 53%), and survival was also similar following both the schedules [12]. Therefore, there is no evidence that better and longer palliation is achieved with a high dose of radiation delivered in multiple small fractions.

Treatment of recurrent carcinoma of the cervix

About 35% of patients treated for cervical cancer will develop recurrent disease, and about 60% of these patients will have a component of failure in the pelvis. Many reports have noted that about 80% of the recurrences occur within the first 2 years following treatment, but long-term failures after more than 5–10 years are also seen. The median survival after recurrence is considerably increased in patients who fail more than 36 months after initial treatment compared with those recurring before 36 months (22.5 months versus 3.8 months, respectively) [13].

Recurrence after definitive radiation

In patients who recur after previous irradiation, surgery in the form of radical hysterectomy or pelvic exenteration is a theoretical option. However, most of these patients are not suitable for this form of surgery, and the mortality and morbidity from this procedure is so high as to preclude its use as a palliative therapy. In addition to radiographic measurement of the extent of recurrent disease, the triad of unilateral leg edema, sciatic pain, and ureteral obstruction almost always indicates unresectable disease on the pelvic sidewall, therefore limiting treatment to palliative interventions. Patients with locally recurrent disease may suffer ureteral obstruction and present with uremia. Urinary diversion may be provided by placement of internal ureteral stents or percutaneous nephrostomy tubes, though the potential merits and drawbacks of these types of interventions need to be discussed with the patient and her family in settings where there are limited means by which to control the recurrent disease.

Re-irradiation may be considered for those who have failed previous radiotherapy courses, though this approach must be limited to those rare circumstances where the lesion causing symptoms is located outside of the high dose region of the previous radiotherapy and exists in a sufficiently small volume to justify the risks of additive doses between initial therapy and re-treatment.

Recurrence after definitive surgery

Radical radiation can salvage approximately 50% of patients with localized pelvic recurrences and no previous radiotherapy. External beam radiation to a dose of 40–50 Gy to the whole pelvis at 1.8–2 Gy per fraction can be delivered with a boost dose given by reduced field external radiation, or, preferably, brachytherapy in the form of either interstitial implant or vaginal cylinder. However, if there is extensive disease with involvement of the lateral pelvic wall, or if the patient has a poor performance status, palliative radiation should be chosen and delivered to 25–30 Gy in 10 fractions or, in patients with short life expectancy, a single fraction of 8–10 Gy delivered at an interval of 4 weeks for a maximum of 3 fractions.

The promise of newer technologies

Intensity modulated radiation therapy (IMRT), image guided radiation therapy (IGRT), sterotactic body radiation therapy (SBRT), and intraoperative radiotherapy (IORT) are newer techniques that are mainly used for radical treatment where the aim is either to increase the dose to the tumor or decrease the normal tissue complications. There is currently little justification for using these expensive modalities, which require extensive planning and longer time for execution, in a palliative care setting. As these newer technologies become more commonly available and data about their use accrue, they may become reasonable to use in settings where improved sparing of normal tissues such as small bowel is required to decrease toxicity risks to this patient group.

Special considerations in developing countries

Worldwide incidence and mortality rates for cervical cancer show a wide geographic variation. Cervical cancer was estimated to account for 8.8% of all new female cancers in 2008 [14]. It remains the most common cancer in women who reside in Eastern Africa, South Central Asia, and Melanesia. However, it is the third most common cancer in women worldwide, preceded only by breast and colorectal cancer. More than 85% of the global burden occurs in developing countries where it accounts for 13% of all female cancers.

Eighty-eight percent of all deaths due to cervical cancer occur in developing countries. The high mortality rates in these countries occur because the major-ity of the patients present for treatment at an advanced clinical stage due to a lack of effective screening programs, insufficient education, and limited awareness of cancer symptoms. There is also lack of access to available and affordable treatment facilities resulting either from poverty or from residing lengthy distances from cancer treatment facilities. Also, generally, the poor socio-economic conditions in these populations further add to the problem. Patients and families generally have to migrate and leave their homes and source of income to seek available treatment. This requirement puts the patient and family under tremendous financial and social stress, and it often serves as a reason for patients not to complete treatment or to forego therapy altogether. Therefore, all of these factors must be taken into account when planning palliative radiation for these patients.

In locales where a large patient load causes throughput issues, such as the tertiary care center where the author works, a single fraction is preferred to the 2-day schedule recommended by the RTOG trial because conventional radical treatment is delivered from Monday to Friday, and Saturday is reserved for palliative treatment. In an unpublished report, 72 patients with advanced cervical carcinoma and poor performance status were treated at our institute between 2006 and 2010 with 3 fractions of 8 Gy at an interval of 4 weeks. As patients come from far off distances, they were advised to come for the second fraction only if they had improvement in their symptoms or their general condition. Forty-six patients received a second fraction, while 38 received the third fraction. Out of the evaluable patients, only 19% had relief of bleeding after the first fraction, though after the second and third fractions hemostasis increased to 54% and 95%, respectively. Some patients whose tumor responded particularly well to the first fraction were then converted to conventional fractionation. Pain relief was noted in 24% and 58% of patients who received second and third fractions, respectively. Long-term toxicity in the form of Grade II proctitis was seen in only 2 patients. Median survival was 9 months, and 10 patients survived beyond one year. A single large fraction was gener-ally followed by acute radiation reactions in the form of vomiting and diarrhea, hence it is deemed important to explain this to the patients and to give them prophylactic treatment for the same.

Conclusion

Palliative radiotherapy may prove safe and effective for relief of pelvic symp-toms caused by locally advanced and recurrent gynecologic malignancies, including bleeding, pain, and ureteral or rectal obstruction. Still, the aim of palliative radiation should follow the principles of good palliative care where the goal of treatment should be to make the patient comfortable by effectively relieving the symptoms in the shortest possible time and most economical way. It is not always necessary to treat every patient with advanced disease, with "no treatment" often being a reasonable pathway for this group. It is well said that, "In oncology, young oncologists learn how to treat, experienced oncologists know when to treat, and mature oncologists know when not to treat."

References

1. Siegel R, Naishadham D, Jemal A. Cancer statistics, 2012. *CA Cancer J Clin* 2012; **62**: 10–29. doi: 10.3322/caac.20138.
2. Friedlander M, Grogan M. Guidelines for the treatment of recurrent and metastatic cervical cancer. *Oncologist* 2002; **7**: 342–347.
3. van Lonkhuijzen L, Thomas G. Palliative radiotherapy for cervical carcinoma, a systematic review. *Radiother Oncol* 2011; **98**: 287–291.
4. Boulware RJ, Caderao JB, Delclos L, et al. Whole pelvis megavoltage irradiation with single doses of 1000 rad to palliate advanced gynecologic cancers. *Int J Radiat Oncol Biol Phys* 1979; **5**: 333–338.
5. Hodson DI, Krepart GV. Once-monthly radiotherapy for the palliation of pelvic gynecological malignancy. *Gynecol Oncol* 1983; **16**: 112–116.
6. Halle JS, Rosenman JG, Varia MA, et al. 1000 cGy single dose palliation for advanced carcinoma of the cervix or endometrium. *Int J Radiat Oncol Biol Phys* 1986; **12**: 1947–1950.
7. Spanos W Jr, Wasserman T, Meoz R, et al. Palliation of advanced pelvic malignant disease with large fraction pelvic radiation and misonidazole final report of RTOG phase I/II study. *Int J Radiat Oncol Biol Phys* 1987; **13**: 1479–1482.
8. Spanos W Jr, Guse C, Perez C, et al. Phase II study of multiple daily fractionations in the palliation of advanced pelvic malignancies: preliminary report of RTOG 8502. *Int J Radiat Oncol Biol Phys* 1989; **17**: 659–661.
9. Mishra SK, Laskar S, Muckaden MA, et al. Monthly palliative pelvic radiotherapy in advanced carcinoma of uterine cervix. *J Cancer Res Ther* 2005; **1**: 208–212.
10. Adelson MD, Wharton JT, Delclos L, et al. Palliative radiotherapy for ovarian cancer. *Int J Radiat Oncol Biol Phys* 1987; **13**: 17–21.
11. May LF, Belinson JL, Roland TA. Palliative benefit of radiation therapy in advanced ovarian cancer. *Gynecol Oncol* 1990; **37**: 408–411.
12. Duchesne GM, Bolger JJ, Griffths T, et al. A randomized trial of hypofractionated schedules of palliative radiotherapy in the management of bladder carcinoma: results of medical research council trial BA09. *Int J Radiat Oncol Biol Phys* 2000; **47**: 379–388.
13. Sommers G, Grigsby PW, Perez CA, et al. Outcome of recurrent cervical carcinoma following definitive irradiation. *Gynecol Oncol* 1989; **35**: 150–155.
14. Ferlay J, Shin HR, Bray F, et al. GLOBOCAN 2008 v1.2, cancer incidence and mortality worldwide: IARC cancer base No. 10 [Internet]. Lyon, France: International Agency for Research on Cancer; 2010. Available at: http://globocan.iarc.fr (accessed February 29, 2012).

CHAPTER 18

Hematologic malignancies and associated conditions

David D. Howell
Department of Radiation Oncology, University of Toledo College of Medicine, Toledo, OH, USA

Introduction

Palliative radiation can be used to relieve active symptoms and to prevent impending problems caused by hematologic malignancies and lymphomas (Box 18.1). Palliative radiation should be delivered with the lowest reasonable dose over the shortest interval to respect the time of both patient and caregivers, and it should be combined with concurrent pharmacologic and non-pharmacologic supportive care measures to give the greatest relief in the shortest period of time for the affected individual. Hematologic malignancies are heterogeneous in their origins, and, as a consequence, different dose-fractionation schemes may be used for similar clinical conditions, depending on the histology and extent of the disease, as well as prior treatment (Figure 18.1). Hematologic malignancies uniformly require lower doses of radiation when compared with their solid tumor counterparts. Since the hematologic malignancies are, as a whole, very sensitive to the effects of cytotoxic systemic therapies, anti-neoplastic pharmacologic solutions and general supportive care should also be considered when faced with the need for symptom relief.

Diagnoses

Acute lymphoblastic leukemia (ALL) is a blood disorder characterized by the uncontrolled growth and proliferation of immature lymphoid cells. The diagnosis of ALL requires the presence of greater than 20% of bone marrow lymphoblasts on evaluation of the bone marrow. Initial treatment for ALL uses various forms of cytotoxic systemic chemotherapy, with the details of the agents and therapy schedule dependent upon the genetic characterization of the tumor cells, the extent of disease, and other patient-related factors.

Radiation Oncology in Palliative Cancer Care, First Edition. Edited by Stephen Lutz, Edward Chow, and Peter Hoskin.
© 2013 John Wiley & Sons, Ltd. Published 2013 by John Wiley & Sons, Ltd.

Box 18.1 Symptoms commonly associated with locally advanced hematologic malignancies, depending upon histology and location of the disease

- Pain
- Fatigue
- Anemia
- Dyspnea
- Urticaria
- Bleeding
- Anorexia
- Obstruction
- Constipation
- Early satiety
- Sweats and chills
- Organ dysfunction

Acute myelogenous leukemia (AML) is a series of blood disorders associated with a failure of certain myeloid stem cells to differentiate and to maintain an appropriate level of proliferation. This diminished regulation manifests as an accumulation of myeloblasts, with the diagnosis of AML defined by the presence of greater than 20% leukemic blasts in the bone marrow. As is true in the setting of ALL, the initial treatment for AML involves various forms of cytotoxic systemic chemotherapy, with the identity of those agents and the therapy schedule dependent upon several factors.

Chronic myelogenous leukemia (CML) is a hematopoietic stem cell disease that is associated with a genetic chromosomal translocation resulting in the formation of what is known as the "Philadelphia chromosome." The diagnosis of CML is made by evaluation of the peripheral blood and bone marrow, with identification of specific genetic, morphologic, and molecular characteristics of the abnormal blood elements. The initial treatment for CML uses medications from a class known as tyrosine kinase inhibitors.

Chronic lymphocytic leukemia (CLL) is a blood disorder characterized by a clonal expansion of small round mature appearing lymphocytes. Patients with this disorder often require no active therapy, though systemic treatments are generally indicated for symptomatic relief of difficulties such as fevers, night sweats, weight loss, or extreme fatigue. Additionally, severe anemia, thrombocytopenia, symptomatic lymphadenopathy, or splenomegaly may also be indications for the use of pharmacologic agents.

Non-Hodgkin lymphomas (NHL) are a class of lymphoproliferative disorders whose origins may arise either in B-lymphocytes (~80%) or T-lymphocytes (~20%). B-cell lymphoma disease categories include diffuse large B-cell

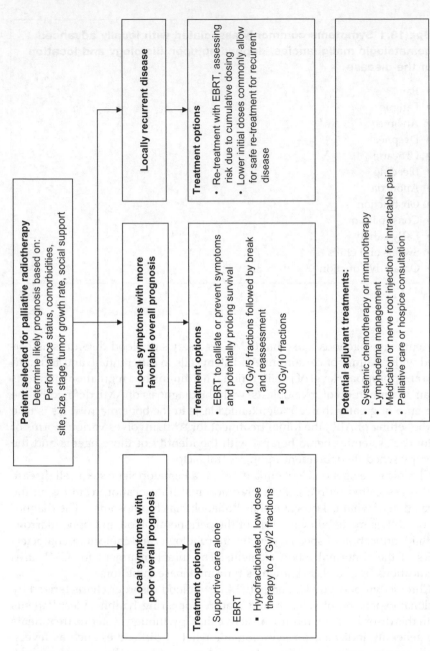

Figure 18.1 Algorithm for use of palliative radiotherapy for patients with hematologic cancer or lymphoma.

lymphoma (DLBCL), follicular lymphoma, mantle-cell lymphoma, lympho-plasmacytic lymphoma, mucosa-associated lymphatic tissue (MALT) lymphoma, and splenic marginal-zone lymphoma. These malignancies generally arise within nodal tissue, though they also may involve extra-nodal sites such as the stomach, orbit, parotid gland, and other anatomic locations. Several histologic classification schemes are commonly used to define NHL, but they can generally be divided into low grade and high grade histologies, which impact on management and prognosis. Treatment of NHL may include observation for low grade lymphomas as well as various cytotoxic systemic agents for both low grade and high grade disease.

Cutaneous lymphomas include mycosis fungoides and cutaneous T-Cell lymphomas. Each of these diagnoses may be treated with various local and systemic therapies at presentation, with radiation therapy utilized to treat symptomatic areas. Occasionally, total skin electron beam therapy may be utilized for areas of disease that are present in several sites over the integument [1–3].

Hodgkin lymphoma (HL) is a lymphoproliferative disorder characterized by the presence of the Reed-Sternberg (R-S) cell. Subtypes are classified by the morphology of the R-S cell as well as the milieu of the reactive cell infiltrate in the tissue around the R-S cells. HL generally arises in and remains within lymph node tissue. The staging of HL is guided by the extent of disease, number, and location of lymph node groups involved, and the presence of certain constitutional symptoms. The initial treatment for HL is cytotoxic systemic therapy, with radiation therapy used as an adjuvant treatment for consolidation of response, or more rarely as primary treatment for early stage disease.

Multiple myeloma (MM) is a hematopoietic disorder of plasma cells that produce a monoclonal protein. Extent of disease is measured by the concentration of the abnormal portion in blood serum, the percentage of bone marrow involvement, and related tissue and/or organ involvement. The initial treatment for MM ranges from observation alone in certain asymptomatic patients to the use of bisphosphonates, cytotoxic systemic therapies, and immunomodulatory drugs in those with symptoms or progressive disease. Radiation may be used as primary treatment in patients who have a solitary collection of abnormal plasma cells without evidence of systemic disease, otherwise known as a "plasmacytoma."

Other hematologic conditions that may require palliative radiation therapy as part of symptom management include polycythemia vera, myelodysplastic syndrome, and myelofibrosis.

Specific clinical circumstances

Large bulky lymph nodes
Symptomatic enlarged lymph nodes can occur in the setting of locally advanced or recurrent lymphomas. Symptoms may include local discomfort

or compressive symptoms due to compression on nerves, blood vessels, visceral organs, an airway, or gastrointestinal structures. The treatment of symptomatic lymph nodes depends on the histology and location of the mass, taking into account current difficulties as well as potential symptoms.

Patients with low grade NHL may develop symptomatic sites from time to time during their disease course. The decision to initiate radiation will depend on type and degree of symptoms experienced. Symptomatic lymph node or nodal aggregates due to low grade lymphomas generally show marked and durable reductions in bulk with the use of 4Gy prescribed to the nodal volume plus a small (e.g. 1–1.5 cm) margin in two 2Gy fractions delivered over 24 hours [4–9].

High grade NHL generally requires a higher total dose to achieve palliation than do low grade lymphomas. So, the high grade lymphomas usually receive total doses of 20 to 36Gy in 10–18 fractions to treatment volumes similar to those described for low grade lymphomas [10]. The radiation course is generally well-tolerated in these situations, though one may need to be mindful of the potential for the tumor lysis syndrome if the bulk of disease treated is substantial, adding allopurinol and maintaining adequate hydration as preventative measures. Alternative treatments for symptomatic lymph nodes in the patient with high-grade lymphoma may include either a hypofractionated scheme such as 30Gy in 10 fractions, 20Gy in 5 fractions, or a lower dose scheme of 10Gy in 5 fractions followed by a break to allow for assessment of treatment response. Single doses of 8–10Gy may also be considered.

Repeat courses of radiation can be delivered to the same volumes from time to time, depending on the total doses delivered to the area as well as the known normal tissue tolerances of adjacent organs.

Enlarged spleen

Symptomatic splenomegaly can occur in various hematologic conditions, including the myeloproliferative disorders such as chronic idiopathic myelofibrosis, CLL, and some of the B-cell and T-cell lymphomas [11]. Symptoms associated with a markedly enlarged spleen may include abdominal or epigastric discomfort or pain, early satiety, difficulty bending at the waist, dyspnea, left upper quadrant fullness, constipation, and others. Many patients with splenomegaly are concurrently noted to suffer anemia or other cytopenias. Options for treatment depend on the hematologic diagnosis, host factors, and prior therapy delivered. Frequently, cytotoxic systemic agents may be useful in this setting. Occasionally, surgical removal of the spleen (splenectomy) might be indicated, especially when patients are presumed to have a life expectancy of at least one year. Radiotherapy is generally utilized when various systemic therapeutic options have failed to control the disease and symptoms, or when performance status and patient prognosis are too limited to justify the risks of surgery.

Several authors [12–29] have outlined their experiences with palliative splenic radiation in an attempt to provide relief. Generally, very low total doses are needed to provide relief. Small fraction sizes should be used (e.g. 0.25 Gy, 0.5 Gy, or 1 Gy per fraction) to a volume that includes the whole spleen with a 1.5 cm margin. Treatment may be given on a two-times-per-week schedule, though some authors recommend delivering 5 fractions per week. It is recommended that patients have a complete blood count prior to each fraction being delivered because anemia and thrombocytopenia may present within a short time frame.

Some authors recommend a set course of treatment for symptomatic splenomegaly, while others monitor the patient's symptoms and radiation effects during treatment, stopping when symptoms have resolved, when the patient has reached an agreeable level of comfort, or when toxicity such as thrombocytopenia requires a break. Some advocate treating for a 2-week course, be it 4 or 10 fractions, considering the patient's clinical and hematopoietic tolerance during the course of treatment, suspending radiation for 1 or 2 weeks, then re-evaluating the patient for symptoms as well as spleen size prior to re-initiating treatment. Frequently, there can be a continued diminution in the bulk of the spleen during a treatment break, which may portend for cessation of radiation.

Also, an assessment of the patient's symptoms and physical examination, including palpation of the spleen, should precede each fraction in order that treatment may be suspended when the patient has achieved a reasonable level of comfort.

Patients are heterogeneous in their disease's response to radiation, as well as to the morbidity of treatment. Cytopenias and anemia are the side effects of greatest concern with splenic radiation, particularly in those with splenomegaly due to chronic idiopathic myelofibrosis, where the spleen serves as the primary extramedullary source of hematopoiesis. Creating a situation where there is too much devitalization of the blood forming elements can create a significant challenge with need for hematopoietic support.

Federico *et al.* [29] showed that for splenomegaly caused by myelofibrosis, a total dose of 1.8 Gy with a median dose of 0.3 Gy /fraction delivered 5 days a week was associated with a 91% reduction in the spleen size and 100% with relief in pain. Howell [28] has shown that a total spleen dose of 1.0–2.0 Gy delivered with 0.25 Gy fractions twice a week can have a 100% chance of reducing spleen size, with 100% relief of pain.

Chloromas (granulocytic sarcoma)

Chloroma is an extramedullary tumor of immature myeloid cells, frequently related to acute myeloid leukemia (AML) or myelodysplastic syndrome. Chloromas are also known as "granulocytic sarcomas." Common sites for chloromas presentation include soft tissue, skin, bone, and lymph nodes. Systemic therapy is generally used as part of treatment for the underlying conditions, though radiation can be used to treat symptomatic chloromas that may or may not be amenable to surgery. There is little in the literature on the use of radiation for chloroma, though the entity appears to be very radiosensitive [30–36]. Bakst *et al.* [30] describe only one local failure out of the patients reported, at a dose of 6 Gy, with over 80% of patients receiving a dose of at least 16 Gy.

Target volumes of the gross chloroma plus a 1 to 2 cm margin can be treated with 2 Gy fractions 5 days a week to a total dose of 10 to 24 Gy. Hypofractionated radiation may also be considered.

Osseous involvement by plasma cell malignancies

While treatment of symptomatic bone metastases is comprehensively addressed in Chapter 20, bone involvement by plasma cell tumors is a unique entity that requires special consideration. The classic treatment of solitary plasmacytoma of bone has ranged from 30 Gy to 50 Gy with various fractionation schemes, with good local control but frequently an unfortunate progression to multiple myeloma may be seen after an interval ranging from several months to 9 years or more.

The presence of plasma cell tumors in multiple skeletal sites defines the diagnosis of multiple myeloma, with radiotherapy playing an important part in the palliative relief of symptomatic lesions. Leigh *et al.* [37] reported on 101 patients treated for palliation of bone involvement by MM. In an analysis of over three hundred treatment courses, with a mean dose of 25 Gy ± 7 Gy, pain responses were complete in 26%, partial in 71%, and absent in only 3%. The rates of pain relief were not shown to increase with increasing total dose. A study by Mill and Griffith [38] showed only 4 pain relapses out of 75 patients who received 15 Gy or less using fraction sizes of 2 Gy or 3 Gy, while only 1 of 26 patients suffered recurrent pain when treated to a total dose of 10 Gy, or less.

Therefore, it would seem that a reasonable approach might be to treat the symptomatic area of bone with a dose of 10 to 15 Gy, using fractionated doses of 2 to 3 Gy, to a volume that encompasses the bone or the lesion with a 1 to 2 cm margin, then monitor for symptom relief and/or a reduced need for analgesics. Further radiation could be added after a suitable interval should symptoms persist.

Locally advanced and recurrent disease

Total body irradiation may be utilized as disease ablative therapy in certain clinical situations in ALL prior to bone marrow or stem cell transplant for rescue, though the other leukemias warrant different systemic therapy regimens prior to bone marrow/stem cell transplant rescue. Radiation to the cranial meningeal spaces may be used as consolidation treatment for certain leukemias. Systemic radiation therapy with radionuclides targeted to CD20 may be indicated for relapsed follicular lymphomas in certain situations [39].

Future directions

Research is ongoing into the use of systemic radionuclides in the treatment of relapsed follicular lymphomas or for diffuse marrow involvement. Given the relatively low doses of radiation used in the treatment of locally advanced hematopoietic disorders, issues about tolerance of adjacent avoidance structures and critical radiosensitive tissues are not as compelling as might be true for the palliative treatment of other categories of malignancy. However, normal tissue dose, and particularly critical tissue radiation tolerance, should always be considered.

Special considerations in developing countries

Most of the clinical situations that require palliative radiation of hematopoietic disorders can be addressed using simple conventional planning. In areas where computerized axial tomographic simulation is unavailable or inconvenient, clinical set ups can generally be employed to manage palpable lymph nodes, visible chloromas, or an enlarged spleen. It would be unusual to find a clinical situation where intensity modulated radiation therapy treatment planning and delivery techniques (or stereotactic radiation treatment planning and delivery) would be mandated or needed in these palliative situations.

Conclusion

Hematologic malignancies and lymphomas are a diverse group of diagnoses that can cause significant and varied symptoms. Radiation therapy can provide symptom relief for several of these circumstances, commonly with low total doses that can be delivered over a short period of time and with a low risk of side effects. The delivery of palliative radiotherapy for these patients should be evaluated in the larger context of patient performance status, overall prognosis, and the availability of useful systemic agents or simple methods for supportive care.

References

1. Funk A, Hensley F, Krempien R, et al. Palliative total skin electron beam therapy (TSEBT) for advanced cutaneous T-cell lymphoma. Eur J Dermatol 2008; **18**: 308–312.
2. Cotter GW, Baglan RJ, Wasserman TH, et al. Palliative radiation treatment of cutaneous mycosis fungoides – a dose response. Int J Radiat Oncol Biol Phys 1983; **9**: 1477–1480.
3. Neelis KJ, Schimmel EC, Vermeer MH, et al. Low-dose palliative radiotherapy for cutaneous B- and T-cell lymphomas. Int J Radiat Oncol Biol Phys 2009; **74**: 154–158.
4. Chan EK, Fung S, Gospodarowicz M, et al. Palliation by low-dose local radiation therapy for indolent non-Hodgkin lymphoma. Int J Radiat Oncol Biol Phys 2011; **81**: 781–786.
5. Luthy SK, Ng AK, Silver B, et al. Response to low-dose involved-field radiotherapy in patients with non-Hodgkin's lymphoma. Ann Oncol 2008; **19**: 2043–2047.
6. Hoskin P. Reduced dose radiotherapy for local control in non-Hodgkin lymphoma: a randomised phase III trial. Radiother Oncol 2011; **100**: 86–92.
7. Haas RL. Low dose radiotherapy in indolent lymphomas, enough is enough. Hematol Oncol 2009; **27**: 71–81.

8. Martin NE, Ng AK. Good things come in small packages: low-dose radiation as palliation for indolent non-Hodgkin lymphomas. *Leuk Lymphoma* 2009; **50**: 1765–1772.

9. Ng M, Wirth A, Ryan G, *et al.* Value of low-dose 2 × 2 Gy palliative radiotherapy in advanced low-grade non-Hodgkin's lymphoma. *Australas Radiol* 2006; **50**: 222–227.

10. NCCN Guidelines. Non-Hodgkin's lymphoma: principles of radiation therapy. 2012. Available at: http://www.nccn.org/professionals/physician_gls/pdf/nhl.pdf (accessed June 18, 2012).

11. Abramson JS, Chatterji M, Rahemtullah A. Case 39-2008. A 51-year-old woman with splenomegaly and anemia. *N Engl J Med* 2008; **359**: 2707–2718.

12. Osorio JI, Watkins JM, Strange C, *et al.* Radiation therapy for palliation of Eisenmenger's syndrome-associated painful splenomegaly. *Radiat Med* 2008; **26**: 84–87.

13. Weinmann M, Becker G, Einsele H, *et al.* Clinical indications and biological mechanisms of splenic irradiation in chronic leukaemias and myeloproliferative disorders. *Radiother Oncol* 2001; **58**: 235–246.

14. Elliott MA, Chen MG, Silverstein MN, *et al.* Splenic irradiation for symptomatic splenomegaly associated with myelofibrosis with myeloid metaplasia. *Br J Haematol* 1998; **103**: 505–511.

15. Shrimali RK, Correa PD, O'Rourke N. Low-dose palliative splenic irradiation in haematolymphoid malignancy. *J Med Imaging Radiat Oncol* 2008; **52**: 297–302.

16. Lavrenkov K, Krepel-Volsky S, Levi I, *et al.* Low dose palliative radiotherapy for splenomegaly in hematologic disorders. *Leuk Lymphoma* 2012; **53**: 430–434.

17. Mesa RA. How I treat symptomatic splenomegaly in patients with myelofibrosis. *Blood* 2009; **113**: 5394–5400.

18. McFarland JT, Kuzma C, Millard FE, *et al.* Palliative irradiation of the spleen. *Am J Clin Oncol* 2003; **26**: 178–183.

19. Paulino AC, Reddy SP. Splenic irradiation in the palliation of patients with lymphoproliferative and myeloproliferative disorders. *Am J Hosp Palliat Care* 1996; **13**: 32–35.

20. Bouabdallah R, Coso D, Gonzague-Casabianca L, *et al.* Safety and efficacy of splenic irradiation in the treatment of patients with idiopathic myelofibrosis: a report on 15 patients. *Leuk Res* 2000; **24**: 491–495.

21. Wagner H Jr, McKeough PG, Desforges J, *et al.* Splenic irradiation in the treatment of patients with chronic myelogenous leukemia or myelofibrosis with myeloid metaplasia. Results of daily and intermittent fractionation with and without concomitant hydroxyurea. *Cancer* 1986; **58**: 1204–1207.

22. Silverstein MN. Control of hypersplenism and painful splenomegaly in myeloid metaplasia by irradiation. *Int J Radiat Oncol Biol Phys* 1977; **2**: 1221–1222.

23. Pardanani A, Brown P, Neben-Wittich M, *et al.* Effective management of accelerated phase myelofibrosis with low-dose splenic radiotherapy. *Am J Hematol* 2010; **85**: 715–716.

24. Greenberger JS, Chaffey JT, Rosenthal DS, *et al.* Irradiation for control of hypersplenism and painful splenomegaly in myeloid metaplasia. *Int J Radiat Oncol Biol Phys* 1977; **2**: 1083–1090.

25. Slanina J, Vondraczek A, Wannenmacher M. Symptomatic irradiation therapy of the spleen in advanced osteomyelosclerosis. *Dtsch Med Wochenschr* 1986; **111**: 1144–1150 [Article in German].

26. Kriz J, Micke O, Bruns F, *et al.* Radiotherapy of splenomegaly: a palliative treatment option for a benign phenomenon in malignant diseases. *Strahlenther Onkol* 2011; **187**: 221–224.

27. Montemagge P, Federico M, Guerrieri P, *et al*. Splenic Irradiation (SI) in Myelofibrosis: Outcome and Toxicity of Three Radiation Schedules. Abstract 2724. Proceedings of the 50th Annual ASTRO meeting September 2008, Boston, MA. Proceedings ASTRO. IJROBP 2008.

28. Howell DD. Radiation Therapy in the Treatment of Symptomatic Splenomegaly. Proceedings of The 2nd Sino-American Network Therapeutic Radiation Oncology Meeting. Hangzhou, Zhejiang, China. October, 2010.

29. Federico M, Pagnucco G, Russo A, *et al*. Palliative splenic irradiation in primary and post PV/ET myelofibrosis: outcomes and toxicity of three radiation schedules. *Hematol Rev* 2009; **1**: e7.

30. Bakst R, Wolden S, Yahalom J. Radiation therapy for chloroma (granulocytic sarcoma). *Int J Radiat Oncol Biol Phys* 2012; **82**: 1816–1822.

31. Bakst RL, Tallman MS, Douer D, *et al*. How I treat extramedullary acute myeloid leukemia. *Blood* 2011; **118**: 3785–3793.

32. Shah DK, Goldwein J, Uri A, *et al*. Granulocytic sarcoma. *Med Pediatr Oncol* 1996; **27**: 132–137.

33. Paydas S, Zorludemir S, Ergin M. Granulocytic sarcoma: 32 cases and review of the literature. *Leuk Lymphoma* 2006; **47**: 2527–2541.

34. Lan TY, Lin DT, Tien HF, *et al*. Prognostic factors of treatment outcomes in patients with granulocytic sarcoma. *Acta Haematol* 2009; **122**: 238–246.

35. Landis DM, Aboulafia DM. Granulocytic sarcoma: an unusual complication of aleukemic myeloid leukemia causing spinal cord compression. A case report and literature review. *Leuk Lymphoma* 2003; **44**: 1753–1760.

36. Chak LY, Sapozink MD, Cox RS. Extramedullary lesions in non-lymphocytic leukemia: results of radiation therapy. *Int J Radiat Oncol Biol Phys* 1983; **9**: 1173–1176.

37. Leigh BR, Kurtts TA, Mack CF, *et al*. Radiation therapy for the palliation of multiple myeloma. *Int J Radiat Oncol Biol Phys* 1993; **25**: 801–804.

38. Mill WB, Griffith R. The role of radiation therapy in the management of plasma cell tumors. *Cancer* 1980; **45**: 647–652.

39. Macklis RM, Pohlman B. Radioimmunotherapy for non-Hodgkin's lymphoma: a review for radiation oncologists. *Int J Radiat Oncol Biol Phys* 2006; **66**: 833–841.

CHAPTER 19

Pediatric palliative radiation oncology

Tamara Vern-Gross
Department of Radiation Oncology, Wake Forest Baptist Health, Winston-Salem, NC, USA

Introduction

Approximately 25% of children diagnosed with cancer will die of their disease, making it the leading cause of non-accidental death in children [1,2]. A 2002 Surveillance Epidemiology and End Results (SEER) review (National Cancer Institute) demonstrated that there were 16.1 new cases of childhood cancers per million each year throughout the world [3]. Palliative care has gained prominence in Pediatrics, emphasizing quality of life, minimizing suffering, optimizing function, and providing opportunities for spiritual, psychosocial, and personal growth [4]. According to the World Health Organization (WHO), Pediatric Palliative Care (PPC) is "the active total care of the child's body, mind, and spirit, and also involves giving support to the family. PPC begins when illness is diagnosed and continues regardless of whether or not a child receives treatment directed at the disease [5]."

Palliative radiotherapy (RT) is often an important adjunctive treatment in the palliative care of a cancer patient. Because of the overwhelming intent to cure in children diagnosed with cancer, palliation to promote comfort for a child often receives less precedence than care aimed at extension of life. On presentation, or throughout the course of their disease, children may develop local symptoms caused by malignant tumor or metastases and may benefit from palliative radiotherapy (Box 19.1). Radiation may also be administered more as a "presumptive palliation" where there is high risk of developing fracture, cord compression, airway obstruction or superior vena cava syndrome (SVCS). Several radiobiologic principles may be less relevant in the application of palliative RT, and treatment should not be longer than necessary to achieve the therapeutic goal, especially in a child who requires daily sedation. The use of lower than definitive doses minimizes the risk of developing acute toxicities such as mucositis, which can have a significant impact on the quality of life of someone who does not have a long life expectancy.

Radiation Oncology in Palliative Cancer Care, First Edition. Edited by Stephen Lutz, Edward Chow, and Peter Hoskin.
© 2013 John Wiley & Sons, Ltd. Published 2013 by John Wiley & Sons, Ltd.

Box 19.1 Symptoms commonly associated with childhood cancers

- Pain from bone or soft tissue metastases causing tissue or nerve root infiltration
- Fungating or ulcerating tumor lesions
- Impending or actual airway obstruction
- Oncologic emergencies including spinal cord compression
- Superior vena cava syndrome and superior mediastinal syndrome
- Obstruction of stomach, gastrointestinal tract, or bladder
- Bleeding in the form of hemoptysis, gastric bleeding, or rectal/vaginal bleeding
- Liver metastases causing pain or decreased infra-diaphragmatic excursion
- Cranial nerve palsies or increased intracranial pressure from brain or leptomeningeal metastases

---

The true number of pediatric cases treated predominately with palliative intent is probably underestimated, given that tumors may be treated with definitive doses to maximize durability of response. For instance, in the setting of recurrent oligometastatic Ewing sarcoma (EWS), a painful metastatic pelvic lesion may be treated to a dose as high as 55.8 Gy. In universally fatal cases such as diffuse infiltrative pontine glioma (DIPG), patients are still offered definitive radiotherapy for palliation of symptoms and hopes of life prolongation. There is no accepted dose that should be prescribed when treating a child with palliative RT. Treatment decisions must be carefully individualized depending on tumor diagnosis, prognosis, patient age, symptoms, and patient/family goals.

Delivery of radiation treatment

Educating the patient and family during the treatment process is important to help them feel familiar and comfortable with the planning and treatment process. Having educational resources available including reading material and video demonstrations of the radiation simulation and treatment may help the child/adolescent and parents feel at ease. Child life therapists are also a beneficial resource to help introduce the child to the CT simulation room, to familiarize them with any set-up material that will be required, and to coach them on exercises or play therapy to help them feel more comfortable with the experience. The child's needs are often determined by patient age, with anesthesia recommended for younger children in order to prevent movement, prevent unnecessary fear, and optimize safety. Whenever possible, the child should be given the decision about whether to have treatment without sedation, both to give them some control over their medical decisions and to help them feel more comfortable with the people caring for them.

Differences between pediatric and adult populations

Approximately half of the population diagnosed with a malignant disease will receive radiation therapy at some time, with only a small percentage of these patients being pediatric [6–8]. Several differences exist between adult and pediatric population including the types of malignancies, disease presentation, response to intervention, and treatment options. For example, adult spinal cord compression (SCC) is most often caused by lung, breast, and prostate primary tumors or metastases [9,10], whereas in children sarcomas are seen in approximately 43 to 65% of cases [11,12]. In the SCC setting, the central nervous system (CNS) can be more forgiving in the pediatric population. Adults who are non-ambulatory at presentation rarely regain function [13,14], while approximately 50% of paraplegic children become ambulatory with appropriate therapy when presenting with symptoms of SCC [15–17].

If a child presents with compressive symptoms without pathologic diagnosis, tissue should be obtained to diagnose the primary malignancy to help differentiate which children may be treated with curative intent. For instance, an adolescent male presenting with obstructive mediastinal mass secondary to a primary Hodgkin lymphoma would require different treatment than a patient with metastatic seminoma. Oncologic emergencies such as SVCS and SCC tend to manifest earlier in the course of disease in children compared to adults, and they may be the presenting symptoms [11,18].

The implications of pain have also been shown to be different in adult and children. One institutional experience noted that refractory pain is often an indication for urgent palliative RT in children, compared to the situation in adults where opioid analgesic usage more commonly precedes palliative RT [19]. Although most long-term toxicities are less relevant when life expectancy is limited, both acute and long-term toxicity risks must match the care goals of the child and patient when long-term survival remains a possibility. Additionally, the risks of radiotherapy-induced acute toxicities such as bone marrow depression must be communicated effectively to the primary medical Pediatric Oncologist to ensure that the child does not become excluded from considerations of phase I clinical trials due to those side effects.

Background

Given that children are often more sensitive to the effects of surgery, chemotherapy, and radiotherapy, treatment must be carefully chosen to minimize long-term toxicities including decreased stature. Radiation therapy and chemotherapy have demonstrated effectiveness for many pediatric tumors, even in the absence of surgery [20–24]. Chemotherapy-sensitive tumors include neuroblastoma, Ewing sarcoma, and lymphoma, so systemic treatment would be the first therapy chosen in patients who present without paraplegia or progressive neurologic impairment [25]. Hodgkin disease is treated by chemotherapy with or without radiotherapy [26].

The prognosis of children suffering from metastatic disease is quite poor, and the development of effective palliative interventions for these patients is limited [27]. The use of palliative RT is often extrapolated from the adult series. There have been no prospective trials evaluating the role of palliative RT in the pediatric population. Although small published series have demonstrated the effectiveness of palliative RT for bone, mediastinum, brain, liver, and painful soft-tissue sites, literature supporting the use of palliative RT for symptom management in the pediatric population is sparse. One of the largest pediatric series comes from the University of Pennsylvania, where 104 children were referred requiring urgent treatment [19]. A total of 115 problems were identified and categorized into five groups: spinal cord, mediastinum, abdomen, brain, and pain (Table 19.1). Forty-five of the problems led to the diagnosis of cancer, and the remaining 70 were relapses of previously known disease. Central nervous system primitive neuroectodermal tumors (PNET), gliomas, and astrocytomas accounted for 20% of the referrals. Neuroblastomas accounted for an additional 20% of referrals. Treatment doses ranged from 1.5 to 4.0 Gy per fraction to total doses ranging from 3.0 to 55.8 Gy. When

Table 19.1 Radiation outcomes of children treated with urgent irradiation.

Group	Site Treated	Number of Patients	Presenting Symptom	Outcomes
I	Spinal cord compression	N = 33	Neurologic symptoms (N = 20)	55% Improvement
			Pain (N = 13)	30% Stabilization
II	Respiratory compromise	N = 18	Thoracic disease (N = 14)	72% Response rate
			Abdominal tumor (N = 5)	
III	Abdominal compromise	N = 8	Renal dysfunction from leukemia (N = 1)	66% Response rate
			Gastrointestinal obstruction (N = 3)	
			Splenomegaly (N = 1)	
			Pain from peritoneal seeding (N = 1)	
			Ureteral obstruction (N = 1)	
IV	Intracranial problems	N = 16	Cranial nerve palsies (N = 10)	63% Response rate
			Respiratory Failure/Obtundation (N = 5)	19% Stabilization
V	Intractable pain	N = 15	Bone metastases (N = 10)	93% Response rate
			Lymph node (N = 4)	

Modified from reference [19]

treated for leukemias and lymphomas, doses in the ranges of 2.2–22.5 Gy were utilized. Of 91 episodes treated, 80% achieved stabilization or improvement, especially for relief of spinal cord compression and pain. Conformal radiotherapeutic techniques were used in order to optimize dose to tumor burden and minimize unnecessary dose to surrounding structures [28].

Clinical indications for palliative radiotherapy

Superior vena cava syndrome and superior mediastinal syndrome

Radiotherapy can have a valuable role in dyspnea secondary to malignant chest disease causing obstruction of the major airways or vessels (Figure 19.1). SVCS was first described as a clinical diagnosis by William Hunter in 1757 [29]. Obstruction from a mediastinal mass causing airway compromise or SVCS is rare in pediatrics, but it can appear at presentation in approximately 12% of pediatric patients with malignant mediastinal tumors [30]. Pediatric SVCS occurs most commonly with T-cell acute lymphoblastic leukemia or Non-Hodgkin lymphoma (NHL), whereas in adults it is more likely a result of lung cancer [31]. While NHL is the leading primary cause of SVCS in children, it occurs in only approximately 6% of children diagnosed with this malignancy [32].

Children have a more compressible trachea than adults, so the presence of a mediastinal mass may cause tracheal compression or "superior mediastinal syndrome" (SMS), which is almost indistinguishable from SVCS in the younger age group [33,34]. Clinical features include headache, tracheal edema, chest pain, cough, hoarseness, respiratory difficulty, swelling of face, neck, arms, and hands, and dizziness. Other less common symptoms of SVCS include syncope, anxiety, confusion, headache, vision problems, and fullness in the ears [33].

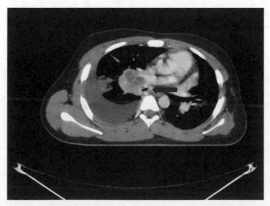

Figure 19.1 16-year-old male with metastatic Ewing sarcoma presenting with obstructive right lung lesion causing dyspnea. He was treated palliatively with 21 Gy in 7 fractions AP/PA followed by 9 Gy in 3 fractions off cord oblique with complete response.

Box 19.2 Differential diagnosis of anterior mediastinal mass in children and adolescents

	Condition
Benign Conditions	Cystic hygroma
	Thymoma
	Tubercular mediastinitis
	Histoplasma capsulatum infection
	Mediastinal abscess or granuloma
	Congenital heart disease and cardiovascular surgery
	Hydrocephalus
	Thrombosis of superior Vena Cava
	Ventriculoatrial shunt for hydrocephalus
Malignant Conditions	Hodgkin lymphoma
	Non-Hodgkin lymphoma
	Acute lymphoblastic leukemia
	Acute non-lymphocytic leukemia
	Neuroblastoma
	Germ cell tumor
	Malignant teratoma
	Osteosarcoma
	Rhabdomyosarcoma
	Ewing sarcoma
	Malignant degeneration of bronchogenic cyst

Tabulated from information available in references [25,26,40–56,63]

Complete history/physical examination and tissue diagnosis is essential in a child presenting with SVCS or SMS, especially since an anterior mediastinal mass may result from either benign or malignant causes (Box 19.2). If a tissue diagnosis cannot be established, urgent radiation may be considered for 2 or 3 fractions to achieve stabilization of the mass and permit initiation of systemic therapy. Unfortunately, in many cases, tissue diagnosis may be unattainable because of anesthesia risk, lack of marrow involvement, or absence of peripheral lymphadenopathy. Radiation is a reasonable treatment option in the emergency setting; however, pre-biopsy radiation therapy may hinder results on subsequent pathologic diagnosis. Loeffler and colleagues reported that 8 of 19 patients who received RT prior to tissue diagnosis were subsequently found to have specimens that were uninterpretable [34].

Extra caution should be used for patients with an anterior mediastinal mass, anticipating potential events that may occur during general anesthesia including airway obstruction and major vessel compression. In situations where radiotherapy is not efficacious, a stent should be considered and indwelling vascular catheters should be removed to diminish the risk of active thrombus. Also, a course of dexamethasone may help alleviate short-term symptoms, particularly in children in whom thoracic symptoms occur late in the course of their disease. However, steroid use in the initial presentation of an undiagnosed malignancy may compromise the diagnosis if the mass is a lymphoma or leukemia [35]. Induction anesthesia should always be approached with caution in this patient population, even in children that present with minimal symptoms such as cough or dyspnea worsening in the supine position. Venous access should be secured in the lower extremity to minimize the risk of complications related to complete SVC obstruction [34,36,37]. In situations where cardiac compromise is present in a patient planned for a cervical lymph node biopsy, anesthesia should be considered in the sitting position [36,38].

Prognostication is a key element when evaluating a child who presents with SVCS. Discussions with the patient and/or their parents are critical in the setting of a new diagnosis or in the setting of recurrent tumor. A St. Jude Children's Research Hospital review of children treated from 1973–1988 described 16 patients who presented initially with SVCS [39]. The median age of patients was 11.5 years (range 1.5–19.4 years), with NHL (all T-cell immunophenotype) being the most frequent malignancy followed by ALL, Hodgkin disease (HD), neuroblastoma, and yolk sac tumor. Median survival time was 92 months (range 5–164 months). Eleven patients presented with SVCS as a late complication during their treatment course: 3 patients (2 with NHL and 1 with HD) had recurrences of their initial mass, and 8 patients (2 with rhabdomyosarcoma, 1 with osteosarcoma, 2 with neuroblastoma) had late initial presentations, 3 of whom (2 with ALL, and 1 with malignant teratoma) were as a result of thrombus formation associated with therapy or tumor hypercoagulability states. Median age for these patients was 11 years, with a range of 8 months to 16 years. Median time to development of SVCS from initial diagnosis with recurrent solid tumors was 10 months (range, 2–15 months). In 5 patients that developed recurrent mediastinal disease, survival was limited, ranging from 2 to 20 weeks despite aggressive salvage treatments.

SVCS and SMS can be treated either with conventional field arrangements or with a more conformal approach such as stereotactic body radiation therapy (SBRT) in an effort to optimize dose to the target volume while minimizing toxicities such as pneumonitis. Although data regarding the use of SBRT in this setting are limited, it may theoretically be a reasonable approach if it safely allows for hypofractionated regimens which minimize the number of treatments and ultimately the number of times a child undergoes anesthesia.

Bone and soft tissue metastases

Palliative RT is effective when bone pain is caused by localized metastatic disease. Even in radioresistant tumors, such as osteosarcoma, a small reduction in size of a lesion can have a significant impact on pain management. The need for palliative RT is commonly seen with Ewing sarcoma, osteosarcoma, neuroblastoma, and rhabdomyosarcoma (Figure 19.2). An older child

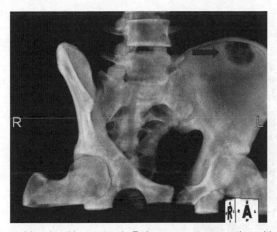

Figure 19.2 16-year-old male with metastatic Ewing sarcoma presenting with pain involving his left hip. He received palliative radiotherapy to the lytic lesion involving the left iliac wing, 30 Gy in 10 fractions with complete resolution of symptoms.

is often able to describe areas of discomfort and to detail the subsequent effective palliation of symptoms. In younger children, treatment decisions will require clinical, radiographic, and parental assessments to make the appropriate correlations. Fractionation schemes are extrapolated from adult literature, including the Radiation Therapy and Oncology Group 9714 trial, the Dutch Bone Metastasis Study, and the Bone Pain Trial Working Party Study [6–8]. Bone metastasis fractionation schemes have not been well-studied in pediatric populations, with most reports having come from single institutions.

Deutsch and Tersak [39] reported their experience at the University of Pittsburgh treating 37 children with RT for symptomatic bone metastases from non-leukemic/lymphomatous primary tumors. The interval from diagnosis of the primary tumor to the first RT treatment for symptomatic metastases ranged from 0 to 163 months (median of 19 months). The most common tumors included neuroblastoma (18), Ewing (5), osteosarcoma (5), squamous cell carcinoma of the lung (2), followed by Wilms tumor, retinoblastoma, medulloblastoma, angiosarcoma, rectal adenocarcinoma, nasopharyngeal, and esthesioneuroblastoma. Of 150 radiotherapy courses, the most common sites treated included the skull (40.5%), hip/femur (43.2%), spine (43.2%), humerus/shoulder (32.4%), and pelvis (29.7%). Younger children were more likely to get fewer fractions if they had difficulty remaining immobilized, if they experienced significant discomfort of daily visits (particularly if travel required long journeys on the road), or if they had rapidly deteriorating clinical conditions with disseminated disease. Prolonged courses were administered to children likely to have a survival of at least several months, with a single fraction or with schedules of 8–10 fractions.

The most common fractionation schedule in this report was a single dose ranging from 3 Gy to 10 Gy (43 courses), followed by 2 fractions and 5

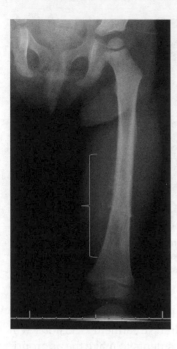

Figure 19.3 2-year-old female with metastatic neuroblastoma presenting with lower extremity swelling. Plain films demonstrate periosteal deposition extending from the proximal third to the distal third of the left femur with extensive soft tissue swelling. She was treated with single fraction 800 cGy × 1 fraction because of sedation requirements.

fractions (22 and 23 courses, respectively). A total of 59 courses in 18 children could be evaluated for response, with 55 of 59 courses producing a rapid relief of pain. Only 10 of the 150 courses administered were delivered in 10 or more fractions. Median survival was 4 months (range 1 to 52 months), with only 11 (29.7%) of the children surviving ≥ 12 months.

For patients who have achieved previous alleviation of symptomatic metastases with palliative RT, repeat treatment may be indicated, especially in the event of intractable or recurrent symptoms [40]. Children may benefit from a shorter course of palliative RT consisting of 1–5 fractions. Single fractionation, such as 800 cGy × 1 fraction is commonly used (Figure 19.3). Single dose treatments tend to be more convenient for the child and family, especially if daily anesthesia is required or if the child has difficulty holding still.

Ewing sarcoma

Not only can radiotherapy palliate symptoms due to bone metastases from Ewing sarcoma, it can also be delivered to definitive doses and provide a chance for cure in some cases of metastatic disease. When treatment is given with curative intent to patients with metastatic Ewing sarcoma, chemotherapy is followed by RT to all gross residual bone tumors with the dose dependent upon the size of gross residual disease [40,41].

Overall, Ewing sarcoma metastasizes to bone, lungs, and bone marrow in approximately 20–25% of patients at the time diagnosis [42]. In a review of 21 patients with metastatic EWS that had 63 irradiated sites treated with palliative radiotherapy [43], pain was the primary indication for treatment in 40 sites (63%). Other indications included neurologic symptoms (6%), palpable mass (3%), and asymptomatic radiologic finding (29%). The median number of sites treated per patient was three with a median dose of 30 Gy (range 4.5–68.5 Gy): spine (11 sites), pelvis/hips (10 sites), and lower extremity (7 sites) were the most common bony sites treated, whereas the lung (8) and the brain (5) were the most common soft tissue sites treated. Patients lived for a median of 349 days from the time of diagnosis. Thirty-five sites had a complete response (56%), and 18 sites had a partial response (29%). The overall response rate was 84%, which is comparable with the adult population response to palliative RT. The median overall duration of treatment response was 81 days (range, 0–1760 days).

Metastatic neuroblastoma

The need for palliation in metastatic neuroblastoma in pediatrics is not uncommon, and these patients often may require more than one course of treatment for different areas of involvement. This disease can spread to the orbit, mediastinum, liver, and brain, causing disruption of vision, respiratory compromise, and neurologic symptoms. These patients often present with both painful bone metastases in addition to soft tissue and organ involvement. The University of Iowa published a series of 29 children with neuroblastoma treated for 53 metastatic sites: soft tissue (n = 26) (median 2000 cGy), bone (n = 19) (median 2000 cGy), brain (n = 5) (median 2400 cGy), and liver (n = 3) (median 450 cGy) [44]. Median survival was 2.5 months after completion of therapy. Duration of response of RT from completion of treatment until death was 90% and 93% in patients with soft tissue and bone metastases, respectively. Complete and partial response was observed in 4% and 73% of patients with soft tissue metastases, and 42% and 37% of patients with bone metastases, respectively. Four of the 5 patients who received cranial irradiation experienced neurologic improvement. Two patients with hepatic metastases had improvement of respiratory status, whereas one patient progressed despite therapy. To emphasize the unpredictable nature of disease, one patient was found to live for 13 years. For this reason, late toxicity should always be taken into consideration, even if the child is receiving palliative RT.

Painful bone metastases can be addressed by other techniques. Historically, sequential hemibody irradiation has shown to be effective in children; however, it is not commonly practiced [45].

Other palliative options

Radioisotopes with medium-energy beta emission and short half-life are attractive targeted radiotherapeutic options, especially in the setting of multiple painful lesions which can frequently be seen in osteosarcoma. Produced form neutron capture, 153-samarium ethylene diamine tetramethylene phosphonate (153 Sm-EDTMP), a tetra phosphonate chelate has a high specific activity for bone uptake. This agent was developed as a pain palliation agent for bone metastases and approved by the FDA in April 1998 with a standard palliative dose of 1 mCi/kg [46]. Although children are also candidates for radioisotope therapy, the bone uptake of this agent should raise concern for those under 12 years of age. Exceptions can be made in the setting of extensive disease and when there is a need for intensive pain palliation. As may be true in adults, toxicity risks include pain flare in the days after the injection and bone marrow suppression several weeks thereafter.

Spinal cord compression

Spinal cord compression is uncommon in children, but it is the most common cause of symptomatic spinal cord disease in pediatric patients diagnosed with cancer [46]. Similar to circumstances in adults, the presenting symptoms of SCC may include motor deficits, back or radicular pain, sensory deficits, gait abnormality, loss of sphincteric control, or abnormal radiographic findings only. Though SCC usually presents in the final phases of a child's disease, it may alternatively present as one of the initial signs of disease [47]. Common causes of pediatric SCC are primitive neuroectodermal tumors (PNET), Ewing sarcoma, soft tissue sarcoma, and neuroblastoma [48]. SCC occurs in about 1–4% of patients with neuroblastoma [47]. Approximately 10–25% of patients with neuroectodermal brain tumors will develop cerebral spinal fluid (CSF) seeding [49]. SCC is rare in children with Hodgkin disease, occurring in 0.2% of those with initial presentation and 5% overall [50].

Bernardi et al. [51] published their experience of 76 children with neuroblastoma who presented with SCC out of a total of 1462 children with previously untreated neuroblastoma (5.2%). With the exception of one patient, all had presented with motor deficits: grade 1 in 43 (57%), grade 2 in 22 (29%), and grade 3 in 10 (13%) of the known deficits. Back and radicular pain often presented with irritability and was present in 47 patients. Sphincteric deficits were present in 30 patients, and sensory loss was evident in 11. The predominant mode of initial therapy was decompressive surgery. However, 11 patients were initially treated with radiotherapy; 2 had resectable disease, and the other 9 had unresectable or disseminated disease at presentation. Of those treated with RT, all but one patient had either stabilization or improvement of symptoms. At the time of analysis, 54 of the 76 children were alive with a median follow-up time of 139 months (range, 2–209 months). Overall survival at 5 years was 70% ± 5.3% for the 76 patients.

Optimal management of SCC involves a multi-disciplinary approach, including a decompressive laminectomy, radiotherapy, and/or chemotherapy, and depends on diagnosis, extent of disease upon presentation, and response to therapies. If SCC is the initial presentation of disease, tissue diagnosis is essential, as the child may benefit more from systemic intervention. Neurosurgical consultation is also crucial in the multi-disciplinary approach of SCC [52]. Neurologic function is the most important factor for recovery, thus in children laminectomy is an appropriate initial move, depending on the malignancy. The role of surgery has been controversial, at times reserved for those few patients who did not have a good response to chemotherapy/ radiotherapy [26]. A recent retrospective review of 2481 children with neuroblastoma identified 99 analyzable children with symptoms of SCC [53]. No significant difference in symptom improvement was noted between treatment modality, whether they received first-line neurosurgery (63.5%) or chemotherapy (55.3%) ($P = 0.42$). After intensive risk-adapted tumor treatment, symptoms of SCC were improved in 81% of patients who had first-line neurosurgery and 72% of patients initially treated with chemotherapy, $P = 0.6$. The 5-year event-free survival (EFS) was not statistically different between those who presented with symptoms of SCC when compared to those who were asymptomatic (69.9% vs 61.9%, respectively ($P = 0.14$)). However, there was a significant difference noted in overall survival at 5 years with 86.2% vs 72.7% favoring patients presenting without symptoms of SCC($p<0.01$).

Despite early intervention, patients continue to be at risk for late sequelae following treatment. In patients with detailed follow-up available, severe motor impairment at diagnosis was associated with a high risk of residual impairment of lower limb motor function ($P = 0.03$), with no differences noted between first-line surgery or chemotherapy ($P = 0.12$). Other factors that did not impact on late effects included age <12 months at diagnosis, use of glucocorticoids, and the interval between first symptoms and start of treatment. Bladder function was still impaired in 26 patients, 14 of whom continued to require self-catheterization. Pain was persistent in 5 patients, and scoliosis noted in 31 patients, 6 of whom required surgery. Unfortunately, the combination of surgery and radiotherapy can result in significant neurologic sequelae, especially in children of younger age [25]. For those with good response to chemotherapy or radiotherapy, surgery should be delayed until progression or worsening of neurologic symptoms.

Brain metastases

Brain metastases are far less common in children than they are in adults, with an incidence in children having solid tumors of approximately 1.5–2.5% [54–59]. The presence of brain metastases correlates with significant symptom burden and a poor prognosis. There have been case reports of patients with brain metastases among most pediatric tumors, including neuroblastoma, osteosarcoma, Ewing sarcoma, Wilms tumor, neuroblastoma, germ cell tumor, retinoblastoma, hepatoblastoma, and other soft tissue sarcoma. Few large series discuss the two patterns of pediatric brain metastases, specifically those that arise from true brain parenchyma and those which invade from adjacent bone metastases [54–59]. Headache, nausea, lateralization, weakness, and seizures are common presenting symptoms.

A review of 31 children who underwent palliative whole brain RT for a variety of tumors showed death from neurologic disease occurred in only 4 of 15 (27%) [60]. Osteogenic sarcoma and rhabdomyosarcoma were the most frequent primary tumors causing brain metastases in children younger than 15 years, while testicular germ cell tumor was the most common cause of

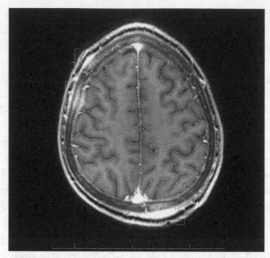

Figure 19.4 16-year-old male with metastatic Ewing sarcoma presenting with seven painful Intramedullary lesions throughout the skull and skull base and multiple soft tissue lesions, who received whole brain radiotherapy 3250 cGy at 250 cGy per fraction.

brain metastases in adolescents and young adults aged 15 to 21 years. After detection of brain metastases, the median survival was 7 months in 6 patients who underwent surgery plus whole brain RT and 4 months in 15 children who were treated with a 30 Gy dose of RT, alone.

There have been a few reports of long-term survivors in patients with Wilms tumor or osteosarcoma and brain metastases, therefore justifying a more individualized approach in these types of cases. Depending on the age, extent of the tumor, tumor histology, and potential for long-term survival, a more protracted course of 30–36 Gy in 1.5–2.5 Gy fractions may be reasonable for selected cases (Figure 19.4). The use of stereotactic radiosurgery (SRS) has not gained full acceptance in these cases, though it may be a reasonable option for circumstances such as when a patient presents with symptomatic recurrent Ewing sarcoma that has previously received full RT dose and is now inoperable. The use of SBRT may be an appropriate treatment option in order to palliate symptoms, gain tumor control, and minimize normal tissue toxicity.

Caring for the pediatric patient

Whether the child and family members are seeking curative therapies, disease-modifying therapy, compassionate care, or "comfort care only," palliative radiotherapy can potentially play a role at several different points in time during a child's illness. It is essential that all dimensions of the medical and psychosocial needs of the child and family are addressed. Without effective communication, the treating team risks falling short of the goals and wishes expressed by the patient and their family [61]. The communication process begins during the initial consultation when the physician delivers the diagnosis, describes treatment options, and identifies the goals of the child and their family. This initial meeting allows time for trust to develop between the caregiver, the child's family, and the referring physician. Children and adolescents should be included in discussions from the time of initial diagnosis. Parents may prefer to not include them in any meetings and decision-making, but this approach often reflects a misplaced attempt to protect their child from hopelessness and fear of dying. When a patient is referred for palliative radiotherapy, the likelihood of long-term survival is minimal; however, with the advent of better salvage therapies for metastatic disease, many children with metastatic disease can survive for lengthy periods of time. This reality impacts on the treatment decisions made, especially with regards to radiation therapy.

Barriers to the use of palliative radiotherapy

Being aware of appropriate indications for palliative RT in children and adolescents is important, since it is often an underutilized treatment modality because of uncertainty and unjustified fear. Tucker *et al.* completed a study evaluating the level of knowledge about the indications for, and utilization of, palliative RT among pediatric oncologists in Canada [62]. Sixty-four of 80 pediatric oncologists responded to a survey about their knowledge of palliative radiation therapy (12 potential indications) and their identification of barriers to their use of palliative RT. Ninety-two percent had provided palliative care for children with cancer within the prior year, and 80% of the physicians had referred a child for palliative radiotherapy. Fifty-nine percent felt that they had appropriate knowledge to identify indications for palliative RT, while 41% responded as "no" or "unsure." Knowledge of the effectiveness of palliative RT for bone metastases, soft-tissue metastasis, and dyspnea were considered adequate in 89%, 61%, and 80%, respectively. Knowledge about the use of palliative RT for bleeding and hemoptysis was adequate in 40% and 22%, respectively, whereas 45% and 64% were unsure of the effectiveness of palliative RT for those indications. Barriers to the use of palliative radiotherapy included patient and family reluctance, fear that the treatment may not improve quality of life, short life expectancy of the child, transportation limitations, fear of perceived or previous side effects, and lack of knowledge about potential benefits of radiotherapy. Some of these concerns were mitigated by giving the families careful explanations about the potential risks and benefits of therapy, especially in cases with a good caregiver–family rapport.

Special considerations in developing countries

The diagnosis of childhood cancer in developing countries might be delayed because of limited access to health-care facilities or outdated diagnostic equipment. Additionally, even where facilities and equipment are available, some countries lack sufficient numbers of clinicians who are properly trained to deal with the special circumstances inherent in the care of children with cancer. The sophistication and experience necessary to deliver radiotherapy for children under anesthesia while also dealing with the emotional needs of a family with a dying child may not be found in countries without dedicated pediatric care facilities.

Conclusion

The care for children and adolescents with life-threatening malignancies is a complex task, requiring support from a multi-disciplinary team. Not only should the child and family weigh the potential benefits of treatment, they should closely assess the long-term side effect risks in situations where the child may live for several years or even decades longer. Although the curative path is often pursued and favored, palliative RT still remains a necessary adjunctive treatment in the pediatric population. Unfortunately, the prognosis of pediatric patients diagnosed with metastatic disease remains poor. It is important to seek optimal quality of life by minimizing symptoms, by maximizing function, and by facilitating communication with the patient, family, and primary care team. Aside from providing palliative RT for relief of a physical symptom, it is essential not to lose sight of the patient's and the family's experience during the treatment process.

References

1. Arias E, MacDorman MF, Strobino DM, *et al.* Annual summary of vital statistics-2002. *Pediatrics* 2003; **112**: 1215–1230.
2. Wolfe J, Grier H, Pizzo PA, Poplack DG. (eds) Care of the dying child. In: *Principles and Practice of Pediatric Oncology*, 4th edn. Philadelphia: Lippincott Williams & Wilkins, 2002, pp. 1477–1503.
3. McNeil DE, Cote TR, Clegg L, *et al.* SEER update of incidence and trends in pediatric malignancies: acute lymphoblastic leukemia. *Med Pediatr Oncol* 2002; **39**: 554–557.
4. Friebert S. National Hospice and Palliative Care Organization. NHPCO facts and figures: pediatric palliative and hospice care in America. 2009. Available at: http://www.nhpco.org (accessed November 16, 2012).
5. World Health Organization. WHO Definition of Palliative Care for Children. Available at: http://www.who.int/cancer/palliative/definition/en/ (accessed November 22, 2012).
6. Steenland E, Leer JW, van Houwelingen H, *et al.* The effect of a single fraction compared to multiple fractions on painful bone metastases: a global analysis of the Dutch Bone Metastasis Study. *Radiother Oncol* 1999; **52**: 101–109.
7. Bone Pain Trial Working Party. 8 Gy single fraction radiotherapy for the treatment of metastatic skeletal pain: randomized comparison with a multifraction schedule over 12 months of patient follow-up. *Radiother Oncol* 1999; **52**: 111–121.
8. Hartsell WF, Scott CB, Bruner DW, *et al.* Randomized trial of short vs long-course radiotherapy for palliation of painful bone metastases. *J Natl Cancer Inst* 2005; **97**: 798–804.

9. Pizzo PA, Horowitz ME, Poplack PG, *et al.* Solid tumors of childhood. In: DeVita VT, Hellmann S, Rosenberg SA. (eds) *Cancer: Principles & Practice of Oncology*, 4th edn. Philadelphia: JB Lippincott, 1993, pp. 1738–1791.

10. Bruckman JE, Bloomer WD. Management of spinal cord compression. *Semin Oncol* 1978; **5**: 135–140.

11. Raffel C, Neave VCD, Lavine S, *et al.* Treatment of spinal cord compression by epidural malignancy malignancy in childhood. *Neurosurgery* 1991; **28**: 349–352.

12. Ch'ien LT, Kalwinsky DK, Peterson G, *et al.* Metastatic epidural tumors in children. *Med Pediatr Oncol* 1982; **10**: 455–462.

13. Gilbert RW, Kim JH, Posner JB. Epidural spinal cord compression from metastatic tumor: diagnosis and treatment. *Ann Neurol* 1978; **3**: 40–43.

14. Rodriguez M, Dinapoli RP. Spinal cord compression: with special reference to metastatic epidural tumors. *Mayo Clin Proc* 1980; **55**: 442–448.

15. Lewis DW, Packer RJ, Raney B, *et al.* Incidence, presentation, and outcome of spinal cord disease in children with systemic cancer. *Pediatrics* 1986; **78**: 438–443.

16. Lange B, D-Angio GJ, Ross AJ, *et al.* Oncologic emergencies. In: Pizzo PA, Poplack DG. (eds) *Principles and Practice of Pediatric Oncology*, 2nd edn. Philadelphia: JB Lippincott, 1993, pp. 951–973.

17. Klein SL, Sanford RA, Muhlbauer MS. Pediatric spinal epidural metastases. *J Neurosurg* 1991; **74**: 70.

18. Ingram L, Rivera GK, Shapiro DN. Superior vena cava syndrome associated with childhood malignancy: anlaysis of 24 cases. *Med Pediatr Oncol* 1990; **18**: 476–481.

19. Bertsch H, Rudoler S, Needle MN, *et al.* Emergent/urgent therapeutic irradiation in pediatric oncology: patterns of presentation, treatment, and outcome. *Med Pediatr Oncol* 1998; **30**: 101–105.

20. Lyding JM, Tseng A, Newman A. Intramedullary spinal cord metastases in Hodgkin's disease: rapid diagnosis and treatment resulting in neurologic recovery. *Cancer* 1987; **60**: 1741–1744.

21. Obviate DL, Kushner HS, Stein RS. Successful chemotherapeutic treatment of epidural compression in non-Hodgkin's lymphoma. *Cancer* 1982; **49**: 2446–2448.

22. Kozlowski K, Bluff G, Masel J, *et al.* Primary vertebral tumours in children: report of 20 cases with brief literature review. *Pediatr Radiol* 1984; **14**: 129–139.

23. Holgersen LO, Santulli TV, Schullinger JN. Neuroblastoma with intraspinal (dumbbell) estension. *J Pediatr Surg* 1983; **4**: 406–411.

24. Ortega JA, Wharam M, Gehan EA, *et al.* Clinical features and results of therapy for children with praspinal soft tissue sarcoma. *J Clin Oncol* 1991; **9**: 796–801.

25. Hayes FA, Thompson EI, Kvizdala E. Chemotherapy as an alternative to laminectomy and radiation in the management of epidural tumor. *J Pediatr* 1984; **2**: 221–224.

26. Fabian CJ, Mansfield CM, Dahlberg S, *et al.* Low dose involved field radiation after chemotherapy in advanced Hodgkin's disease: a Southwest Oncology Group Randomized study. *Ann Intern Med* 1994; **120**: 903–912.

27. Little J. Epidemiology of Childhood Cancer. IARC Scientific Publication No 149. Lyon, France: International Agency for Research on Cancer; 1999.

28. Taylor RE. Cancer in children: radiotherapeutic approaches. *Br Med Bull* 1996; **52**: 873–886.

29. Arya LS, Narain S, Tomar S, *et al.* Superior vena cava syndrome. *Indian J Pediatr* 2002; **69**: 293–237.

30. King RM, Telander RL, Smithson WA. Primary mediastinal tumors in children. *J Pediatr Surg* 1982; **17**: 512–520.

31. D'angio GJ, Mitus A, Evans AE. The superior mediastinal syndrome in children with cancer. *Am J Roentgenol Radium Ther Nucl Med* 1975; **93**: 537.

32. Rheingold SR, Lange BJ. Oncologic emergencies. In: Pizzo PA, Poplack DG. (eds) *Principles and Practice of Pediatric Oncology*, 4th edn. Philadelphia: Lippincott Williams and Wilkins, 2002, pp. 1177–1203.

33. Ferrari LR, Bedofrd RF. General anesthesia prior to treatment of anterior mediastinal masses in pediatric cancer patients. *Anesthesiology* 1990; **72**: 991–995.

34. Loeffler JS, Leopold KA, Recht A, *et al.* Emergency prebiopsy radiation for mediastinal masses: impact on subsequent pathologic diagnosis and outcome. *J Clin Oncol* 1986; **4**: 716–721.

35. Claman HN. Corticosteroids and lymphoid cells. *N Engl J Med* 1972; **287**: 388–397.

36. Kumari I, Gupta S, Singhal PP. Superior vena caval syndrom in children – a case report. *Middle East J Anesthesiol* 2006; **18**: 933–938.

37. Stanley TH, Weidauer HE. Anesthesia for the patient with cardiac Tamponade. *Anesth Analg* 1973; **52**: 110–114.

38. Ingram L, Rivera GK, Shapiro DN. Superior vena cava syndrome associated with childhood malignancy: analysis of 24 cases. *Med Pediatr Oncol* 1990; **18**: 476–481.

39. Deutsch M, Tersak JM. Radiotherapy for symptomatic metastases to bone in children. *Am J Clin Oncol* 2004; **27**: 128–131.

40. Grier HE, Krailo MD, Tarbell NJ, *et al.* Addition of ifosfomide and etoposide to standard chemotherapy for Ewing's sarcoma and primitive neuroectodermal tumor of bone. *N Engl J Med* 2003; **348**: 694–701.

41. Crist WM, Anderson JR, Meza JL, *et al.* Intergroup rhabdomyosarcoma study-IV: results for patients with nonmetastatic disease. *J Clin Oncol* 2001; **19**: 3091–3102.

42. Aparicio J, Munarriz B, Pastor M, *et al.* Long-term follow-up and prognostic factors in Ewing's sarcoma. A multivariate analysis of 116 patients from a single institution. *Oncology* 1998; **55**: 20–26.

43. Koontz BF, Clough RW, Halperin EC. Palliative radiation therapy for metastatic Ewing sarcoma. *Cancer* 2006; **106**: 1790–1793.

44. Paulino AC. Palliative radiotherapy in children with neuroblastoma. *Pediatr Hematol Oncol* 2003; **20**: 111–117.

45. Jenkin RD, Berry MP. Sequential half-body irradiation in childhood. *Int J Radiat Oncol Biol Phys* 1983; **9**: 1969–1971.

46. Baten M, Vannucci RC. Intraspinal metastatic disease in childhood cancer. *J Pediatr* 1977; **90**: 207–212.

47. Punt J, Putchard J, Pincott JR, *et al.* Neuroblastoma: a review of 21 cases presenting with spinal cord compression. *Cancer* 1980; **45**: 3095–3101.

48. Pollono D, Drut R, Ibanez O, *et al.* Spinal cord compression: a review of 70 pediatric patients. *Pediatr Hematol Oncol* 2003; **20**: 457–466.

49. Shyin PB, Campbell GA, Guinto FC, *et al.* Primary intracranial ependymoblastoma presenting as apinal cord compression due to metastasis. *Childs Nerv Syst* 1986; **2**: 323–325.

50. Gupta V, Srivastava A, Bhatia B. Hodgkin disease with spinal cord compression. *J Pediatr Hematol Oncol* 2009; **31**: 771–773.

51. Bernardi BD, Pianca C, Pistomiglio P, *et al.* Neuroblastoma with symptomatic spinal cord compression at diagnosis: treatment and results with 76 cases. *J Clin Oncol* 2001; **19**: 183–190.

52. Tchdjian M, Matson DD. Orthopaedic aspects of intraspinal tumors in infants and children. *J Bone Joint Surg* 1965; **47**: 223–248.

53. Simon T, Niemann CA, Hero B, *et al.* Short- and long-term outcome of patients with symptoms of spinal cord compression b neuroblastoma. *Dev Med Child Neurol* 2012; **54**: 347–352.

54. Kebudi R, Gorgun O, Ağaoğlu FY, *et al.* Brain metastasis in pediatric extracranial solid tumors: survey and literature review. *J Neurooncol* 2005; **71**: 43–48.

55. Allen JC. Brain metastases. In: Deutsch M. (ed.) *Management of Childhood Brain Tumors.* Boston: Kluwer Academic Publishers, 1990, pp. 457–464.

56. Deutsch M, Albo V, Wollman MR. Radiotherapy for cerebral metastases in children. *Int J Radiat Oncol Biol Phys* 1982; **8**: 1441–1446.

57. Bouffet E, Doumi N, Thiesse P, *et al.* Brain metastases in children with solid tumors. *Cancer* 1997; **79**: 403–410.

58. Deutsch M, Orlando S, Wolmann M. Radiotherapy for metastases to the brain in children. *Med Pediatr Oncol* 2002; **39**: 60–62.

59. Vannucci RC, Baten M. Cerebral metastatic disease in childhood. *Neurology* 1974; **24**: 981–985.

60. Graus F, Walker RW, Allen JC. Brain metastases in children. *J Pediatr* 1983; **103**: 558–561.

61. Vern-Gross T. Establishing communication within the field of pediatric oncology: a palliative care approach. *Curr Probl Cancer* 2011; **35**: 337–350.

62. Tucker MD, Samant RS, Fitzgibbon EJ. Knowledge and utilization of palliative radiotherapy by pediatric oncologists. *Curr Oncol* 2010; **17**: 48–55.

63. Anderson PM, Wiseman GA, Dispenzieri A, *et al.* High-dose samarium-153 ethylene diamine tetramethylene phosphonate: low toxicity of skeletal irradiation in patients with osteosarcoma and bone metastases. *J Clin Oncol* 2002; **20**: 189–196.

PART 4

Metastatic disease

CHAPTER 20

Bone metastases

Yvette van der Linden[1], Dirk Rades[2]
[1]Department of Clinical Oncology, University Medical Centre, Leiden,
The Netherlands
[2]Department of Radiotherapy, University Hospital, Lübeck, Germany

Introduction

In approximately half of the patients who are faced with cancer, metastatic spread of tumor cells has occurred at the diagnosis of cancer, or will eventually occur during follow-up after an initial period of remission. For the patient this signifies a catastrophic event: it means that the malignant process is incurable and treatment is no longer directed towards cure. Only optimal palliation of disease-related symptoms is achievable. Bone is the third most frequent site of tumor metastasis, after lung and liver. The malignant tumors that frequently metastasize to the skeleton also affect patients most commonly: breast cancer, prostate cancer, and lung cancer. The incidence and prevalence of bone metastases in cancer patients are difficult to determine with accuracy: studies report a frequency of 10–47% of all patients with breast cancer developing metastases to the bone during their illness [1–3]. In autopsy studies, more than 70% of breast cancer patients had tumor deposits in the bone [4,5]. For the radiotherapy department and its employees, care for patients with painful bone metastases comprises a large percentage of the daily workload: up to 10–15%.

Clinical implications and treatment modalities

For the patient, bone metastases may cause a range of complications (Box 20.1), varying from mild to severe pain at the site of the metastasis, pathologic fracturing of bone, spinal cord compression or nerve root compression syndromes, and hypercalcemia. The intensity of these symptoms is mostly dependent on the localization and extent of the lesion in the skeleton [6,7].

A variety of palliative treatment modalities is available for bone metastases ranging from local to systemic, and from non-invasive to invasive. The

Radiation Oncology in Palliative Cancer Care, First Edition. Edited by Stephen Lutz,
Edward Chow, and Peter Hoskin.
© 2013 John Wiley & Sons, Ltd. Published 2013 by John Wiley & Sons, Ltd.

Box 20.1 Symptoms commonly associated with bone metastases

- Pain
- Pathologic fracture
- Spinal cord compression
- Nerve root compression
- Hypercalcemia

---

majority of treatments are directed towards optimum palliation with minimum treatment related morbidity. Choice for a certain treatment is dependent on the complaints, life expectancy, and personal wishes of the patient, which earlier treatments have been applied, and whether comorbidity exists that opposes this treatment. Other influencing factors are the localization of the metastasis in the skeleton, and whether the metastasis is solitary or multiple bone lesions exist.

Clinical symptoms

Pain

The mechanisms that underlie the sensation of pain caused by metastasis are poorly understood. The presence of pain does not seem to be correlated with the type of tumor, location, number, or size of the metastases [8]. It is thought that when tumor cells grow, the periosteum, which is the highly innervated connective tissue sheath that covers the external surface of the bone, is stretched. Pain receptors (nociceptors) are subsequently activated and may show sensitization, which is manifest as a decreased threshold of activation after injury and the emergence of spontaneous activity [9,10]. This may explain why some lesions cause such a deep, dull, aching sensation without even minimal contact [11]. In addition, chemical mediators of pain such as prostaglandins are thought to play a role [8]. Treatment strategies are focused on these above-mentioned mechanisms.

Analgesic drugs that inhibit certain pathways are generally available and relatively simple to administer. Most analgesics are effective in treating pain, although some patients respond poorly. Depending on the quantity and duration of analgesics intake the patient may suffer from serious side effects. For example, opioids cause nausea, constipation, and drowsiness. Non-steroidal anti-inflammatory drugs may cause gastrointestinal ulceration with subsequent bleeding. If pain is caused mainly by edema subsequent to metastatic involvement, steroids such as dexamethasone may also be helpful. Steroids should be administered for as short a period as possible, because they may cause drug dependency and induce diseases like diabetes and Cushing syndrome.

For localized bone pain and for pain with a radiating component, neuropathic pain, radiotherapy is considered the standard treatment modality. Overall pain relief with a 60–80% response was reported within 3 to 4 weeks, with these data coming from pooled results arising from the results of numerous randomized clinical trials [12–15] (Table 20.1). Response calculations were performed in different ways in the multiple trials, with different endpoints and definitions. Therefore, in 2000, a consensus meeting was held and regulations were written to improve consistency in future trials [16]. The precise analgesic mechanism of radiotherapy remains unknown. Because in some patients the onset of pain relief is rapid, within days, it is not credible to link the anesthetic effect to tumor shrinkage alone, which will take several weeks [17]. More probable, a response mechanism through chemical mediators such as prostaglandins is the cause of less pain within days after radiotherapy.

There is worldwide evidence-based consensus that a single fraction of 8 Gy is the standard treatment for localized bone pain, regardless of primary tumor type, expected survival, or skeletal localization, with no additional benefit to response from higher total radiotherapy doses [12,18]. Single dose radiotherapy reduces the number of visits to the hospital for the patient and is considered cost-effective and easy to implement in the radiotherapy department schedule [19,20]. Even in patients with an observed minimum survival of one year, results from a randomized trial showed in a subgroup of 320 patients no additional benefit of higher total doses [21]. On the other hand, almost 50% of 247 patients in the same trial with an observed limited survival of less than 12 weeks after randomization achieved a meaningful pain response [22,23]. One trial reported no differences in the net pain relief (NPR), that is, the duration of benefit measured by dividing the period of pain relief by the period of survival in days and multiplying the result by 100. For the 30 Gy arm the NPR was 71%, and for the 8 Gy arm 68% [24]. The general consensus is that higher total doses up to 20–30 Gy are appropriate for bone metastases with extensive soft tissue involvement on the CT scan, or for large osteolytic lesions with impending pathologic fracturing (see later). The principle in these cases is to achieve more tumor control and hence induce remineralization. However, since these additional effects on top of just pain control may take up to several months, the expected survival of patients must be relatively favorable to justify more time consuming treatments.

For neuropathic pain, a single trial so far showed that 20 Gy in 5 fractions was not superior to 8 Gy single fraction, although the response duration was slightly better after multiple fractions [25]. Therefore, for neuropathic pain, these results should optimally be repeated in another trial [26].

Dependent on which part of the body is irradiated, treatment volume, and total radiotherapy dose, transient side effects of radiotherapy that may occur are tiredness, flare up of pain, skin reactions, or gastrointestinal complaints such as nausea or diarrhea. Trials report only mild to moderate side effects with a moderate higher incidence after multiple fractions when compared to

Table 20.1(a) Radiotherapy for painful bone metastases: outcome of meta-analyses of randomized clinical trials comparing different fractionation regimens.

Initial radiotherapy	Number of trials / patients	Radiotherapy doses	Assessable patients	Overall response (%)*	OR†	Complete pain relief (%)	OR
Sze et al. 2004[14]	11 / 3435	SF 1 × 8–10 Gy	Dropout range 0–69%	60	1.03 (0.89–1.19)	34	1.11 (0.94–1.30)
-SF vs MF		MF 3 × 5 Gy, 5–6 × 4 Gy, 10 × 3 Gy		59		32	
Wu et al. 2003 [13]	7/3260 (SF vs MF trials only)	SF 1 × 8–10 Gy	Dropout range 0–63%	62.1	1.05 (1.00–1.11)	33.4	1.03 (0.94–1.14)
-SF vs SF		MF 5–6 × 4 Gy, 10 × 3 Gy		58.7		32.3	
-SF vs MF							
-MF vs MF							
Chow et al. 2007[12]	16/5000	SF 1 × 8–10 Gy	81% of patients assessable	58	0.99 (0.95–1.03)	23	0.97 (0.88–1.06)
-SF vs MF		MF 3 × 5 Gy, 5–6 × 4 Gy, 10 × 3 Gy		59		24	
Additional							
Foro Arnalot et al. 2008[24]	1/160	SF 1 × 8 Gy	Not mentioned	75	Not mentioned	15	Not mentioned
		MF 10 × 3 Gy		86		13	
Retreatment							
Huisman et al. 2012[34]	7/2694	SF 4–6–8 Gy MF	65–100% (of 527 retreated patients)	36–100%		16–40%	

Note: the paper by Foro Arnalot has not been part of any review so far.

Note: Huisman et al. studied retreatment data from both retrospective and prospective studies, as from subgroup analyses from randomized clinical trials.

*responses are calculated according to the intention to treat principle

†OR, odds ratio with 95% confidence intervals between brackets

Response duration (months)	Re-irradiation rates (%)	OR	Pathologic fracture rate (%)	OR	SCC (%)	OR	Remarks
ns	21.5	3.44 (2.67–4.43)	3	1.82 (1.06–3.11)	1.9	1.41 (0.72–2.75	Repeated measurements excluding
ns	7.4		1.6		1.4		dropouts similar results
ns	21	ns	2.75	ns	2.1	ns	No dose response relationship when comparing
ns	6.4		2.2		1.5		outcome MF vs. MF studies
4–13	20	2.5 (1.76–3.56)	3.2	1.10 (0.61–1.99)	2.8	1.44 (0.9–2.3)	
6–14	8		2.8		1.9		
5.4	28	Not mentioned	Not mentioned		Not mentioned		Net pain relief reported
5.4	2						
5–22	11–42%		Not mentioned		Not mentioned		

Table 20.1(b) Radiotherapy for painful bone metastases: outcome of meta-analyses of randomized clinical trials comparing different fractionation regimens.

Initial radiotherapy	References	Primary tumor (%)	Localization (%)	Follow-up	Pain assessment tools
Sze et al. 2002	[14]	Breast 39.3 Prostate 23.5 Lung 19.9	Spine 34 Pelvis 32	Weekly to monthly	11 point numerical 4 point Likert scale VAS
Wu et al. 2003	[13]	Not mentioned	Not mentioned	Weekly to monthly	11 point numerical 4 point Likert scale VAS
Chow et al. 2007	[12]	Not mentioned	Not mentioned	Weekly to monthly	11 point numerical 4 point Likert scale VAS
Additional					
Foro Arnalot et al. 2008	[24]	Breast 27 Prostate 26 Lung 27	Spine 6 Pelvis 34	Week 3, 12, 24, 48	11 point numerical
Retreatment					
Huisman et al. 2012	[34]	Breast 33 Prostate 21 Lung 23 Other 23	Spine 36 Pelvis 38 Proximal long bones 12 Other 14	Not mentioned	4 point Likert scale 11 point numerical

Who assessed pain	Response	Net pain relief	Survival	QOL data	Side effects
Mostly patient	Best score at any time	Not mentioned	Not mentioned	Not mentioned	Similar, or > when MF
Mostly patient	Best score at any time	Not mentioned	Not mentioned	Not mentioned	Similar, or > when MF
Mostly patient	Best score at any time or fixed at 1 month	Not mentioned	Not mentioned	Not mentioned	Similar, or > when MF
Patient	At 3 and 12 weeks	SF 68%	SF 28 weeks	Not mentioned	12% after SF, 18% after MF
		MF 71%	MF 33 weeks		
Patient	Best score at any time or fixed at 1 month	Not mentioned	Not mentioned	Not mentioned	Mostly grade 1–2

single fractions [24,27,28]. In studies looking at transient pain flare after radiotherapy, percentages varying from 20–40% were observed [29–31]. The use of oral dexamethasone to prevent pain flare from occurring is the topic of two current placebo controlled randomized trials – one in Canada and one in the Netherlands.

In the meta-analysis presented by Chow *et al.*, 20% retreatment during follow-up was noted after initial single fraction radiotherapy, compared to only 8% after initial multiple fractions [12]. Whether a retreatment was given to patients in the randomized trials was at the discretion of the treating physician, making these results likely biased. Both doctors and patients were probably more willing to irradiate after single dose radiotherapy [32]. Therefore, in the consensus meetings that were held to promote consistency in conducting clinical trials, the minimum interval to apply retreatment was set at 4 weeks from initial radiotherapy treatment [33]. In general, palliative radiotherapy is a relatively safe treatment that can be applied repetitively. For progressive pain after initial response or non-responsive pain to radiotherapy, a second or even third radiotherapy treatment is delivered with responses varying from 50–70%, coming from mostly retrospective or prospective cohort data [34]. The results from a large international collaborative randomized trial are awaited eagerly [35]. In this trial, pain response and duration of response in patients retreated with either 8 Gy or 20 Gy in 5 fractions are being studied. Patients are stratified by initial treatment dose and their response to the first treatment with radiotherapy.

Another local treatment for pain is a surgical intervention. If a patient suffers from painful osteolytic metastases in the femur or humerus with cortical involvement and rising instability, osteosynthesis may cause immediate relief of pain and, in addition, prevent pathologic fracture. The treating physician should weigh the morbidity of a surgical procedure against the stabilizing capability of prophylactic surgery. Relatively new minimal invasive procedures such as vertebroplasty in osteolytic spinal metastases when polymethylmethacrylate is injected into the vertebra to immediately strengthen the affected bone. may be appropriate to treat back pain [36,37].

A number of new treatments have been developed in the past years that perhaps are useful in patients who do not gain a valuable response to radiotherapy. Radiofrequency ablation (RFA) utilizes a high-frequency alternating current that is passed from the needle electrode into surrounding tissue, resulting in frictional heating and necrosis. A decrease of pain in 95% of treated patients was reported with this technique [38]. Percutaneous cryoablation is a minimally invasive technique that induces necrosis by alternately freezing and thawing a target tissue [39]. Another non-invasive treatment is MRI-HIFU, using high frequency focused ultrasound to ablate bone metastases for mostly lesions in the pelvic region [40]. Unfortunately, for all these treatment options, prospective randomized trials with comparison to standard radiotherapy are lacking.

If a patient has diffuse pain arising from numerous metastases in the skeleton, a systemic treatment is considered more beneficial than a local treatment, provided of course that the primary tumor is sensitive to any of the available systemic therapies. A variety of effective chemotherapeutic agents, hormonal therapies [41], and radionuclides is available [15,42,43]. Mostly, patients with breast cancer, prostate cancer, or lung cancer benefit from these treatments. When using radionuclides, best pain relief results are achieved in osteoblastic lesions, achieved from inhibition of pain mediators derived from normal bone cells, not from a direct effect on the tumor. Strontium-89 and samarium-153 are radioisotopes that are effective in providing pain relief with a 40–95% response rate. Pain relief starts from 1 to 4 weeks after the initiation of treatment. Thrombocytopenia and neutropenia are the most common toxic effects but are generally mild and reversible; therefore repeated use of radionuclides is possible. For patients with multiple sites of painful bone metastases that are not predominately osteoblastic, single fraction hemibody radiotherapy can provide good rates of relief with acceptable rates of toxicity.

Another treatment option is regular infusions with potent inhibitors of osteoclastic bone resorption such as bisphosphonates to decrease the number of skeleton related events and bone pain in patients with breast cancer and prostate cancer [44–46], as well as in patients with lung cancer and other solid tumors [47]. Relatively new is the use of the monoclonal antibody Denosumab to prevent the occurrence of skeletal related events [48,49]. At the moment, combinations of different treatments are the focus of clinical trials in order to achieve higher response percentages.

Impending or pathologic fracturing

Progressive involvement of the bone cortex weakens the axial strength of the bone and gives rise to instability. To minimize the chance of a pathologic fracture in weight-bearing bones it is important to search for lesions at risk of fracturing and treat them assertively. An advantage of elective surgery is that patients with a relatively good performance are easier to operate with less morbidity and even mortality than after pathologic fracturing has occurred. Unfortunately, it is difficult to predict which lesions are at risk using radiographic imaging and clinical information [50,51]. Most indications for prophylactic treatment come from retrospective surgical studies. Prediction of fracture based on lesional characteristics is therefore still not very accurate and leads to surgical overtreatment [52]. Results from the randomized Dutch Bone Metastasis Study showed that patients with femoral metastases and an axial cortical involvement (Lcort) exceeding 30 mm have a 23% chance of fracturing during follow-up. The negative predictive value of Lcort <30 mm was 97%. Therefore, for femoral lesions with Lcort <30 mm radiotherapy provides safe pain treatment [52,53]. Ongoing research on the use of computer finite element modeling to predict fracture risk based on CT data is showing promising results for the future [54].

Pathologic fractures can occur spontaneously or following only trivial injury, particularly in osteolytic lesions. Even in bed-ridden patients long bones tend to fracture due to torsional forces when patients turn in their beds. Fracture mostly arises in weight-bearing bones, such as the femur, humerus, and vertebrae of the spinal column. Dependent on the localization of the fracture the patient faces direct immobilization with considerable pain and morbidity. Pathologic fractures in long bones require stabilizing osteosynthesis to restore mobility and to treat pain [50]. Based on observations only, radiotherapy to 20–30 Gy is administered afterwards to induce remineralization of the fractured bone and stabilize the osteosynthetic prosthesis [55,56].

Technical considerations

Radiotherapy is usually delivered with two opposed treatment fields using 6–10 MV photons from a linear accelerator. Relatively superficial lesions such as rib metastases can also be treated with electrons. For both the patient and the radiotherapy department, these techniques provide easy and swift treatment. Most optimal for patients not living in the vicinity of a radiotherapy facility is when the assessment, treatment simulation, and actual treatment can take place on the same day. For lesions in already heavily irradiated parts of the body where normal tissues or so-called "organs at risk," such as the spinal cord, are limiting factors for delivering optimal doses of radiotherapy, the use of highly conformal techniques with tight margins such as intensity modulated radiation therapy (IMRT) and stereotactic body radiation therapy (SBRT) provide the possibility of reaching further pain control [57,58]. These techniques, however, are more costly and time consuming, and therefore their exact place in palliative radiotherapy for bone metastasis remains controversial and is a topic for further research. In RTOG 0631 for example, 8 Gy single dose conventional radiotherapy is being compared to 16 Gy using SBRT for painful spinal metastases. In addition, the question arises whether, in the case of true oligometastatic disease, treatment should be more aggressive aiming at ablation of the metastasis. The use of highly conformal radiotherapy techniques may achieve this with the ability to spare surrounding normal tissues far better than with conventional radiotherapy; however, good evidence for this is currently lacking.

Prognosis and choice for treatment

Duration of survival after the clinical manifestation of bone metastases depends on a number of patient-related factors. First, the clinical condition of the patient is of importance, with comorbidities hampering the application of systemic treatments. Next, the metastatic burden: is the bone metastasis a solitary lesion or do multiple metastases exist throughout the skeleton. If a patient also has visceral metastases, his prognosis is generally worse. In addition, the type of primary tumor affects the disease outcome. Patients with breast cancer or prostate cancer may have a prolonged survival, sometimes stretching over several years. Improvements in systemic therapy and the relatively long clinical course of these primary tumors underline this observation. In the literature, the median survival after radiotherapy for bone metastases ranged from 15–16 months for patients with breast cancer, 9–10 months for patients with prostate cancer, and 3–4 months for patients with lung cancer [21,59].

Proactive approach

Although, in general, small lesions give few symptoms and large lesions may cause severe problems, there is no linear correlation between size of the metastasis and severity of the symptoms. It is therefore important to monitor patients carefully and choose diagnostic imaging tools and subsequent treatments individually for each patient. In addition, patients and their relatives should be informed of the symptoms of bone metastases. During their illness, many patients receive one or more different treatments, sometimes concomitantly or consecutively. Optimally, the treating physicians and health-care workers cooperate in a multi-disciplinary setting to discuss the right choice of treatment for each patient, taking into account life expectancy and expected outcome after palliative treatment (Figure 20.1). Quality of life assessments, both on an individual patient basis and of entire groups of bone metastases patients, are imperative for appropriate ongoing care.

Special considerations in developing countries

Patients in developing countries may have limited access to health-care centers with radiographic equipment to diagnose bone metastases. Furthermore, insufficient access to radiopharmaceuticals for the treatment of widespread bone disease or to qualified surgeons for management of impending or completed pathologic fractures may create suboptimal care scenarios. In geographic locales with high throughput on linear accelerators or cobalt-60 treatment machines, time constraints may demand single fraction treatment. Finally, poorly developed or even completely absent palliative care programs may limit the availability of necessary adjuvant treatments such as narcotic analgesics and end-of-life care planning.

Conclusion

Bone metastases are a common clinical problem that is associated with the potential for significant symptoms such as pain, pathologic fracture, spinal cord compression, and hypercalcemia. External beam radiation therapy

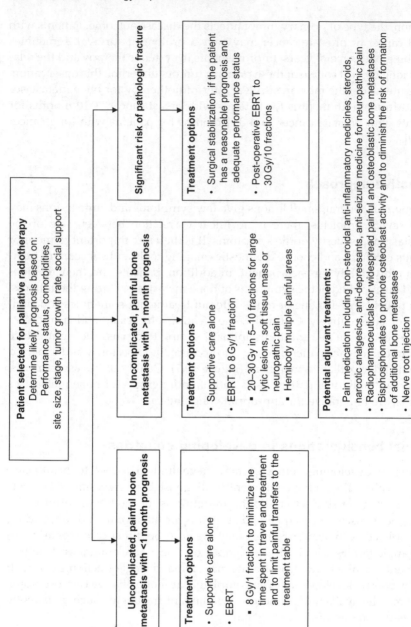

Figure 20.1 Algorithm for use of palliative radiotherapy for patients with bone metastases.

provides effective and time efficient palliative relief of pain. Adjuvant treatments may include surgical intervention for impending or completed pathologic fracture or systemic therapies such as chemotherapy, osteoclast inhibitors, or radiopharmaceuticals. The proper management of painful bone metastases requires well-coordinated, multi-disciplinary care that honors palliative care principles and seeks to maximize quality of life.

References

1. Wedin R, Bauer H, Rutqvist LE. Surgical treatment for skeletal breast cancer metastases. A population-based study of 641 patients. *Cancer* 2001; **92**: 257–262.
2. Miller F, Whitehill R. Carcinoma of the breast metastatic to the skeleton. *Clin Orthop* 1984; **Apr (184)**: 121–127.
3. Kamby C, Vejborg I, Daugaard S, et al. Clinical and radiologic characteristics of bone metastases in breast cancer. *Cancer* 1987; **60**: 2524–2531.
4. Galasko CS. The anatomy and pathways of bone metastases. In: Weiss L, Gilbert A. (eds) *Bone Metastases*. Boston: GK Hall, 1981, pp. 49–63.
5. Lee YT. Breast carcinoma: pattern of metastasis at autopsy. *J Surg Oncol* 1983; **23**: 175–180.
6. Adami S. Bisphosphanates in prostate carcinoma. *Cancer* 1997; **80**: 1674–1679.
7. Ang KK, Jiang GL, Feng Y, et al. Extent and kinetics of recovery of occult spinal cord injury. *Int J Radiat Oncol Biol Phys* 2001; **50**: 1013–1020.
8. Hoskin PJ. Scientific and clinical aspects of radiotherapy in the relief of bone pain. *Cancer Surv* 1988; **7**: 69–86.
9. Payne R. Mechanisms and management of bone pain. *Cancer* 2003; **80**: 1608–1613.
10. Mercadante S. Malignant bone pain: pathophysiology and treatment. *Pain* 1997; **69**: 1–18.
11. Coleman RE. Skeletal complications of malignancy. *Cancer* 1997; **80**: 1588–1594.
12. Chow E, Harris K, Fan G, et al. Palliative radiotherapy trials for bone metastases: a systematic review. *J Clin Oncol* 2007; **25**: 1423–1436.
13. Wu JS, Wong R, Johnston M, et al. Meta-analysis of dose-fractionation radiotherapy trials for the palliation of painful bone metastases. *Int J Radiat Oncol Biol Phys* 2003; **55**: 594–605.
14. Sze WM, Shelley M, Held I, et al. Palliation of metastatic bone pain: single fraction versus multifraction radiotherapy – a systematic review of the randomised trials. *Cochrane Database Syst Rev* 2004; **(2)**: CD004721.
15. Falkmer U, Jarhult J, Wersall P, et al. A systematic overview of radiation therapy effects in skeletal metastases. *Acta Oncol* 2003; **42**: 620–633.
16. Chow E, Wu J, Hoskin P, et al. International consensus on palliative radiotherapy endpoints for future clinical trials in bone metastases. *Radiother Oncol* 2002; **64**: 275–280.
17. Vakaet LA, Boterberg T. Pain control by ionizing radiation of bone metastasis. *Int J Dev Biol* 2004; **48**: 599–606.
18. Lutz S, Berk L, Chang E, et al. Palliative radiotherapy for bone metastases: an ASTRO evidence-based guideline. *Int J Radiat Oncol Biol Phys* 2011; **79**: 965–976.
19. van den Hout WB, van der Linden YM, Steenland E, et al. Single- versus multiple-fraction radiotherapy in patients with painful bone metastases: cost-utility analysis based on a randomized trial. *J Natl Cancer Inst* 2003; **95**: 222–229.

20. Konski A, James J, Hartsell W, *et al.* Economic analysis of radiation therapy oncology group 97-14: multiple versus single fraction radiation treatment of patients with bone metastases. *Am J Clin Oncol* 2009; **32**: 423–428.
21. van der Linden YM, Steenland E, van Houwelingen H, *et al.* Patients with a favourable prognosis are equally palliated with single and multiple fraction radiotherapy: results on survival in the Dutch Bone Metastasis Study. *Radiother Oncol* 2006; **48**: 245–253.
22. Meeuse JJ, van der Linden YM, van Tienhoven G, *et al.* Efficacy of radiotherapy for painful bone metastases during the last 12 weeks of life: results from the Dutch Bone Metastasis Study. *Cancer* 2010; **116**: 2716–2725.
23. Dennis K, Wong K, Zhang L, *et al.* Palliative radiotherapy for bone metastases in the last 3 months of life: worthwhile or futile? *Clin Oncol (R Coll Radiol)* 2011; **23**: 709–715.
24. Foro AP, Fontanals AV, Galceran JC, *et al.* Randomized clinical trial with two palliative radiotherapy regimens in painful bone metastases: 30 Gy in 10 fractions compared with 8 Gy in single fraction. *Radiother Oncol* 2008; **89**: 150–155.
25. Roos DE, Turner SL, O'Brien PC, *et al.* Randomized trial of 8 Gy in 1 versus 20 Gy in 5 fractions of radiotherapy for neuropathic pain due to bone metastases (Trans-Tasman Radiation Oncology Group, TROG 96.05). *Radiother Oncol* 2005; **75**: 54–63.
26. Dennis K, Chow E, Roos D, *et al.* Should bone metastases causing neuropathic pain be treated with single-dose radiotherapy? *Clin Oncol (R Coll Radiol)* 2011; **23**: 482–484.
27. Gaze MN, Kelly CG, Kerr GR, *et al.* Pain relief and quality of life following radiotherapy for bone metastases: a randomised trial of two fractionation schedules. *Radiother Oncol* 1997; **45**: 109–116.
28. Hartsell WF, Scott C, Bruner DW, *et al.* Phase III randomized trial of 8 Gy in 1 fraction vs. 30 Gy in 10 fractions for palliation of painful bonemetastases: preliminary results of RTOG 97-14. *Int J Radiat Oncol Biol Phys* 2003; **57**: S124.
29. Chow E, Loblaw A, Harris K, *et al.* Dexamethasone for the prophylaxis of radiation-induced pain flare after palliative radiotherapy for bone metastases: a pilot study. *Support Care Cancer* 2007; **15**: 643–647.
30. Loblaw DA, Wu JS, Kirkbride P, *et al.* Pain flare in patients with bone metastases after palliative radiotherapy – a nested randomized control trial. *Support Care Cancer* 2007; **15**: 451–455.
31. Hird A, Chow E, Zhang L, *et al.* Determining the incidence of pain flare following palliative radiotherapy for symptomatic bone metastases: results from three Canadian cancer centers. *Int J Radiat Oncol Biol Phys* 2009; **75**: 193–197.
32. van der Linden YM, Lok JJ, Steenland E, *et al.* Single fraction radiotherapy is efficacious: a further analysis of the Dutch Bone Metastasis Study controlling for the influence of retreatment. *Int J Radiat Oncol Biol Phys* 2004; **59**: 528–537.
33. Chow E, Hoskin P, Mitera G, *et al.* Update of the international consensus on palliative radiotherapy endpoints for future clinical trials in bone metastases. *Int J Radiat Oncol Biol Phys* 2012; **82**: 1730–1737.
34. Huisman M, van den Bosch MA, Wijlemans JW, *et al.* Effectiveness of reirradiation for painful bone metastases: a systematic review and meta-analysis. *Int J Radiat Oncol Biol Phys* 2012; **84**: 8–14.
35. Chow E, Hoskin PJ, Wu J, *et al.* A phase III international randomised trial comparing single with multiple fractions for re-irradiation of painful bone metastases: National Cancer Institute of Canada Clinical Trials Group (NCIC CTG) SC 20. *Clin Oncol (R Coll Radiol)* 2006; **18**: 125–128.

36. Lieberman I, Reinhardt MK. Vertebroplasty and kyphoplasty for osteolytic vertebral collapse. *Clin Orthop* 2003; Oct **(415 Suppl)**: S176–S186.

37. Kallmes DF, Jensen ME. Percutaneous vertebroplasty. *Radiology* 2003; **229**: 27–36.

38. Goetz MP, Callstrom MR, Charboneau JW, *et al*. Percutaneous image-guided radiofrequency ablation of painful metastases involving bone: a multicenter study. *J Clin Oncol* 2004; **22**: 300–306.

39. Masala S, Schillaci O, Bartolucci AD, *et al*. Metabolic and clinical assessment of efficacy of cryoablation therapy on skeletal masses by 18F FDG positron emission tomography/ computed tomography (PET/CT) and visual analogue scale (VAS): initial experience. *Skeletal Radiol* 2011; **40**: 159–165.

40. Kurup AN, Callstrom MR. Ablation of skeletal metastases: current status. *J Vasc Interv Radiol* 2010; **21**: S242–S250.

41. Harvey HA. Issues concerning the role of chemotherapy and hormonal therapy of bone metastases from breast carcinoma. *Cancer* 1997; **80**: 1646–1651.

42. Finlay IG, Mason MD, Shelley M. Radioisotopes for the palliation of metastatic bone cancer: a systematic review. *Lancet Oncol* 2005; **6**: 392–400.

43. Quilty PM, Kirk D, Bolger JJ. A comparison of the palliative effects of strontium-89 and external beam radiotherapy in metastatic prostate cancer. *Radiother Oncol* 1994; **31**: 33–40.

44. Hortobagyi GN, Theriault RL, Porter L, *et al*. Efficacy of pamidronate in reducing skeletal complications in patients with breast cancer and lytic bone metastases. Protocol 19 Aredia Breast Cancer Study Group. *N Engl J Med* 1996; **335**: 1785–1791.

45. Rogers MJ, Watts DJ, Russell RG. Overview of bisphosphanates. *Cancer* 1997; **80**: 1652–1657.

46. Lipton A. Bisphosphanates and metastatic breast carcinoma. *Cancer* 2003; **97**: 848–853.

47. Rosen LS, Gordon D, Simon Tchekmedyian N, *et al*. Long term efficacy and safety of Zoledronic acid in the treatment of skeletal metastases in patients with nonsmall cell lung carcinoma and other solid tumors. A randomized, phase III, double-blind, placebo-controlled trial. *Cancer* 2004; **100**: 2613–2621.

48. Stopeck AT, Lipton A, Body JJ, *et al*. Denosumab compared with zoledronic acid for the treatment of bone metastases in patients with advanced breast cancer: a randomized, double-blind study. *J Clin Oncol* 2010; **28**: 5132–5139.

49. Fizazi K, Carducci M, Smith M, *et al*. Denosumab versus zoledronic acid for treatment of bone metastases in men with castration-resistant prostate cancer: a randomised, double-blind study. *Lancet* 2011; **377**: 813–822.

50. Springfield DS. Pathologic fractures. In: Bucholz RW, Heckman JD. (eds) *Rockwood & Green's Fractures in Adults*. Philadelphia: Lippincott Williams & Wilkins, 2001, pp. 557–583.

51. Nielsen OS, Munro AJ, Tannock IF. Bone metastases: pathophysiology and management policy. *J Clin Oncol* 1991; **9**: 509–524.

52. van der Linden YM, Dijkstra PD, Kroon HM, *et al*. Comparative analysis of risk factors for pathological fracture with femoral metastases. Results based on a randomised trial of radiotherapy. *J Bone Joint Surg Br* 2004; **86-B**: 566–573.

53. van der Linden YM, Kroon HM, Dijkstra PD, *et al*. Simple radiographic parameter predicts fracturing in metastatic femoral bone lesions: results from a randomized trial. *Radiother Oncol* 2003; **69**: 21–31.

54. Tanck E, van Aken JB, van der Linden YM, *et al*. Pathological fracture prediction in patients with metastatic lesions can be improved with quantitative computed tomography based computer models. *Bone* 2009; **45**: 777–783.

55. Koswig S, Budach V. [Remineralization and pain relief in bone metastases after different radiotherapy fractions (10 times 3 Gy vs. 1 time 8 Gy). A prospective study]. *Strahlenther Onkol* 1999; **175**: 500–508.

56. Townsend PW, Smalley SR, Cozad SC, *et al.* Role of postoperative radiation therapy after stabilization of fractures caused by metastatic disease. *Int J Radiat Oncol Biol Phys* 1995; **31**: 43–49.

57. Gerszten PC, Burton SA, Ozhasoglu C, *et al.* Radiosurgery for spinal metastases: clinical experience in 500 cases from a single institution. *Spine (Phila Pa 1976)* 2007; **32**: 193–199.

58. Wang XS, Rhines LD, Shiu AS, *et al.* Stereotactic body radiation therapy for management of spinal metastases in patients without spinal cord compression: a phase 1–2 trial. *Lancet Oncol* 2012; **13**: 395–402.

59. Kaasa S, Brenne E, Lund JA, *et al.* Prospective randomised multicenter trial on single fraction radiotherapy (8 Gy × 1) versus multiple fractions (3 Gy × 10) in the treatment of painful bone metastases. *Radiother Oncol* 2006; **79**: 278–284.

CHAPTER 21

Spinal cord compression

Ernesto Maranzano, Fabio Trippa

Radiation Oncology Centre, Santa Maria Hospital, Terni, Italy

Introduction

Definition and incidence

The definition of metastatic spinal cord compression (MSCC) has changed over the last few decades. It has both clinical and radiographic criteria and encompasses the anatomy of the cord as well as the cauda equina. The Princess Margaret Hospital of Canada defines MSCC as: "compression of the dural sac (spinal cord and/or cauda equina) and its content by an extradural tumor mass. The minimum evidence for cord compression is indentation of the theca at the level of clinical features (i.e. local or radicular pain, weakness, sensory disturbance, and/or sphincter dysfunction)." Spinal cord compression is one of the most dreaded complications of metastatic cancer, occurring in 5–10% of all cancer patients during the course of their disease requiring urgent oncologic care [1]. Autopsy studies suggest that approximately one-third of patients with solid tumors may have metastases to the spine, but clinical evidence of MSCC is found in 3 to 7% of patients [2]. Approximately 50% of MSCC cases in adults arise from breast, lung, or prostate cancer, but MSCC has also been described in patients with lymphoma, melanoma, renal cell carcinoma, thyroid carcinoma, sarcoma, and myeloma. In children, the most common tumors are sarcoma, neuroblastoma, and lymphoma [2]. The most frequently involved site is the thoracic spine (59–78%), followed by the lumbar spine (16–33%) and the cervical spine (4–13%) [3]. Several studies have shown that MSCC arises at multiple non-contiguous levels in 10 to 38% of cases and the tumoral mass is usually located in the anterior or antero-lateral spinal canal [4].

Pathophysiology

In the majority of cases, vertebral body metastases can produce spinal cord compression in two ways. The first results from continued growth and obliteration of the marrow space with expansion into the epidural space,

Radiation Oncology in Palliative Cancer Care, First Edition. Edited by Stephen Lutz, Edward Chow, and Peter Hoskin.
© 2013 John Wiley & Sons, Ltd. Published 2013 by John Wiley & Sons, Ltd.

producing impingement on the anterior thecal sac and its surrounding venous plexus. Alternatively, destruction of cortical bone by the tumor can result in vertebral body collapse with posterior displacement of bony fragments into the epidural space and epidural venous plexus. The pathophysiology of MSCC is vascular in nature because the compression of the epidural venous plexus leads to venous stasis, consequent hypoxia, and increased vascular permeability. This edema impairs spinal cord function which results in weakness and sensory impairment. In more advanced stages, the increased interstitial edema combined with progressive direct physical pressure on the spinal cord by the expanding mass ultimately leads to ischemia of white matter and permanent neurologic loss [5].

Clinical presentation and diagnosis

Spinal cord compression, once established, is usually highly symptomatic (Box 21.1). Pain accompanies spinal cord compression in approximately 95% of adults and 80% of children with MSCC, and usually precedes the diagnosis by days to months. Pain can be local, radicular, or both. Local pain (i.e. back or neck pain) depends on expansion, destruction, or fracture of the involved vertebral elements and radicular pain is caused by compression of the nerve roots or cauda equina. Several characteristics distinguish it from the pain of degenerative joint disease. The first may arise at any level, whereas the second one rarely occurs outside the low cervical or low lumbar spine. Recumbence alleviates the pain of degenerative joint disease but frequently aggravates that of MSCC [2]. Weakness, the second most common symptom at presentation, usually follows the development of local or radicular pain and generally progresses to plegia over a period of hours or days [2]. Other symptoms of MSCC are sensory loss and incontinence, which typically develop after the pain. Urinary retention (a common occurrence in patients who receive narcotics) is an atypical presentation without spinal pain or neurologic signs [3]. Unfortunately, plegic patients have a poor prognosis, regardless of treatment administered. For this reason, MSCC should be suspected in cancer patients with back pain, and osteolysis and/or bone scan positivity even in the absence of neurologic deficits.

It is worth noting that magnetic resonance imaging (MRI) diagnoses MSCC in 32 to 35% of patients with back pain, bone metastases, and a normal

---

Box 21.1 Symptoms commonly associated with spinal cord compression

- Pain
- Weakness
- Sensory loss
- Incontinence
- Urinary retention

neurologic examination [6]. In the pre-MRI era, myelography and computed tomography (CT) were the imaging modalities of choice for the diagnosis of MSCC, and CT remains the best exam when MRI is not available. MRI has a sensitivity of 93%, a specificity of 97%, and an overall diagnostic accuracy of 95% in detecting MSCC [7]. The advantages of MRI include its non-invasive ability to image soft tissue anatomy in detail, its ability to image multiple levels of cord impingement in one examination, and consequently, its usefulness in planning local treatment.

Survival rates and life expectancy

Prognosis is above all related to early diagnosis and therapy. The speed of neurologic deficit onset can condition functional outcome, which is significantly better with slower development of motor dysfunction before RT. One study evidenced that ambulatory recovery occurred in 86% and 35% of patients with a history of >14 days compared with 1–7 days, respectively [8]. Survival after MSCC is related to primary tumor type ranging from 17–20 months for breast, prostate, and myeloma to only 4 months for lung [9]. If untreated, the majority of patients with MSCC become paraplegic. Early detection and treatment when the patient is still able to walk result in the highest chance of ambulation [10].

Treatment

In MSCC the aim of treatment is to improve the patient's quality of life through control of back pain and preservation or recovery of motor and sphincter functions. Although it could be questioned whether local treatment increases patients' survival, there is a tight relationship between survival time and functional status. In fact, MSCC patients who have no motor dysfunction live longer than paraparetic and paraplegic ones, and generally die of systemic tumors rather than local progression at the spine. Considering that treatment success is related to the severity of the epidural disease and to the patient's clinical condition at the time of diagnosis, it is important to confirm diagnosis early and to begin treatment before significant myelopathy develops [4,11,12]. Treatment of spinal cord compression can be surgery followed by radiotherapy (RT) or RT alone. The choice of treatment depends on patient selection according to specific factors reported in Figure 21.1 and discussed below. When a diagnosis of MSCC is made, the first intervention is generally steroids to control edema and lessen pain.

Surgery

Surgery plays an important role in selected cases. Patchell *et al.* published the results of a trial that randomized patients to surgery and post-operative RT or RT alone [13]. The study aimed to recruit 200 patients but was prematurely closed after a planned interim analysis demonstrated significant improvement in ambulatory rate in the combined surgery and RT arm. The published

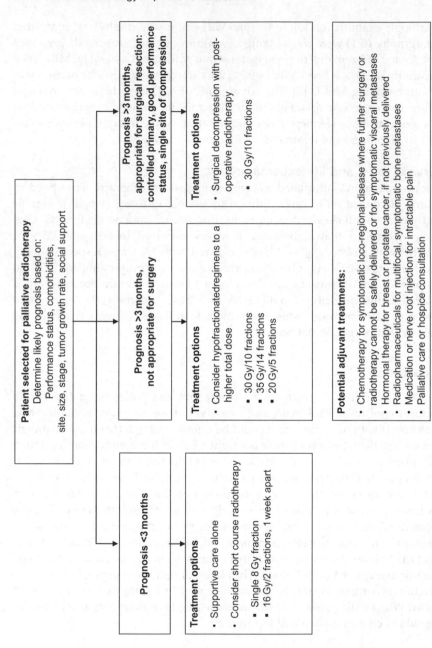

Figure 21.1 Algorithm for use of palliative radiotherapy for patients with spinal cord compression.

results are therefore based on 101 patients accrued from seven centers over a 10-year period with 70 of the patients recruited from one centre. The study has been criticized because of the poor results in the RT-alone arm which contrast with published RT data and, furthermore, since mechanical causes of cord compression were not stipulated as an exclusion criteria some patients may have been treated inappropriately with RT alone [1,14]. A secondary data analysis of this study published in 2009 looked at age stratification and demonstrated a tight interaction between age and treatment effect, such that as age increases, the benefit of surgery is diminished. Statistical analysis showed that there was no difference in outcome between treatments for patients aged 65 years or above [15].

A meta-analysis of surgery versus RT for MSCC published in 2005 found a statistically significant difference between surgery and RT in the ambulatory success rates [16]. Overall, the surgical patients were 1.3 times more likely to be ambulatory after treatment compared with the RT patients. However, the surgical data used in this meta-analysis contain primarily uncontrolled cohort studies and preceded the Patchell *et al.* publication. Conversely, an analysis performed retrospectively on 122 patients treated with surgery followed by RT matched 11 known prognostic factors to 244 patients submitted to RT alone and found that treatment approach had no impact on outcome and survival [17]. On the basis of the literature evidence, it can be concluded that initial surgical resection followed by RT should be considered for a carefully selected group of patients that are affected by single-level MSCC and neurologic deficits and controlled or absent primary and metastatic disease elsewhere. Other possible indications for surgery include stabilization, vertebral body collapse causing bone impingement on the cord or nerve root, compression recurring after RT, and an unknown primary requiring histologic confirmation for diagnosis [1,3,18]. However, when there are diagnostic doubts, CT-guided percutaneous vertebral biopsy can be an alternative to open surgery to avoid surgical side effects, and reduce incisional pain and recovery period [19].

Regarding the surgical approach, laminectomy should be abandoned in favor of a more aggressive surgery (i.e. posterior, anterior, and/or lateral approach, tumor mass resection, and stabilization of the spine). In fact, laminectomy does not remove the neoplastic mass and, when there is vertebral body collapse, it may also cause post-surgery spinal instability [1,3,18]. Moreover, the indication for surgery is also related to performance status and life expectancy of patients and to the extent of disease. Radiotherapy must be administered generally 7–10 days after surgery, either after no grossly complete resection or as an adjuvant treatment after a macroscopic radical ablative surgical procedure.

Radiotherapy

Although RT is an effective approach for the majority of MSCC patients, the optimal radiation schedule remains unknown. Except in particular circumstances, the use of conventional fractionated RT (2 Gy per day to a total dose of 30–50 Gy in 3–5 weeks) has been abandoned in favor of RT regimens requiring a smaller number of fractions. Since 2005, two phase III randomized multi-center Italian trials have been published [20,21]. The first compared a short-course regimen (i.e. 8 Gy repeated after one week to a total dose of 16 Gy) to a split-course regimen (i.e. 5 Gy × 3, 4 days rest, and then 3 Gy × 5) [20]. The second compared the same short-course regimen to 8 Gy in a single fraction [21]. It is worth noting that both of these studies were performed on patients with short life expectancy (6 months), and that responders maintained function until death. While both hypofractionated RT regimens adopted were effective, the authors concluded that 8 Gy single fraction is the best option considering that it is well-tolerated, effective, and convenient in this setting of patients. Published retrospective and prospective non-randomized data support the above randomized data in that no dose-fractionation schedule has demonstrated a higher ambulation rate [20,22] (Table 21.1). However, some experience suggested that in MSCC patients, duration of local control is superior, and consequently the rate of in-field recurrences is lower

Table 21.1 Clinical response comparing different radiotherapy regimens in metastatic spinal cord compression.

Author	Number of patients	Short-course RT regimens (number of fractions)	Long-course RT regimens (number of fractions)	Ambulation response rate
Randomized trials				
Maranzano et al. 2005 [20]	300	16 Gy (2)	15 Gy (3) + 15 Gy (5)	68% vs 71% (NS)
Maranzano et al. 2009 2009 [21]	327	16 Gy (2)	8 Gy (1)	69% vs 62% (NS)
Non-randomized trials				
Rades et al. 2004 [23]	214	30 Gy (10)	40 Gy (20)	68% vs 71% (NS)
Rades et al. 2005 [24]	1304	8 Gy (1) 20 Gy (5)	30 Gy (10) 37.7 Gy (15) 40 Gy (20)	68.5% vs 67% (NS)
Rades et al. 2011 [25]	231	8 Gy (1) 20 Gy (5)	30 Gy (10) 37.7 Gy (15) 40 Gy (20)	84% vs 84% (NS)

RT, radiotherapy; NS, not significant; vs, versus.

following long-course RT regimens; these data add further weight to the argument for selecting patient treatment based on prognosis [23–25].

Recently, Rades *et al.* published a score predicting post-RT ambulatory status [26]. It was developed based on 2,096 retrospectively evaluated MSCC patients and considered six prognostic factors (i.e. tumor type, interval between tumor diagnosis and MSCC, presence of other bone or visceral metastases at the time of RT, pre-treatment ambulatory status, and duration of motor deficits). This scoring system has been validated prospectively for the endpoints survival and ambulatory function [26]. In conclusion, evidence suggests that until further randomized data are available, short-course/single fraction regimens (e.g. $5 \times 4\,Gy$, $2 \times 8\,Gy$, or $1 \times 8\,Gy$) can be used for patients with short life expectancy, while fractionated, higher dose schedules (e.g. $10 \times 3\,Gy$ or greater) should be considered for patients with better prognosis.

Radiotherapy planning is optimal when an MRI is available. With MRI, vertebral and paravertebral involvement can be better defined with respect to all other radiologic procedures. Radiation portals should be centered on the site of epidural compression and accurate 3D-conformal RT should be used in the majority of cases. In the 16 to 25% of cases who develop recurrent MSCC after RT, 64% of early recurrences are within two vertebral bodies of the site of initial compression [3]. Therefore, radiation portals should be extended two vertebral bodies above and two vertebral bodies below the site of compression. Adjacent sites of bony involvement and paravertebral masses should also be encompassed in the treatment portal.

Adjuvant treatment modalities

Steroids
Generally, in MSCC patients RT is administered with concomitant steroids to lessen back pain, prevent progressive neurologic symptoms, and reduce radiation-induced spinal edema [3]. Steroids should be given immediately when the clinical-radiologic diagnosis of MSCC is obtained. Dexamethasone is the most frequently used drug, although the use of methylprednisolone is also reported [26,27]. The dexamethasone dose ranges from moderate (16 mg/die in two-four-times daily parenteral or oral divided doses) to high (36–96 mg/die) preceded by a bolus of 10–100 mg intravenously [26,27]. The steroids are usually tapered over 2 weeks. No study has been published comparing high-dose to moderate dexamethasone dose. There is only one randomized clinical trial comparing high-dose dexamethasone to no drug in 57 patients with MSCC treated with RT [27]. This trial evidenced that high dose dexamethasone significantly improves post-treatment ambulation but is accompanied by a certain probability (11%) of high toxicity [28]. A phase II trial showed the feasibility of treating patients with MSCC, no neurologic

deficits, or only radiculopathy, and no massive invasion of the spine at MRI or CT, with RT ($3\,Gy \times 10$) without steroids [29]. However, in clinical practice, considering that published studies have shown no difference in outcome between high-dose and moderate dose dexamethasone, and the relatively high incidence of side effects from steroids, above all in patients with diabetes mellitus, hypertension, and peptic ulcer [30], a moderate dexamethasone dose (e.g. 16–32 mg/total daily dose) is suggested for symptomatic MSCC patients.

Chemotherapy and hormone therapy

For treatment of MSCC, chemotherapy or hormone therapy can be used in combination with RT, or alone in adults who are not surgical or radiation candidates but who have sensitive tumors such as lymphoma, small cell lung carcinoma, myeloma, breast, prostate, or germ cell tumors. In children, chemotherapy is the primary treatment for chemo-responsive tumors [3].

Promise of newer technologies

The majority of MSCC patients have low performance status, paraparesis, paraplegia, and/or other prognostic factors associated with a short life expectancy. In these cases palliative short course or single fraction RT regimens represent the standard treatment. A more aggressive palliative RT may eventually be justifiable for patients selected according to good performance status, oligometastatic disease, and longer life expectancy. In this subset of patients a higher RT dose can be prescribed using techniques to avoid excessive dose to surrounding critical normal tissue organs. Linear accelerator technology has evolved with multi-leaf collimation, intensity modulated irradiation, systems of image guidance, and robotic technology. Radiosurgery (SRS) and stereotactic body radiation therapy (SBRT) have emerged as new treatment options in the multi-disciplinary management of metastases located within or adjacent to the vertebrae and spinal cord. They provide attractive options to deliver high dose per fraction radiation, typically in single dose (e.g. of SRS, 10–16 Gy) or in hypofractionation (e.g. of SBRT, $9\,Gy \times 3$ fractions or $6\,Gy \times 5$ fractions) [31].

In contrast to other RT techniques, SRS and SBRT allow treatment to the involved vertebrae and spinal cord with a high radiation dose, reducing irradiated volume, and sparing uninvolved segments [31,32]. The role of SRS and SBRT for epidural decompression in selected groups of MSCC patients is under evaluation. These techniques are unlikely to be able to be used as an emergency procedure given the time taken for planning and treatment verification. The need for sophisticated radiation units which are offered only in a few specialized centers that are more expensive, and can be associated with a higher risk of radiation induced myelopathy, must also be considered [33–35]. Radiosurgery is to be compared to conventional RT as upfront treatment for spinal metastases in a randomized trial. This study is being conducted by the Radiation Therapy Oncology Group and will include patients with a limited number (1–3) of vertebral metastases, with or without minimal spinal cord compression.

Re-irradiation

Patients should be followed clinically and/or radiologically to determine whether a local relapse or a subsequent MSCC episode develops in a non-irradiated spine. Although few data are available in the literature, in patients with MSCC, the incidence of an in-field recurrence can vary from 2.5 to 11% of cases and can occur 2–40 months after the first RT cycle [3,7].

In the majority of cases, RT remains the only treatment option, even if radiation oncologists are reluctant to give re-irradiation to the spinal cord. Radiation-induced myelopathy (RIM) is a relevant late toxicity, because it may result in severe neurologic dysfunction. Higher RT doses, larger doses per fraction, and previous exposure to radiation could be associated with a higher probability of developing RIM [36]. The dose and technique of radiation should be chosen to keep the cumulative biologically effective dose of RT less than $120\,\mathrm{Gy_2}$ [18]. In fact, in the case of re-irradiation with the aim to facilitate the comparison of different fractionation schedules, the total doses of the first and second treatment were transformed to the biologically effective dose using the linear-quadratic model. The following equation was used:

$$\text{biologically effective dose} = \text{total dose} \times (1 + \text{single dose} / \alpha / \beta \text{ value})$$

where α is the linear (first-order dose-dependent) component of cell killing, β is the quadratic (second-order dose-dependent) component of cell killing, and the α/β ratio is the dose at which both components of cell killing are equal. Generally, the α/β ratio suggested for RIM is $2\,\mathrm{Gy}$. Using this biologic threshold, no myelopathy was observed in 24 of Maranzano's patients and 124 of Rades' patients [36,37]. As with the first presentation of MSCC diagnosis, prognosis, probability of neurologic recovery, and time to neurologic recovery are highly dependent on pre-treatment neurologic status [1,7].

The new RT techniques can be used to minimize cord dose, while the tumor receives higher dose; recent experiences have been published [38,39]. In Figure 21.2 an example of re-irradiation with SBRT in a MSCC patient who relapsed after primary RT is shown.

Special considerations in developing countries

Patients in developing countries may present for management of spinal cord compression in a time frame with lower chances for preventing or reversing paralysis, especially given that a difference of merely a few hours can alter

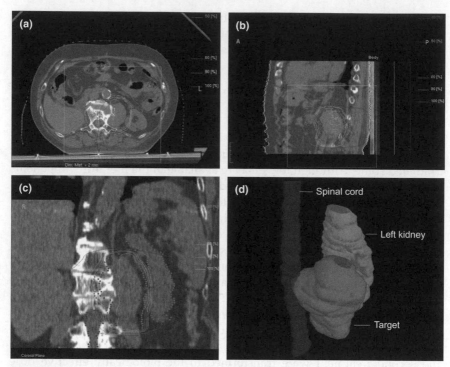

Figure 21.2 Re-irradiation with stereotactic body radiation therapy of left paravertebral mass involving omolateral radicular root: treatment planning and elaboration in axial (a), sagittal (b) and coronal (c) planes. The planning target volume (PTV) and the curve of isodose which encompasses the target are shown. In 3D-reconstruction (d) it shows the PTV (nearmost) and the near organ at risk (spinal cord and left kidney) volumes (see Plate 21.1).

those odds a great deal. Furthermore, access to qualified surgeons or appropriately equipped radiotherapy facilities may be limited in some geographic locales, to the detriment of the patient. Simple radiotherapy techniques using direct fields with cobalt can be effective and may need to be applied based on clinical diagnoses in this setting.

Conclusion

Early diagnosis and prompt therapy are powerful predictors of outcome in MSCC. Generally, RT is accepted as the first line treatment for the majority of patients with metastasis at the spinal cord or nerve roots, and surgery should be considered for a carefully selected group of patients, specifically with single-level MSCC and neurologic deficits. Although RT is an effective treatment for MSCC patients, the optimal radiation schedule remains unknown. As suggested by many prospective clinical trials, a hypofractionated RT regimen can be considered the regimen of choice, while more protracted RT schedules (e.g. 3 Gy × 10 fractions) can be used in selected MSCC patients with a predicted long life expectancy. The new technologies of irradiation provide an interesting opportunity for patients relapsing after a previous RT, though it is much more expensive and can be administered only in highly specialized radiation centers.

References

1. Loblaw DA, Perry J, Chambers A, *et al.* Systematic review of the diagnosis and management of malignant extradural spinal cord compression: the Cancer Care Ontario Practice Guidelines Initiative's Neuro-Oncology Disease Site Group. *J Clin Oncol* 2005; **23**: 2028–2037.
2. Byrne TN. Spinal cord compression from epidural metastases. *N Engl J Med* 1992; **327**: 614–619.
3. Maranzano E, Trippa F, Chirico L, *et al.* Management of metastatic spinal cord compression. *Tumori* 2003; **89**: 469–475.
4. Gilbert HS, Kim JB, Posner JB. Epidural spinal cord compression from metastatic tumor: diagnosis and treatment. *Ann Neurol* 1978; **3**: 40–51.
5. Arguello F, Baggs RB, Duerst RE, *et al.* Pathogenesis of vertebral metastasis and epidural spinal cord compression. *Cancer* 1990; **65**: 98–106.
6. Bayley A, Milosevic M, Blend R, *et al.* A prospective study of factors predicting clinically occult spinal cord compression in patients with metastatic prostate carcinoma. *Cancer* 2001; **92**: 303–310.
7. Maranzano E, Bellavita R, Floridi P, *et al.* Radiation-induced myelopathy in long-term metastatic spinal cord compression patients after hypofractionated radiotherapy: a clinical and magnetic resonance imaging analysis. *Radiother Oncol* 2001; **60**: 281–288.
8. Rades D, Heidenreich F, Karstens JH. Final results of a prospective study of the prognostic value of the time to develop motor deficits before irradiation in metastatic spinal cord compression. *Int J Radiat Oncol Biol Phys* 2002; **53**: 975–979.
9. Prewett S, Venkitaraman R. Metastatic spinal cord compression: review of the evidence for a radiotherapy dose fractionation schedule. *Clin Oncol* 2010; **22**: 222–230.
10. Prasad D, Schiff D. Malignant spinal-cord compression. *Lancet Oncol* 2005; **6**: 15–24.
11. Maranzano E, Latini P. Effectiveness of radiation therapy without surgery in metastatic spinal cord compression: final results from a prospective trial. *Int J Radiat Oncol Biol Phys* 1995; **32**: 959–967.
12. Rades D, Blach M, Bremer M. Prognostic significance of the time of developing motor deficits before radiation therapy in metastatic spinal cord compression: one-year results of a prospective trial. *Int J Radiat Oncol Biol Phys* 2000; **48**: 1403–1408.
13. Patchell RA, Tibbs PA, Regine WF, *et al.* Direct decompressive surgical resection in the treatment of spinal cord compression caused by metastatic cancer: a randomised trial. *Lancet* 2005; **366**: 643–648.
14. Maranzano E, Trippa F. Be careful in getting cost-effectiveness conclusions from a debatable trial! *Int J Radiat Oncol Biol Phys* 2007; **68**: 314.
15. Chi JH, Gokaslan Z, McCormick P, *et al.* Selecting patients for treatment for metastatic epidural spinal radiosurgery cord compression: does age matter?: results from a randomized trial. *Spine* 2009; **35**: 431–435.

16. Klimo P Jr, Thompson CJ, Kestle JR, *et al*. A meta-analysis of surgery versus conventional radiotherapy for the treatment of metastatic spinal epidural disease. *Neuro Oncol* 2005; 7: 64–76.

17. Rades D, Huttenlocher S, Dunst J, *et al*. Matched pair analysis comparing surgery followed by radiotherapy and radiotherapy alone for metastatic spinal cord compression. *J Clin Oncol* 2010; 28: 3597–3604.

18. Holt T, Hoskin P, Maranzano E, *et al*. Malignant epidural spinal cord compression: the role of external beam radiotherapy. *Curr Opin Support Palliat Care* 2012; 6: 103–108.

19. Adapon BD, Legenda BD Jr, Lim EV, *et al*. CT-guided closed biopsy of the spine. *J Comput Assist Tomogr* 1981; 5: 73–78.

20. Maranzano E, Bellavita R, Rossi R, *et al*. Short-course versus split-course radiotherapy in metastatic spinal cord compression: results of a phase III, randomized, multicenter trial. *J Clin Oncol* 2005; 23: 3358–3365.

21. Maranzano E, Trippa F, Casale M, *et al*. 8Gy single-dose radiotherapy is effective in metastatic spinal cord compression: results of a phase III randomized multicentre Italian trial. *Radiother Oncol* 2009; 93: 174–179.

22. Venkitaraman R, Sohaib SA, Barbachano Y, *et al*. Frequency of screening magnetic resonance imaging to detect occult spinal cord compromise and to prevent neurological deficit in metastatic castration-resistant prostate cancer. *Clin Oncol* 2010; 22: 147–152.

23. Rades D, Fehlauer F, Stalpers LJ, *et al*. A prospective evaluation of two radiotherapy schedules with 10 versus 20 fractions for the treatment of metastatic spinal cord compression: final results of a multicenter study. *Cancer* 2004; 101: 2687–2692.

24. Rades D, Stalpers LJ, Veninga T, *et al*. Evaluation of five radiation schedules and prognostic factors for metastatic spinal cord compression. *J Clin Oncol* 2005; 23: 3366–3375.

25. Rades D, Lange M, Veninga T, *et al*. Final results of a prospective study comparing the local control of short-course and long-course radiotherapy for metastatic spinal cord compression. *Int J Radiat Oncol Biol Phys* 2011; 79: 524–530.

26. Rades D, Douglas S, Huttenlocher S, *et al*. Validation of a score predicting post-treatment ambulatory status after radiotherapy for metastatic spinal cord compression. *Int J Radiat Oncol Biol Phys* 2011; 79: 1503–1506.

27. Loblaw A, Laperriere NJ. Emergency treatment of malignant extradural spinal cord compression: an evidence-based guideline. *J Clin Oncol* 1998; 16: 1613–1624.

28. Sorensen S, Helweg-Larsen S, Mouridsen H, *et al*. Effect of high-dose dexamethasone in carcinomatous metastatic spinal cord compression treated with radiotherapy: a randomized trial. *Eur J Cancer* 1994; 1: 22–27.

29. Maranzano E, Latini P, Beneventi S, *et al*. Radiotherapy without steroids in selected metastatic spinal cord compression patients. A phase II trial. *Am J Clin Oncol* 1996; 19: 179–184.

30. Weissman DE. Glucocorticoid treatment for brain metastases and epidural spinal cord compression: a review. *J Clin Oncol* 1988; 6: 543–551.

31. Saghal A, Larson DA, Chang EL. Stereotactic Body radiosurgery for spinal metastases: a critical review. *Int J Radiat Oncol Biol Phys* 2008; 71: 652–665.

32. Regine W, Ryu S, Chang EL. Spine radiosurgery for spinal cord compression: the radiation oncologist's perspective. *Jour. of Radiosurgery and SBRT* 2011; 1: 55–61.

33. Chang EL, Shiu AS, Mendel E, *et al*. Phase I/II study of stereotactic body radiotherapy for spinal metastasis and its pattern of failure. *J Neurosurg Spine* 2007; 7: 151–160.

34. Gerszten PC, Burton SA, Ozhasoglu C, *et al*. Radiosurgery for spinal metastases: clinical experience in 500 cases from a single institution. *Spine* 2007; 32: 193–199.

35. Macbeth F, Wheldom TE, Girling DJ, *et al.* Radiation myelopathy: estimates of risk in 1048 patients in three randomised trials of palliative radiotherapy for non-small cell lung cancer. The Medical Research Council Lung Cancer Working Party. *Clin Oncol* 1996; **8**: 176–181.

36. Maranzano E, Trippa F, Casale M, *et al.* Reirradiation of metastatic spinal cord compression: definitive results of two randomized trials. *Radiother Oncol* 2011; **98**: 234–237.

37. Rades D, Rudat V, Veninga T, *et al.* Prognostic factors for functional outcome and survival after reirradiation for in-field recurrences of metastatic spinal cord compression. *Cancer* 2008; **113**: 1090–1096.

38. Ryu S, Rock J, Jain R, *et al.* Radiosurgical decompression of metastatic epidural compression. *Cancer* 2010; **116**: 2250–2257.

39. Mancosu P, Navarria P, Bignardi M, *et al.* Re-irradiation of metastatic spinal cord compression: a feasibility study by volumetric-modulated arc radiotherapy for in-field recurrence creating a dosimetric hole on the central canal. *Radiother Oncol* 2010; **94**: 67–70.

CHAPTER 22

Brain metastases

May Tsao
Department of Radiation Oncology, University of Toronto; Sunnybrook Odette
Cancer Centre, Toronto, ON, Canada

Introduction

Incidence, prevalence, and symptoms

Brain metastases are a significant cause of morbidity and mortality in the cancer population. Up to approximately 40% of patients diagnosed with cancer will develop one or more brain metastases during the course of their illness [1]. Lung, breast, and melanoma are the most frequent to develop brain metastases and account for 67–80% of all cancers [2]. Symptoms from brain metastases vary from general neurologic symptoms such as those caused by increased intracranial pressure to specific neurologic deficits dependent on the site of the brain metastases to no symptoms, whatsoever (Box 22.1).

Survival rates/life expectancy

Although several prognostic indices have been reported in the literature [3–11] for survival duration in patients with newly diagnosed brain metastases, three prognostic characteristics (namely age, performance status, and extracranial disease status) are consistently included among all the prognostic indices. The Radiation Therapy Oncology Group (RTOG) reported on three prognostic groups using recursive partitioning analysis (RPA) [3,4]. Based on 1200 patients treated in prospective trials of whole brain radiation therapy (WBRT) alone or with the addition of radiosensitizers, the three prognostic groups were the following: Class I, patients with Karnofsky performance status (KPS) ≥ 70, age less than 65 years and controlled primary (3 month stability on imaging or newly diagnosed), and no extracranial metastases; Class III, KPS <70 and Class II, all others. Median survivals were 7.1 months, 4.2 months, and 2.3 months for Class I, II, and III respectively.

The graded prognostic assessment (GPA) [5,10,11] identified statistically significant diagnosis-specific prognostic factors in an updated era (1985–2007) as compared to the RTOG RPA. The scoring system is based on pathologic

Radiation Oncology in Palliative Cancer Care, First Edition. Edited by Stephen Lutz,
Edward Chow, and Peter Hoskin.
© 2013 John Wiley & Sons, Ltd. Published 2013 by John Wiley & Sons, Ltd.

Box 22.1 Symptoms commonly associated with brain metastases

- General neurologic symptoms associated with increased intracranial pressure
  - ○ Headaches
  - ○ Nausea and vomiting
  - ○ Seizures
  - ○ Decreased memory
  - ○ Confusion
  - ○ Lethargy
- Focal neurologic deficits dependent upon the site of brain metastases
  - ○ Weakness due to involvement of the motor cortex
  - ○ Numbness due to involvement of the sensory cortex
  - ○ Decreased balance due to involvement of the cerebellum
  - ○ Aphasia due to involvement of speech areas
  - ○ Visual disturbance due to involvement of optic tracts or occipital lobe
  - ○ Personality changes due to involvement of the frontal lobe
- Asymptomatic, found by radiographic studies during work-up or follow-up

---

cancer diagnosis, statistically significant prognostic factors such as age, KPS, presence or absence of extracranial metastases, and number of brain metastases (Table 22.1). Median survival is estimated from the summed score (Table 22.2). Estimated survivals range from 2.8 months to 25.3 months. The addition of pathologic diagnosis to the GPA versus the RPA allows for both a better estimate of the potential worth of stereotactic radiosurgery or surgical resection for "radioresistant" metastases as well as a means by which to estimate the potential for systemic disease response to chemotherapy. Though there are insufficient data to conclusively recommend protracted WBRT schedules or single high dose radiosurgery for brain metastases due to malignant melanoma or renal cell carcinoma, the theoretical advantages to these approaches may be proven with further research.

These prognostic instruments are useful tools when educating patients about their prognosis, when separating patients into appropriate treatment categories (Figure 22.1), for predicting the results of therapeutic interventions, and for comparison of treatment results between research trials.

Radiotherapy treatment

There are various treatment modalities available to care for those with brain metastases, including WBRT, surgical resection, stereotactic radiosurgery (SRS), and supportive care including the use of dexamethasone with the goal

Table 22.1 Diagnosis specific graded prognostic assessment (GPA) [5,10,11].

GPA	Significant prognostic factors	GPA scoring criteria				
Non-small cell lung cancer / small cell lung cancer		**0**	**0.5**	**1**		
	Age	>60	50–60	<50		
	KPS	<70	70–80	90–100		
	ECM	Present	—	Absent		
	# BM	>3	2–3	1		
Melanoma/ Renal cell cancer		**0**	**1**	**2**		
	KPS	<70	70–80	90–100		
	# BM	>3	2–3	1		
Breast cancer		**0**	**0.5**	**1.0**	**1.5**	**2.0**
	KPS	<60	60	70–80	90–100	
	ER/PR/Her2	Triple negative		ER/PR + Her2 −	ER/PR − Her2 +	Triple Positive
	Age	≥70	<70			
Gastrointestinal		**0**	**1**	**2**	**3**	**4**
	KPS	<70	70	80	90	100

GPA, graded prognostic assessment; KPS, Karnofsky performance status; ECM, extra-cranial metastases; #BM, Number of brain metastases; ER, estrogen receptor; PR, progesterone receptor; Her2, human epidermal growth factor receptor 2.

Table 22.2 Median survivals stratified by diagnosis and diagnosis specific graded prognostic assessment (GPA) score for patients with newly diagnosed brain metastases [10,11,15].

Diagnosis	Overall median survival (months)	Diagnosis specific (GPA)			
		GPA: 0–1 median survival (months)	GPA: 1.5–2.0 median survival (months)	GPA: 2.5–3.0 median survival (months)	GPA: 3.5–4.0 median survival (months)
Non-small cell lung cancer	7.0	3.0	5.5	9.4	14.8
Small cell lung cancer	4.9	2.8	4.9	7.7	17.1
Melanoma	6.7	3.4	4.7	8.8	13.2
Renal Cell	9.6	3.3	7.3	11.3	14.8
Gastrointestinal	5.4	3.1	4.4	6.9	13.5
Breast	13.8	3.4	7.7	15.1	25.3
TOTAL	7.2	3.1	5.4	9.6	16.7

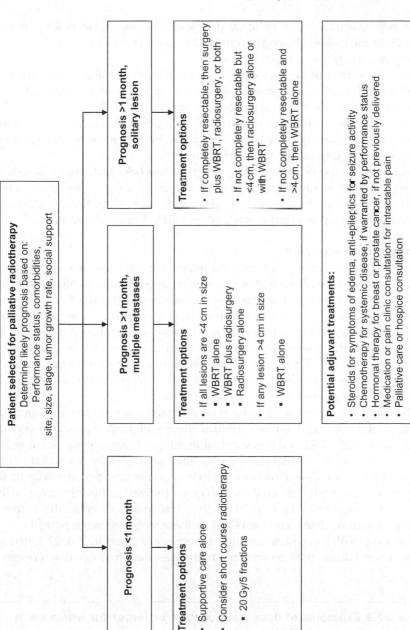

Patient selected for palliative radiotherapy
Determine likely prognosis based on:
Performance status, comorbidities,
site, size, stage, tumor growth rate, social support

Prognosis <1 month

Treatment options
- Supportive care alone
- Consider short course radiotherapy
  - 20 Gy/5 fractions

Prognosis >1 month, multiple metastases

Treatment options
- If all lesions are <4 cm in size
  - WBRT alone
  - WBRT plus radiosurgery
  - Radiosurgery alone
- If any lesion >4 cm in size
  - WBRT alone

Prognosis >1 month, solitary lesion

Treatment options
- If completely resectable, then surgery plus WBRT, radiosurgery, or both
- If not completely resectable but <4 cm, then radiosurgery alone or with WBRT
- If not completely resectable and >4 cm, then WBRT alone

Potential adjuvant treatments:
- Steroids for symptoms of edema, anti-epileptics for seizure activity
- Chemotherapy for systemic disease, if warranted by performance status
- Hormonal therapy for breast or prostate cancer, if not previously delivered
- Medication or pain clinic consultation for intractable pain
- Palliative care or hospice consultation

Figure 22.1 Algorithm for use of palliative radiotherapy for patients with brain metastases.

of decreasing intracranial swelling and pressure. The management for patients with brain metastases depends on the following factors:

Patient factors: age, performance status

Tumor factors: type of primary cancer, status of extracranial disease, number of metastatic lesion(s) to brain (single or multiple), size of brain metastases, presence of mass effect or symptomatic edema

Treatment factors: availability of radiation facilities, radiosurgery, neurosurgery, aims of therapy (survival prolongation, brain control, neurocognition preservation, improvement of symptoms)

So, through the use of the available prognostic indices and other associated factors, patients can roughly be separated into those with poor prognoses due to the extent of their intracranial or systemic disease versus those with more favorable prognoses and either single or multiple brain metastases.

Poor prognosis patients

Patients with poor prognosis (e.g. estimated survival less than 3 months) may be managed with palliative comfort measures alone (with the use of dexamethasone), or such patients may be managed with WBRT and dexamethasone. These patients often have progressive systemic disease either due to chemotherapy-insensitive tumor or a performance status so poor that it does not even allow for systemic therapy. For these patients with poor prognosis, the use of WBRT may or may not significantly improve symptoms from brain metastases. Comfort measures only with or without the use of WBRT are reasonable options.

There has only been one (outdated) randomized controlled trial performed in the pre-CT era [12] that has examined the use of prednisone alone versus prednisone and WBRT. Median survival in the prednisone alone arm was 10 weeks compared to 14 weeks in the combined arm (p value not stated). The results of a Medical Research Council trial that randomizes patients to optimal supportive care with dexamethasone versus optimal supportive care with dexamethasone plus WBRT to 20 Gy in 5 fractions will hopefully further clarify the appropriate niche for WBRT in these poor prognosis patients.

Common WBRT dose fractionation schemes are listed in Box 22.2. There are no known differences in survival among these dose fractionation schemes.

Box 22.2 Examples of dose fractionation schemes for whole brain radiation therapy (WBRT)

- 30 Gy in 10 daily fractions
- 20 Gy in 5 daily fractions
- 37.5 Gy in 15 daily fractions
- 40 Gy in 20 daily fractions
- 40 Gy in 20 twice daily fractions

There is a suggestion that 40 Gy in 20 fractions given twice per day of WBRT is associated with better brain control as compared to 20 Gy in 4 to 5 daily fractions. It is unclear whether there are differences in quality of life or neurocognitive outcomes among these different WBRT fractionation schemes, so the poorer prognosis patients would best be treated with hypofractionated courses over 4 to 5 days.

Good prognosis patients

Management of patients with good prognosis (e.g. estimated survival more than 3 months) depends on whether the patient harbors (contrast-enhanced MRI diagnosed) single brain metastasis or multiple brain metastases.

Good prognosis patients and single brain metastasis

For good prognosis patients with a single brain metastasis which is surgically amenable to complete resection, surgery improves survival and the use of post-operative WBRT improves brain control [13–17]. Noordijk et al. [13] reported a median survival of 10 months in those patients treated with surgery and WBRT versus 6 months in those patients treated with WBRT, $P = 0.04$. Patchell et al. [17] reported a median survival of 40 weeks in patients treated with surgery and WBRT versus 15 weeks in patients treated with WBRT alone, $P < 0.01$. Recurrence at the site of the original metastasis was also less frequent in the surgery and WBRT group versus the WBRT alone group, 20% vs 52%, $P < 0.02$.

The survival benefit for surgery is lost in patients with greater systemic involvement. Noordijk et al. [13] reported a 5 month median survival in patients with progressive systemic disease in both the WBRT plus surgery versus WBRT alone arms. Patients with stable systemic disease had a median of 12 month survival with WBRT and surgery versus 7 months with WBRT alone. Mintz et al. [16] reported a significant difference ($P = 0.009$) in the Cox regression analysis of mortality in patients having extracranial metastases versus no evidence of primary tumor (risk ratio 2.3).

Patchell et al. [15] reported that recurrence of tumor anywhere in the brain was less frequent in the post-operative WBRT arm compared to the surgery alone arm (18% vs 70%, $p < 0.001$). Patients in the post-operative WBRT arm were also less likely to die of neurologic causes than patients in the surgery alone arm (14% vs 44%, $P = 0.003$). There was no difference, however, in survival or length of time that patients remained functionally independent between the two arms.

The European Organization for Research and Treatment of Cancer (EORTC) 22952-26001 trial [18] found that the use of post-operative WBRT reduced 2-year relapse at the initial site of surgery from 59% to 27%, $p < 0.001$ and at new brain sites from 42% to 23%, $P = 0.008$. In addition, salvage brain therapies were used more frequently after surgery alone as compared to surgery and post-operative WBRT.

For patients with a single brain metastasis which is smaller than 4 cm in the largest dimension, radiosurgery and WBRT has been found to improve survival as compared to WBRT alone [19]. Based on the randomized controlled trial, RTOG 95-08 (19), median survival was significantly improved in patients with single brain metastasis treated with radiosurgery and WBRT (6.5 months) as compared to WBRT alone (4.9 months), $P = 0.01$.

Three trials [18,20,21] examined the use of radiosurgery alone versus WBRT and radiosurgery for selected patients with single brain metastasis. Overall, there was no survival difference among those treated with radiosurgery alone versus radiosurgery and WBRT. One trial [21] reported better neurocognitive outcomes in patients treated with radiosurgery alone. The use of postoperative WBRT significantly reduced intracranial relapse.

Some practitioners are offering use of surgery and radiation boost to the surgical cavity (with or without WBRT) in selected patients with single brain metastasis. There is a lack of randomized controlled evidence supporting this strategy. There is, however, a lower level of evidence supporting radiation boost (using radiosurgery or conformal radiation) to the surgical cavity [22–37]. The rationale of surgery and radiation boost to the surgical cavity is to improve local control to the surgical cavity and perhaps avoid neurocognitive decline by avoiding WBRT. The rationale of surgery, radiation boost, and WBRT is to maximize local control at the surgical site and overall brain control.

Good prognosis patients and multiple brain metastases

For patients with good prognosis and multiple brain metastases (all smaller than 4 cm in size), patients may be managed with radiosurgery alone, radiosurgery and WBRT, or WBRT alone [18–21,38]. There is no survival difference among these three management options. The rationale of radiosurgery and WBRT is to maximize brain control as compared to radiosurgery alone or WBRT alone. The rationale of radiosurgery alone is to avoid or delay the use of WBRT. Radiosurgery alone has been reported in one trial [21] to be associated with less neurocognitive decline as compared to radiosurgery and WBRT. The radiosurgery trials have examined selected patients with 1–4 brain metastases (all less than 4 cm in size). The optimal number of brain metastases best suited for radiosurgery remains unknown. The appropriate approaches to treatment for each of the aforementioned clinical circumstances are detailed in the guidelines publication from the American Society for Radiation Oncology (ASTRO) [39].

Side effects

Whole brain radiation therapy

The acute side effects of WBRT include hair loss, mild scalp irritation (such as dryness, mild itchiness), fatigue, and risk of increased brain edema requiring increased dexamethasone use.

The possible late side effects of WBRT include neurocognitive decline, prolonged fatigue, and chronic hair thinning.

Radiosurgery

The acute side effects of radiosurgery include pain at the pin placement sites for the stereotactic frame, small risk of seizure induction, and risk of brain edema requiring increased dexamethasone use. In most cases, radiosurgery patients can resume all of their normal activities within 1 or 2 days.

The late side effects of radiosurgery include a small chance of symptomatic radiation necrosis. Several studies have reported symptomatic radiation necrosis in 2–14% of patients and neuroradiologic changes in up to 46% of patients treated with radiosurgery [40–43]. Often, it is difficult to differentiate between recurrent brain metastasis versus radiation necrosis based on imaging alone as the appearance of central necrosis, increased contrast enhancement, and increased perilesional edema, can occur in progressive brain metastasis and in radiation necrosis. Some investigators [44] have reported that many radiographic features have a low sensitivity and predictive value for necrosis. Although pathologic examination is the gold standard for the diagnosis of radiation necrosis, the tissue retrieved may show a combination of viable tumor and radiation-induced necrotic tissue.

Radiotherapy limitations

The only scenario where survival is improved in the management of brain metastases (based on level 1 evidence) is in the situation of good prognosis patients with a single brain metastasis treated with surgery [13,14,17] or radiosurgery [19]. For all other scenarios, the use of WBRT or radiosurgery is to improve either whole brain control or targeted brain metastases control, respectively. Ultimately, these patients will succumb to uncontrolled systemic disease or uncontrolled brain metastases. Based on the GPA, survival for patients with brain metastases may be as short as 2.8–3 months for lung cancer patients with poor prognostic features or as long as 25.3 months for breast cancer patients and good prognostic features [5,10,11].

Particularly in patients with poor survival, questions arise as to whether there is value in treating brain metastases. A longitudinal observational prospective study of patients receiving WBRT (20 Gy in 5 daily fractions) for symptomatic brain metastases reported that the median survival for the 75 patients was 86 days. At 1 month, 19% of patients showed an improvement or resolution of the presenting symptoms, 23% were stable, and 55% had progressed or died. The authors concluded that many patients with brain metastases have a short life expectancy and may not benefit even from short duration radiation schedules [45].

Promise of newer technologies and areas of ongoing research

Though patients with brain metastases may not survive long enough to suffer from the late side effects of WBRT, those who do live sufficiently lengthy periods of time face some risk of diminished short-term memory as a side effect of treatment. Some studies in rodents have suggested that avoiding radiotherapy dose to the hippocampus of the brain may minimize the neuro-cognitive side effects of WBRT and that metastases only rarely affect that part of the brain. These findings have led to exciting new research approaches in which the hippocampus may be spared through the use of highly conformal therapy that treats the rest of the brain [46–48]. Additionally, the use of novel systemic therapies (including molecular targeted therapies) and stem-cell associated therapies either alone or combined with brain radiation may hold promise in the future treatment of these patients [49–66].

International patterns of care and special considerations in developing countries

An international survey was undertaken to evaluate patterns of practice for the management of metastatic disease to brain [67]. A total of 445 individuals responded to the survey over a 3 month period (April to June 2010). Forty-eight percent of respondents were from Europe, 17% from Australia/New Zealand, 10% from USA, 15% from Canada, and 10% from other countries. 91% of respondents indicated that neurosurgery facilities were available to them (9% did not have available neurosurgery services). Seventy-four percent of respondents indicated that radiosurgery services were available, whereas 26% did not have radiosurgery access. Seventy-one percent of respondents had multi-disciplinary meetings for brain metastases patients, 30% did not. Special considerations for developing countries include limited access to radiotherapy centers and lack of access to neurosurgery and radiosurgery resources. It has been estimated that only 20–25% of patients in developing countries that need radiotherapy can access it [68].

Conclusion

The management of brain metastases has historically included whole brain radiotherapy and supportive care with interventions such as dexamethasone. While these approaches still effectively palliate symptoms due to brain metastases, newer data prove the usefulness of surgery and highly conformal radiotherapy techniques in selected patients. Supportive care remains essential to the care of this group, while the choice for more aggressive therapies depends upon patient, tumor, and treatment factors. Given that virtually all of these patients will die from their brain disease or systemic manifestations of their malignancy, quality of life is a critical endpoint to be taken into account along with local control and survival duration. Studies completed to date have rarely accounted for quality of life measures, and those which have measured quality of life have been plagued by incomplete follow-up due to patient drop out due to declining functional status or death. Novel approaches are needed to address the quality of life needs of patients with brain metastases.

References

1. Gavrilovic IT, Posner JB. Brain metastases: epidemiology and pathophysiology. *J Neurooncol* 2005; **75**: 5–14.

2. Nayak L, Lee EQ, Wen PY. Epidemiology of brain metastases. *Curr Oncol Rep* 2012; **14**: 48–54.

3. Gaspar LE, Scott C, Rotman M, *et al*. Recursive partitioning analysis (RPA) of prognostic factors in three Radiation Therapy Oncology Group (RTOG) brain metastases trials. *Int J Radiat Oncol Biol Phys* 1997; **37**: 745–751.

4. Gaspar LE, Scott C, Murray K, *et al*. Validation of the RTOG recursive partitioning analysis (RPA) classification for brain metastases. *Int J Radiat Oncol Biol Phys* 2000; **47**: 1001–1006.

5. Sperduto PW, Berkey B, Gaspar LE, *et al*. A new prognostic index and comparison to three other indices for patients with brain metastases: an analysis of 1960 patients in the RTOG database. *Int J Radiat Oncol Biol Phys* 2008; **70**: 510–514.

6. Weltman E, Salvajoli JV, Brandt RA, *et al*. Radiosurgery for brain metastases: a score index for predicting prognosis. *Int J Radiat Oncol Biol Phys* 2000; **46**: 1155–1161.

7. Lorenzoni J, Devriendt D, Massager N, *et al*. Radiosurgery treatment of brain metastases: estimation of patient eligibility using three stratification systems. *Int J Radiat Oncol Biol Phys* 2004; **60**: 218–224.

8. Golden DW, Lamborn KR, McDermott MW, *et al*. Prognostic factors and grading systems for overall survival in patients treated with radiosurgery for brain metastases: variation by primary site. *J Neurosurg* 2008; **109**(Suppl): 77–86.

9. Rades D, Dunst J, Schild SE. A new scoring system to predicting the survival of patients treated with whole brain radiotherapy for brain metastases. *Strahlenther Onkol* 2008; **184**: 251–255.

10. Sperduto PW, Chao ST, Sneed PK, *et al*. Diagnosis-specific prognostic factors, indexes, and treatment outcomes for patients with newly diagnosed brain metastases: a multi-institutional analysis of 4259 patients. *Int J Radiat Oncol Biol Phys* 2010; **77**: 655–661.

11. Sperduto PW, Xu Z, Sneed P, *et al*. The graded prognostic assessment for women with brain metastases from breast cancer (GPA-Breast): a Diagnosis-specific Prognostic Index. *Int J Radiat Oncol Biol Phys* 2010; **78**(Suppl): S6–S7.

12. Horton J, Baxter DH, Olson KB. The management of metastases to the brain by irradiation and corticosteroids. *Am J Roentgenol Radium Ther Nucl Med* 1971; **111**: 334–336.

13. Noordijk EM, Vecht CJ, Haaxma-Reiche H, *et al*. The choice of treatment of single brain metastasis should be based on extracranial tumor activity and age. *Int J Radiat Oncol Biol Phys* 1994; **29**: 711–717.

14. Vecht CJ, Haaxma-Reiche H, Noordijk EM, *et al*. Treatment of single brain metastasis: radiotherapy alone or combined with neurosurgery? *Ann Neurol* 1993; **33**: 583–590.

15. Patchell RA, Tibbs PA, Regine WF, *et al*. Postoperative radiotherapy in the treatment of single brain metastasis to the brain. *JAMA* 1998; **280**: 1485–1489.

16. Mintz AH, Kestle J, Rathbone MP, *et al*. A randomized trial to assess the efficacy of surgery in addition to radiotherapy in patients with single brain metastasis. *Cancer* 1996; **78**: 1470–1476.

17. Patchell RA, Tibbs PA, Walsh JW, *et al*. A randomized trial of surgery in the treatment of single metastasis to the brain. *N Engl J Med* 1990; **322**: 494–500.

18. Kocher M, Soffietti R, Abacioglu U, *et al*. Adjuvant whole-brain radiotherapy versus observation after radiosurgery or surgical resection of one to three cerebral metastases: results of the EORTC 22952-26001 study. *J Clin Oncol* 2011; **29**: 134–142.

19. Andrews DW, Scott CB, Sperduto PW, *et al.* Whole brain radiation therapy with or without stereotactic radiosrugery boost for patients with one to three brain metastases: phase III results of the RTOG 9508 randomised trial. *Lancet* 2004; **363**: 1665–1672.

20. Aoyama H, Shirato H, Tago M, *et al.* Stereotactic radiosurgery plus whole-brain radiation therapy versus stereotactic radiosurgery alone for the treatment of brain metastases: a randomized controlled trial. *JAMA* 2006; **295**: 2483–2491.

21. Chang EL, Wefel JS, Hess KR, *et al.* Neurocognition in patients with brain metastases treated with radiosurgery or radiosurgery plus whole-brain irradiation: a randomized controlled trial. *Lancet Oncol* 2009; **10**: 1037–1044.

22. Roberge D, Petrecca KI, El Refae M, *et al.* Whole brain radiotherapy and tumour bed radiosurgery following resection of solitary brain metastasis. *J Neurooncol* 2009; **95**: 95–99.

23. Soltys SG, Adler JR, Lipani JD, *et al.* Stereotactic radiosurgery of the postoperative resection cavity for brain metastases. *Int J Radiat Oncol Biol Phys* 2008; **70**: 187–193.

24. Jagannathan J, Yen CP, Ray DK, *et al.* Gamma knife radiosurgery to the surgical cavity following resection of brain metastases. *J Neurosurg* 2009; **111**: 431–438.

25. Do L, Pezner R, Radany E, *et al.* Resection followed by stereotactic radiosurgery to resection cavity for intracranial metastases. *Int J Radiat Oncol Biol Phys* 2009; **73**: 486–491.

26. Quigley MR, Fuhrer R, Karlovits B, *et al.* Single session stereotactic radiosurgery boost to the post-operative site in lieu of whole brain radiation in metastatic brain disease. *J Neurooncol* 2008; **87**: 327–332.

27. Mathieu D, Knodziolka D, Flickinger JC, *et al.* Tumor bed radiosurgery after resection of cerebral metastases. *Neurosurgery* 2008; **62**: 817–823.

28. Bahl G, White G, Alksne J, *et al.* Focal radiation therapy of brain metastases after complete surgical resection. *Med Oncol* 2006; **23**: 317–324.

29. Hwang SW, Abozed MM, Hale A, *et al.* Adjuvant Gamma Knife radiosurgery following surgical resection of brain metastases: a 9-year retrospective cohort study. *J Neurooncol* 2010; **98**: 77–82.

30. Tolentino PJ. Brain metastases secondary to breast cancer: treatment with surgical resection and stereotactic radiosurgery. *Mo Med* 2009; **106**: 428–431.

31. Karlovits BJ, Quigley MR, Karlovits SM, *et al.* Stereotactic radiosurgery boost to the resection bed for oligometastatic brain disease: challenging the tradition of adjuvant whole-brain radiotherapy. *Neurosurg Focus* 2009; **27**: E7.

32. Lindvall P, Bergstrom P, Lofroth PO, *et al.* A comparison between surgical resection in combination with WBRT or hypofractionated stereotactic irradiation in the treatment of solitary brain metastases. *Acta Neurochir (Wien)* 2009; **151**: 1053–1059.

33. Limbrick DD Jr, Lusis EA, Chicoine MR, *et al.* Combined surgical resection and stereotactic radiosurgery for treatment of cerebral metastases. *Surg Neurol* 2009; **71**: 280–288.

34. Iwai Y, Yamanaka K, Yasui T. Boost radiosurgery for treatment of brain metastases after surgical resections. *Surg Neurol* 2008; **69**: 181–186.

35. Iwadate Y, Namba H, Yamaura A. Whole brain radiation therapy is not beneficial as adjuvant therapy for brain metastases compared with localized irradiation. *Anticancer Res* 2002; **22**: 325–330.

36. Coucke PA, Zouhair A, Ozsahin M, *et al.* Focalized external radiotherapy for resected solitary brain metastasis: does the dogma stand? *Radiother Oncol* 1998; **47**: 99–101.

37. Roberge D, Souhami L. Tumor bed radiosurgery following resection of brain metastases: a review. *Technol Cancer Res Treat* 2010; **9**: 597–602.

38. Kondziolka D, Patel A, Lunsford LD, et al. Stereotactic radiosurgery plus whole brain radiotherapy versus radiotherapy alone for patients with multiple brain metastases. Int J Radiat Oncol Biol Phys 1999; **45**: 427–434.

39. Tsao MN, Rades D, Wirth A, et al. Radiotherapeutic and surgical management for newly diagnosed brain metastasis(es): an American Society for Radiation Oncology evidence-based guideline. Pract Radiat Oncol 2012; **2**: 210–225.

40. Petrovich Z, Yu C, Giannotta SL, et al. Survival and pattern of failure in brain metastases treated with stereotactic Gamma Knife radiosurgery. J Neurosurg 2002; **97**: 499–506.

41. Blonigen BJ, Steinmetz RD, Levin L, et al. Irradiated volume as a predictor of brain radionecrosis after linear accelerator stereotactic radiosurgery. Int J Radiat Oncol Biol Phys 2010; **77**: 996–1001.

42. Lutterback J, Cyron D, Henne K, et al. Radiosurgery followed by planned observation in patients with one to three brain metastases. Neurosurgery 2003; **52**: 1066–1074.

43. Flickinger JC, Lunsford LD, Kondziolka D, et al. Radiosurgery and brain tolerance: an analysis of neurodiagnostic imaging changes after Gamma Knife radiosurgery for arteriovenous malformation. Int J Radiat Oncol Biol Phys 1992; **23**: 19–26.

44. Desquesada BS, Quisling RG, Yachnis A, et al. Can standard magnetic resonance imaging reliably distinguish recurrent tumor from radiation necrosis after radiosurgery for brain metastases? A radiographic-pathological study. Neurosurgery 2008; **63**: 898–903.

45. Bezjak A, Adam J, Barton R, et al. Symptom response after palliative radiotherapy for patients with brain metastases. Eur J Cancer 2002; **38**: 487–496.

46. Gondi V, Tome WA, Mehta MP. Why avoid the hippocampus? A comprehensive review. Radiother Oncol 2010; **97**: 370–376.

47. Kirby N, Chuang C, Pouliot J, et al. Physics strategies for sparing neural stem cells during whole-brain radiation treatments. Med Phys 2011; **38**: 5338–5344.

48. van Kesteren Z, Belderbos J, van Herk M, et al. A practical technique to avoid the hippocampus in prophylactic cranial irradiation for lung cancer. Radiother Oncol 2012; **102**: 225–227.

49. Olson JJ, Paleologos NA, Gaspar LE, et al. The role of emerging and investigational therapies for metastatic brain tumors: a systematic review and evidence-based clinical practice guideline of selected topics. J Neurooncol 2010; **96**: 115–142.

50. Hotta K, Kiura K, Ueoka H, et al. Effect of gefitinib ("Iressa", ZD 1839) on brain metastases in patients with advanced non-small cell lung cancer. Lung Cancer 2004; **46**: 255–261.

51. Namba Y, Kijima T, Yokota S, et al. Geftinib in patients with brain metastases from non-small cell lung cancer: review of 15 clinical cases. Clin Lung Cancer 2004; **6**: 123–128.

52. Shimato S, Mitsudomi T, Kosaka T, et al. EGFR mutations in patients with brain metastases from lung cancer: association with the efficacy of gefitinib. Neuro Oncol 2006; **8**: 137–144.

53. Ceresoli GL, Cappuzzo F, Gregore V, et al. Gefitinib in patients with brain metastases from non-small cell lung cancer: a prospective trial. Ann Oncol 2004; **15**: 1042–1047.

54. Chiu CH, Tsai CM, Chen YM, et al. Gefitinib is active in patients with brain metastases from non-small cell lung cancer and response is related to skin toxicity. Lung Cancer 2005; **47**: 129–138.

55. Wu C, Li YL, Wang ZM, et al. Gefitinib as palliative therapy for lung adenocarcinoma metastatic to the brain. Lung Cancer 2007; **57**: 359–364.

56. Hirsch FR, Herbst RS, Olsen C, et al. Increased EGFR gene copy number detected by fluorescent in situ hybridization predicts outcome in non-small cell lung cancer patients treated with cetuximab and chemotherapy. J Clin Oncol 2008; **26**: 3351–3357.

57. Yano S, Shinohara H, Herbst RS, *et al*. Expression of vascular endothelial growth factor is necessary but not sufficient for production and growth of brain metastasis. *Cancer Res* 2000; **60**: 4959–4967.

58. Sandler A, Gray R, Perry MC, *et al*. Paclitaxel-carboplatin alone or with bevacizumab for non-small cell lung cancer [erratum appears in *N Engl J Med* 356(3): 318, 2007]. *N Engl J Med* 2006; **355**: 2542–2550.

59. Akerley WL, Langer CJ, Oh Y, *et al*. Acceptable safety of bevacizumab therapy in patients with brain metastases due to non-small cell lung cancer. *J Clin Oncol* 2008; **26**: 8043.

60. Arsian C, Dizdar O, Altundag K. Systemic treatment in breast cancer patients with brain metastases. *Expert Opin Pharmacother* 2010; **11**: 1089–1100.

61. Lin NU, Dieras V, Paul D, *et al*. Multicenter phase II study of lapatinib in patients with brain metastases from HER2-positive breast cancer. *Clin Cancer Res* 2009; **15**: 1452–1459.

62. Tevaarwerk AJ, Kolesar JM. Lapatinib: a small molecule inhibitor of epidermal growth factor receptor and human epidermal growth factor receptor-2 tyrosine kinases used in the treatment of breast cancer. *Clin Ther* 2009; **31**: 2332–2348.

63. Aboody KS, Brown A, Rainov NG, *et al*. Neural stem cells display extensive tropism for pathology in adult brain: evidence from intracranial gliomas. *Proc Natl Acad Sci U S A* 2000; **97**: 12846–12851.

64. Schmidt NO, Przylecki W, Yang W, *et al*. Brain tumor tropism of transplanted human neural stem cells is induced by vascular endothelial growth factor. *Neoplasia* 2005; **7**: 623–629.

65. Aboody KS, Najbauer J, Schmidt NO, *et al*. Targeting of melanoma brain metastases using engineered neural stem/progenitor cells. *Neuro Oncol* 2006; **8**: 119–126.

66. Joo KM, Park IH, Shin JY, *et al*. Human neural stem cells can target and deliver therapeutic genes to breast cancer brain metastases. *Mol Ther* 2009; **17**: 570–575.

67. Tsao MN, Rades D, Wirth A, *et al*. International practice survey on the management of brain metastases: third international consensus workshop on palliative radiotherapy and symptom control. *Clin Oncol* 2012; **24**: e81–92.

68. Bhadrasain V. Radiation therapy for the developing countries. *J Cancer Res Ther* 2005; **1**: 7–8.

CHAPTER 23

Liver metastases

Sean Bydder
Department of Radiation Oncology, Sir Charles Gairdner Hospital and School of
Surgery, University of Western Australia, Perth, Australia

Introduction

Incidence/prevalence, at-risk populations

Liver metastases are the most common visceral metastases. In a series of 9700
consecutive autopsies performed at one cancer center, liver metastases were
found with 41.4% of non-hepatic primary malignancies. These were more
frequent than lung (39.7%), bone (35%), or adrenal (20.3%) metastases [1].
Almost any primary malignancy site or type can metastasize to the liver.
Common primaries include colorectal cancers (CRC), breast, and lung cancers
[1]. Metastases from CRC are of particular interest, because they are so
common (probably due to portal venous drainage directly to the liver) but
also because a significant proportion are detected when metastases are still
limited to the liver – where surgery may have an important role. The risk of
liver metastases is highest with ocular melanomas, breast, and gastrointestinal cancers [1]. In non-cirrhotic livers, metastases are much more common
than primary liver malignancies [1,2]. In cirrhotic livers, metastases are rare
and the majority of malignant liver tumors are primary [3,4].

Symptoms

Diffuse liver metastases can cause both local and systemic symptoms [5–7]
(Box 23.1). This clinical circumstance can often be associated with impaired
performance. Liver metastases can also cause liver dysfunction on blood
tests or clinically (i.e. jaundice or other signs of liver failure). Liver metastases from gastrointestinal neuro-endocrine tumors (NET) can be associated
with the "carcinoid syndrome": episodic flushing, wheezing, diarrhea,
and eventual right-sided valvular heart disease. Liver metastases may be
asymptomatic and discovered on imaging at the time of diagnosis or at
follow-up [2].

Radiation Oncology in Palliative Cancer Care, First Edition. Edited by Stephen Lutz,
Edward Chow, and Peter Hoskin.
© 2013 John Wiley & Sons, Ltd. Published 2013 by John Wiley & Sons, Ltd.

Box 23.1 Symptoms commonly associated with widely disseminated liver metastases

- Pain
- Nausea
- Vomiting
- Anorexia
- Abdominal distension
- Night sweats
- Fever

Survival rates/life expectancy

Liver metastases are generally associated with poor survival. In one series of 484 patients with untreated liver metastases from CRC, the median survival was 7.5 months and the 5-year survival rate was 0.9% [8]. With modern chemotherapy, metastatic CRC has median survivals of 20 months [9]. For other primary malignancies, liver metastases may be associated with even worse survival rates (e.g. ocular melanoma) [10]. In a series of patients with liver metastases treated with palliative whole liver radiation treatment, therefore symptomatic and typically heavily pre-treated, median survival following radiotherapy was typically only 8–17 weeks [10]. In Pickren's autopsy series, hepatic failure was the cause of death in 10% of the cases with liver metastases, highlighting the seriousness of this disease state [1]. Aggressive treatment may substantially improve survival in a subset of patients with limited liver metastases. Resection of liver metastases from CRC is associated with 5-year overall survival rates of 25–47% [8,11–16].

Radiotherapy treatment

Systemic therapy is often preferred for patients with liver metastases, using the same treatment as might be used for disease elsewhere in the body. Unfortunately liver metastases commonly have lower response rates than metastases elsewhere. Patients with "carcinoid syndrome" can be treated with octreotide [17]. Regional chemotherapy, such as hepatic artery infusion (HAI), has also been used, especially for CRC metastases localized to the liver. Radiotherapy may have a role in symptom control and also in more aggressive treatment [7]. Whole-liver radiation therapy (WLRT) is uncommonly used but can improve quality of life. Conformal RT, selective internal radiation therapy (SIRT), and brachytherapy may have roles in some patients. Surgical resection should be considered for selected patients with limited liver involvement, to both improve time to progression and overall survival. Other techniques of focal ablation, including stereotactic body radiation therapy (SBRT), may be alternatives if surgery is not possible (Figure 23.1).

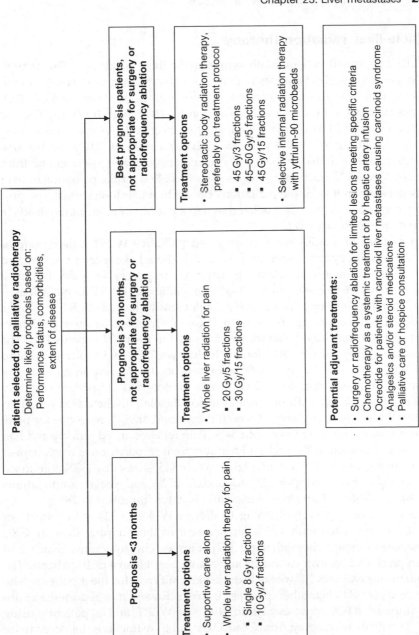

Patient selected for palliative radiotherapy
Determine likely prognosis based on:
Performance status, comorbidities,
extent of disease

Prognosis <3 months

Treatment options
• Supportive care alone
• Whole liver radiation therapy for pain
  ▪ Single 8 Gy fraction
  ▪ 10 Gy/2 fractions

**Prognosis >3 months,
not appropriate for surgery or
radiofrequency ablation**

Treatment options
• Whole liver radiation for pain
  ▪ 20 Gy/5 fractions
  ▪ 30 Gy/15 fractions

**Best prognosis patients,
not appropriate for surgery or
radiofrequency ablation**

Treatment options
• Stereotactic body radiation therapy,
  preferably on treatment protocol
  ▪ 45 Gy/3 fractions
  ▪ 45–50 Gy/5 fractions
  ▪ 45 Gy/15 fractions
• Selective internal radiation therapy
  with yttrium-90 microbeads

Potential adjuvant treatments:
• Surgery or radiofrequency ablation for limited lesions meeting specific criteria
• Chemotherapy as a systemic treatment or by hepatic artery infusion
• Ocreotide for patients with carcinoid liver metastases causing carcinoid syndrome
• Analgesics and/or steroid medications
• Palliative care or hospice consultation

Figure 23.1 Algorithm for use of palliative radiotherapy for patients with liver metastases.

Whole-liver radiation therapy

WLRT can benefit patients with symptomatic liver metastases. This is typically given using short-courses to deliver relatively low total doses. Common fractionation schedules and symptom response rates are shown in Table 23.1. These range from 8 Gy in a single fraction to 30 Gy in 15 fractions. The 1–2 fraction courses shown have a Biologically Effective Dose (calculated using the linear-quadratic model with an alpha-beta ratio of 10 Gy for tumors) approximately half that of the 5 and 7 fraction courses and just over one-third that of 30 Gy in 15 fractions. RT is used far less often for the palliation of liver metastases than it is for the palliation of bone, brain, or lung metastases, possibly because of an incorrect belief that hepatic irradiation inevitably leads to radiation liver toxicity [7].

A number of studies have investigated palliative WLRT either alone or combined with systemic therapy [5,6,18–27]. These have mostly been carried out using 2-dimensional planning. Reported responses for pain, the most common symptom, range from 55–80% in studies on WLRT alone. A Radiation Therapy Oncology Group (RTOG) pilot study allowed WLRT in a range of dose-fractionation schedules, from 21 Gy in 7 fractions to 30 Gy in 15 fractions (and in some cases also localized boosts) to treat 109 patients [23]. The most commonly used WLRT alone, schedule was 25.6 Gy in 16 fractions and this was given to just over one-third of patients. Useful response rates were seen for a range of symptoms. Leibel et al. randomized 214 patients to 21 Gy in 7 fractions WLRT with or without misonidazole [5]. There was no difference between the study arms. Overall they found an 80% response for pain, which was a complete response in 54%. Pain relief occurred quickly and had a median duration of 13 weeks. Other symptom response rates were: nausea or vomiting (49%), fever and night sweats (45%), ascites (33%), anorexia (28%), abdominal distension (27%), jaundice (27%), and weakness and fatigue (19%). In addition, Karnofsky performance status improved in 28%.

Yeo et al. used 3D-CT planning to deliver WLRT of 21 Gy in 7 fractions to 10 patients, each with >75% replacement of their normal liver by CRC metastases despite chemotherapy [27]. Further chemotherapy, which had been precluded by liver dysfunction, became possible in 4 of 10 patients. The median survival was 7.7 weeks but the *mean* survival for the 4 patients who received post-RT chemotherapy was 20 weeks. Russell et al. reported a multi-institutional RTOG dose-escalation study of WLRT in 173 patients, using WLRT with doses ranging from 27 to 33 Gy in 1.5 Gy fractions delivered twice daily [26]. Higher total doses did not increase the median survival or decrease how often liver metastases were the cause of death. However, the 33 Gy dose-level was associated with a 10% incidence of late liver injury.

Symptom control can be achieved with hypofractionated WLRT given over a few fractions. The Trans Tasman Radiation Oncology Group (TROG) study used 10 Gy in 2 fractions WLRT and achieved symptom improvements for one-half to two-thirds of patients [6]. Single fraction courses may also be useful.

Table 23.1 Common fractionation schemes for whole liver radiation therapy to treat liver metastases.

Series	RT schedule (Gy/fraction #)	No. of patients	Design	Outcomes / comments	Median survival
	8/1	–			
Bydder et al. 2003 [6]	10/2	28	Prospective, multi-institutional TROG	Improvement in baseline symptoms in ~50–66%	10 wk
				Pain relief in 65%	
				7% Acute Grade 3/4 toxicity	
				No late toxicity	
	20/5	–			
Leibel et al. 1987 [5]	21/7*	214 (187 evaluable)	Randomized ± misonidazole*, multi-institutional RTOG	Pain relief in 80% (complete in 54%)	17 wk
				Performance status improved in 28%	
				Worsening of nausea in 6%	
				No difference with misonidazole	
Yeo et al. 2010 [27]	21/7†	10†		Further chemotherapy became possible in 40%	8 wk
	(30/10)	–		May exceed 5% risk of RILD and delivery in 15 fractions may be safer [28]	
	30/15	–		Estimated <5% risk of RILD [28]	
Russell et al. 1993 [26]	27 – 30 / 18 –20 †*	173	Dose escalation, multi-institutional RTOG	6% Acute Grade 3/4 toxicity	17 wk
	(1.5 Gy per fxn bid)	–		10% late liver injury at 33 Gy	
				No advantage with higher dose	

Abbreviations: RT = radiotherapy; TROG = Trans Tasman Radiation Oncology Group; wk = week; RTOG = Radiation Therapy Oncology Group; ECOG = Eastern Cooperative Oncology Group; fxn = fraction; RILD = radiation-induced liver disease

*21 Gy in 7 fxn and 27–33 Gy in 1.5 Gy fxn bid are now not commonly used but are included because of their use in large trials; 30 in 15 fxn is not commonly used, but WLRT to 30 Gy may be more safely delivered in 15 fxn (28)

*33 Gy in 22 fxn was also used, but was felt to be "unsafe"

†Liver metastases replacing >75% of normal liver and advanced hepatic dysfunction, 1 patient received 30 Gy in 10 fxn

Side effects of WLRT

Acute effects of WLRT can include nausea, diarrhea, and a temporary exacerbation of pain. Supportive medication such as high-dose steroids and anti-emetic drugs should be administered prior to therapy. The tolerance of the liver to radiation depends on dose and volume. The tolerance of the whole liver is relatively low. The dose per fraction may be important – for most organs smaller doses per fraction increase tolerance – but this is poorly characterized for liver [28]. Tolerance may be reduced with impaired liver reserve, hepatitis B infection, or concurrent chemotherapy. Radiation induced liver disease (RILD) is similar to post-transplant veno-occlusive disease [28]. When it occurs, it usually does so 2–12 weeks after irradiation. It can cause ascites, hepatomegaly, altered liver function tests, and may progress to liver failure. The whole liver tolerates RT in doses up to 30 Gy in 15 fractions [23,28], 21 Gy in 7 fractions [6], or 10 Gy in 2 fractions [5]. A dose-level of 33 Gy in 1.5 Gy fractions delivered twice daily was associated with a 10% rate of late liver injury and was considered unsafe [26]. Partial liver irradiation allows higher doses [28]. Doses used for palliation may be high enough to cause kidney damage, so at least one (functioning) kidney should be excluded from the treatment volumes.

Conformal radiation therapy

Conformal radiation treatment with three-dimensional planning (3D-CRT) allows targeting of tumors and the avoidance of normal tissues. This can be combined with other sophisticated techniques such as intensity modulated radiation therapy (IMRT) and image guided radiation therapy (IGRT). Partial liver irradiation allows higher doses to be delivered safely, depending on the volume of liver treated. A group from the University of Michigan treated 128 patients with primary or secondary liver cancers (47 with CRC metastases) using 3D-CRT concurrently with regional chemotherapy, in consecutive phase 1 and 2 studies [29,30]. The radiation doses used were limited to an individual 10–15% risk of RILD, based on a model of normal-tissue complication probability. The median radiation dose delivered was 60.75 Gy (24–90 Gy) in 1.5 Gy fractions given twice daily. The response rate for CRC liver metastases was 60%. The median survival was 17 months, which was longer than for historical controls [30]. Higher doses appeared more effective and total dose was the only significant predictor of survival. In the overall group 39 patients (30%) developed grade 3–4 toxicity (including 4% RILD). There was one treatment-related death.

Systemic or regional chemotherapy in conjunction with WLRT or CRT

A number of small, non-randomized reports describe attempts to improve the results of WLRT with the use of concurrent chemotherapy or radiosensitizers [22,24,31–38]. The outcomes with concurrent systemic or regional chemotherapy appear modestly superior to RT alone but also associated with increased toxicity [7]. A randomized, multi-institutional RTOG study with 187 patients treated with WLRT with 21 Gy in 7 fractions with or without miso-nidazole, a hypoxic cell radiosensitizer, did not find any difference in outcomes [5].

Limitations of WLRT and conventional conformal external beam radiation therapy (EBRT)

WLRT does not offer a survival advantage and it should be reserved for symptom control [7]. The duration of benefits may be short, symptoms may recur or new symptoms develop [6]. Despite high response rates after CRT, there is no proven survival advantage. Most patients with symptomatic liver metastases have a short life expectancy – so any benefit may be small. There are risks of nausea, and kidney and liver toxicity, but these can generally be avoided with pre-medication and attention to radiation dose and technique.

Brachytherapy

Brachytherapy can be delivered after insertion of needles into the liver (by CT-guidance or at laparatomy) with high-dose rate 192-iridium sources later sent down the needles using after-loading techniques. Alternatively iodine seeds can be implanted surgically. This can give a good radiation dose distribution (i.e. a high tumor dose while sparing normal liver) [39]. It has been used for metastases from CRC and breast cancers with good local control [39–42]. Brachytherapy is invasive. Severe complications, such as intrahepatic bleeding, abscess, pneumothorax, or pleural effusion can occur [42]. It should be limited to experienced centers [7].

Selective internal radiation therapy

Selective internal RT (SIRT) is performed by embolization of 90-yttrium-containing microbeads into the hepatic arterial supply. These emit beta radiation locally. It has been used in therapy of focal and diffuse liver metastases. A randomized Phase III trial of 74 patients with liver metastases from CRC comparing Hepatic Arterial Infusion (HAI) of chemotherapy ± SIRT showed an increased hepatic progression-free survival from 9.7 months to 15.9 months for the combined treatment but no difference in overall survival [43]. Hendlisz *et al.* randomized 46 patients with unresectable, chemotherapy-refractory liver-limited CRC metastases to intravenous chemotherapy ± SIRT. Combined treatment improved the median time to tumor progression from 2.1 to 4.5 months [44]. A multicenter Phase II study using SIRT as salvage therapy for inoperable CRC liver metastases showed a median survival of 12.6 months and a 2-year survival of 19.6% [45]. These studies are poorly statistically powered [46]. Toxicities can include neutropenic sepsis, liver abscess, gastric perforation, and RILD [47]. There may also be a role for SIRT in metastases from other primary sites and for primary liver cancers.

Surgery for liver metastases

Surgery is often used for selected patients with limited liver metastases from CRC and results in 5-year survival rates of 25–47% [11–16]. However, there are no randomized studies comparing resection to no resection in patients with potentially resectable liver metastases. Multiple prognostic factors have been identified. These include the number and size of lesions, the presence of satellite lesions or extra-hepatic disease, surgical margins, age, pre-operative carcinoembryonic antigen (CEA) levels, primary tumor stage, and the disease-free interval between the resection of the primary tumor and the appearance of metastases [7,11–13,15]. Surgery for CRC liver metastases is often combined with post-operative or pre-operative chemotherapy. Surgical resection of non-CRC liver metastases has been used in selected indolent non-CRC cases. A series of hepatic resection of neuroendocrine (NET) liver metastases reported survival better than for a contemporaneous CRC cohort [48]. A large multi-institutional, retrospective study of 1452 patients with non-CRC, non-NET liver metastases showed a 5-year survival rate of 36% and a 10-year survival rate of 23%. Patients with breast primaries had the best survival with melanoma and squamous cell cancers the poorest [49]. Patients unsuitable for surgical resection for technical or medical reasons may be treated by radiofrequency ablation (RFA), cryotherapy, laser-induced thermotherapy, high-intensity focal ultrasound, or SBRT.

Radiofrequency ablation

Radiofrequency Ablation can be given via a needle inserted into tumors under radiographic guidance. Radiofrequency waves are used to generate heat. The European Organisation for Research and Treatment of Cancer (EORTC) randomized 119 patients with non-resectable CRC liver metastases on a Phase II trial to systemic treatment ± RFA [50]. Combined therapy was associated with improved median progression-free survival from 10 to 17 months. There was no overall survival advantage but the statistical power of the study was low. An American Society of Clinical Oncology review of RFA for CRC liver metastases found a large variability in local tumor recurrence rates (3.6–60%) and 5-year survival rates (14–55%) [51]. Tumor size >3 cm or location close to large vessels was associated with reduced local control, while multiple or extra-hepatic metastases were associated with poor survival.

Promising new radiotherapy techniques

Stereotactic body radiation therapy

Stereotactic body radiation therapy (SBRT) involves patient immobilization and precise delivery of highly conformal, high-dose RT in a limited number of fractions [7]. Table 23.2 illustrates prospective [52–58] and Table 23.3 retrospective [59–63] studies of SBRT for liver metastases [7]. There are significant

Table 23.2 Stereotactic body radiation therapy for liver metastases – prospective studies.

Series	RT schedule (Gy/fraction #)	No. of patients	Primary site	Toxicity	Outcomes
Herfarth et al. 2004 [52]	14–26/1 Dose escalation	35	NR	No significant toxicity	1-y LC, 71%; 1-y OS, 72%
Mendez Romero et al. 2006 [53]	30–37.5/3	25 (17 LM)	CRC (14) Lung (1) Breast (1) Carcinoid (1)	2 G3 liver toxicities	2-y LC, 86%; 2-y OS, 62%
Hoyer et al. 2006 [54]	45/3	64	CRC (44)	1 liver failure 2 late GI toxicities	2-y LC, 79% 2-y LC (by patient), 64%
Rusthoven et al. 2009 [55]	30–60/3, Dose escalation	47	CRC (15) Lung (10) Breast (4) Ovarian (3) Esophageal (3) HCC (2) Other (10)	No RILD <2% Late G3/4 toxicty	1-y LC, 95%; 2-y LC, 92%; Med survival, 20.5 mo
Lee et al. 2009 [56]	27.7–60/6, Individualized dose	68	CRC (40) Breast (12) Gallbladder (4) Lung (2) Anal canal (2) Melanoma (2) Other (6)	No RILD 10% G3/4 acute toxicity No G3/4 late toxicity	1-y LC, 71%; Med survival, 17.6 mo
Ambrosino et al. 2009 [57]	25–60/3	27	CRC (11) Other (16)	No serious toxicity	Crude LC rate, 74%
Goodman et al. 2010 [58]	18–30/1, Dose escalation	26	CRC (6) Pancreatic (3) Gastric (2) Ovarian (2) Other (6)	No dose-limiting toxicity 2 G2 late GI toxicity 2 G2 late soft tissue/ rib toxicity	1-y local failure, 23%; 2-y OS, 49%

Abbreviations: RT, radiotherapy; NR, not reported; 1-y, 1-year; 2-y, 2-year; LC, local control; OS, overall survival; Med survival, median survival; mo, months; HCC, hepatocellular carcinoma; CRC, colorectal; LM, Liver metastases; RILD, radiation-induced liver disease; GI, gastrointestinal; G, Grade

Table 23.3 Stereotactic body radiation therapy for liver metastases – retrospective studies.

Series	RT schedule (Gy/fraction #)	No. of patients	Primary site	Toxicity	Outcomes
Blomgren et al. 1995 [59]	7.7–45/1–4	14	CRC (11) Anal Canal (1) Kidney (1) Ovarian (1)	2 Hemorrhagic gastritis	50% response rate
Wada et al. 2004 [60]	45/3	5	NR	No serious toxicity	2-y LC, 71.2%
Wulf et al. 2006 [61]	30–37.5/3 26/1	44 (39 LM)	CRC (23) Breast (11) Ovarian (4) Other (13)	No G2–4 toxicity	1-y LC, 92%; 2-y LC, 66% 1-y %; 2-y OS, 32%OS, 72
Katz et al. 2007 [62]	30–55 / 5–15	69	CRC (20) Breast (16) Pancreas (9) Lung (5) Other (19)	No G3/4 toxicity	1-y LC, 92%; 2-y LC, 66% 1-y OS, 72%; 2-y OS, 32%
van der Pool et al. 2010 [63]	30–37.5/3	20	CRC (20)	2 G3 late LFT changes 1 G2 rib fracture	10-mo LC, 76%; 2-y LC, 74%, Med survival, 34 mo

Abbreviations: RT = radiotherapy; CRC = colorectal; NR = not reported; 1-y = 1-year; 2-y = 2-year; LC = local control; LM= Liver metastases; OS = overall survival; mo = months; Med survival = median survival; LFTs = Liver Function Tests; G = Grade

differences between the reported studies – in patient selection, primary malignancies treated, tumor volumes, total dose, dose per fraction, and dosimetric planning criteria. In general, most SBRT studies used doses ranging from 30 to 60 Gy delivered in 1–6 fractions, to <5 metastases, <6 cm [7]. Most treated metastases were from CRC primaries, but there were an increasing numbers of patients with breast and lung cancer included in more recent series. No randomized trials have been reported.

Reported local control of liver metastases with SBRT ranges from 70–100% at 1 year and 60–90% at 2 years (Tables 23.2 and 23.3) [52–63]. Prognostic factors related to improved local control include smaller tumor volumes [55,56], metachronous liver metastases [54], no previous chemotherapy [54], non-CRC metastases [52,56] (perhaps because most patients with CRC liver metastases have been heavily pre-treated), and radiation dose [7]. There appears to be a dose response for local control and a total prescription dose

>48 Gy in 3 fractions has been recommended when possible [7,56,61,64,65]. Reported median overall survival after SBRT for liver metastases ranges from 10 to 34 months, with 2-year overall survival rates ranging from 30–83%. There are occasional long-term survivors [63]. Patients included in Phase I/ II SBRT studies have generally been heavily pre-treated, and therefore it is difficult to compare survival outcomes with other local modalities used for liver metastases [7]. Ideal candidates for liver metastasis SBRT have a good performance status (Eastern Cooperative Oncology Group Performance: 0–1), possess adequate hepatic function, have no extra-hepatic disease, and have an uninvolved liver volume >700 mL [7].

Side effects of stereotactic body radiation therapy
Although grade 1–2 toxicities are common after SBRT, severe toxicity (grade 3) is not [7]. Toxicity is more likely in patients receiving a high dose to the bowel or to large volumes of the liver. The risk of RILD in SBRT is low [54]. In the study by Lee *et al.*, with a median mean liver dose of 16.9 Gy in 6 fractions, no RILD was seen in 68 patients [56]. In a Phase I/II study by Rusthoven *et al.*, where >700 mL of uninvolved liver was limited to <15 Gy in 3 fractions, no RILD was seen in 47 patients [55]. There has, however, been a reported death from hepatic failure 7 weeks after SBRT, possibly related to RT [54]. Duodenal ulceration (2 patients), colonic perforation (1 patient), grade 3 soft-tissue toxicity (1 patient), and non-traumatic rib fractures (2 patients) have been seen [54–56].

Limitations of SBRT
A multi-disciplinary team approach in the management of patients with liver metastases is important [7]. Correct patient selection is important. SBRT is technically demanding and resource intensive. There are significant risks, although these can be minimized by careful application. Out-of-field metastatic progression develops in a substantial proportion of patients, and effective systemic treatments are still required.

Practice variation among different countries

An international survey was undertaken to evaluate patterns of practice for the radiotherapeutic management of metastatic disease to liver [66]. Common palliative regimens included 8 Gy in 1 fraction, 10 Gy in 2 fractions, 20 Gy in 5 fractions. 30 Gy in 10 fractions was also commonly used, although this may exceed a 5% risk of RILD (and delivering the same dose in 15 fractions would be preferred) [28]. The majority of referrals were for radical RT. The most common technologies used were 4D-CT, SBRT, IGRT, and/or IMRT. The most commonly employed radical regimens were 45 Gy in 3 fractions, 40–50 Gy in 5 fractions, and 45 Gy in 15 fractions. There was no uniform treatment approach.

Conclusion

Liver metastases commonly occur in patients with a variety of solid tumors and can cause both localized and systemic symptoms. Systemic treatment is the mainstay for the management of the majority of patients with liver metastases, though good performance status patients with favorable prognosis may be treated with surgical resection or radiofrequency ablation in an effort to maximize local control or even prolong survival. Patients with painful liver lesions and a poor prognosis may receive hypofractionated EBRT as an end-of-life palliative measure. Newer technologies such as SBRT and SIRT with yttrium-90 have created hope that radiotherapy will come to play a more useful role in the management of this patient group.

Acknowledgments

This chapter is based in part on a systematic review of radiation treatment for liver metastases [7]. Sean Bydder would like to acknowledge his co-authors of that review.

References

1. Pickren JW, Tsukada Y, Lane WW. Liver metastases: analysis of autopsy data. In: Weiss L, Gilbert HA (eds) *Liver Metastases*. Boston: Hall Medical Publishers, 1982, pp. 2–18.
2. Imam K, Bluemke DA. MR imaging in the evaluation of hepatic metastases. *Magn Reson Imaging Clin N Am* 2000; **8**: 741–776.
3. Melato M, Laurino L, Mucli E, *et al.* Relationship between cirrhosis, liver cancer, and hepatic metastases. An autopsy study. *Cancer* 1989; **64**: 445–455.
4. Uetsuji S, Yamamura M, Yamamichi K, *et al.* Absence of colorectal cancer metastasis to the cirrhotic liver. *Am J Surg* 1992; **164**: 176–177.
5. Leibel SA, Pajak TF, Massullo V, *et al.* A comparison of misonidazole sensitized radiation therapy to radiation therapy alone for the palliation of hepatic metastases: results of a Radiation Therapy Oncology Group randomized prospective trial. *Int J Radiat Oncol Biol Phys* 1987; **13**: 1057–1064.
6. Bydder S, Spry NA, Christie DR, *et al.* A prospective trial of short-fractionation radiotherapy for the palliation of liver metastases. *Australas Radiol* 2003; **47**: 284–288.
7. Hoyer M, Swaminath A, Bydder S, *et al.* Radiotherapy for liver metastases: a review of evidence. *Int J Radiat Oncol Biol Phys* 2012; **82**: 1047–1057.
8. Stangl R, Altendorf-Hofmann A, Charnley RM, *et al.* Factors influencing the natural history of colorectal liver metastases. *Lancet* 1994; **343**: 1405–1410.
9. Goldberg RM, Rothenberg ML, Van Cutsem E, *et al.* The continuum of care: a paradigm for the management of metastatic colorectal cancer. *Oncologist* 2007; **12**: 38–50.
10. Kim IK, Lane AM, Gragoudas ES. Survival in patients with presymptomatic diagnosis of metastatic uveal melanoma. *Arch Ophthalmol* 2010; **128**: 871–875.
11. Nordlinger B, Guiguet M, Vaillant JC, *et al.* Surgical resection of colorectal carcinoma metastases to the liver. A prognostic scoring system to improve case selection, based on 1568 patients. Association Francaise de Chirurgie. *Cancer* 1996; **77**: 1254–1262.

12. Fong Y, Fortner J, Sun RL, *et al.* Clinical score for predicting recurrence after hepatic resection for metastatic colorectal cancer: analysis of 1001 consecutive cases. *Ann Surg* 1999; **230**: 309–318.

13. Wei AC, Greig PD, Grant D, *et al.* Survival after hepatic resection for colorectal metastases: a 10-year experience. *Ann Surg Oncol* 2006; **13**: 668–676.

14. Robertson DJ, Stukel TA, Gottlieb DJ, *et al.* Survival after hepatic resection of colorectal cancer metastases: a national experience. *Cancer* 2009; **115**: 752–759.

15. Smith MD, McCall JL. Systematic review of tumour number and outcome after radical treatment of colorectal liver metastases. *Br J Surg* 2009; **96**: 1101–1113.

16. House MG, Ito H, Gonen M, *et al.* Survival after hepatic resection for metastatic colorectal cancer: trends in outcomes for 1,600 patients during two decades at a single institution. *J Am Coll Surg* 2010; **210**: 744–745.

17. Rinke A, Muller HH, Schade-Brittinger C, *et al.* Placebo controlled, double-blind, prospective, randomized study on the effect of octreotide LAR in the control of tumor growth in patients with metastatic neuroendocrine midgut tumors: a report from the PROMID study group. *J Clin Oncol* 2009; **27**: 4656–4663.

18. Phillips R, Karnofsky DA, Hamilton LD, *et al.* Roentgen therapy of hepatic metastases. *Am J Roentgenol Radium Ther Nucl Med* 1954; **71**: 826–834.

19. Turek-Maischeider M, Kazem I. Palliative irradiation for liver metastases. *JAMA* 1975; **232**: 625–628.

20. Prasad B, Lee MS, Hendrickson FR. Irradiation of hepatic metastases. *Int J Radiat Oncol Biol Phys* 1977; **2**: 129–132.

21. Sherman DM, Weichselbaum R, Order SE, *et al.* Palliation of hepatic metastasis. *Cancer* 1978; **41**: 2013–2017.

22. Webber BM, Soderberg CH, Leone LA, *et al.* A combined treatment approach to management of hepatic metastasis. *Cancer* 1978; **42**: 1087–1095.

23. Borgelt BB, Gelber R, Brady LW, *et al.* The palliation of hepatic metastases: results of the Radiation Therapy Oncology Group pilot study. *Int J Radiat Oncol Biol Phys* 1981; **7**: 587–591.

24. Leibel SA, Order SE, Rominger CJ, *et al.* Palliation of liver metastases with combined hepatic irradiation and misonidazole. Results of a Radiation Therapy Oncology Group Phase I-II study. *Cancer Clin Trials* 1981; **4**: 285–293.

25. Wiley AL, Wirtanen GW, Stephenson JA, *et al.* Combined hepatic artery 5-fluorouracil and irradiation of liver metastases. A randomized study. *Cancer* 1989; **64**: 1783–1789.

26. Russell AH, Clyde C, Wasserman TH, *et al.* Accelerated hyperfractionated hepatic irradiation in the management of patients with liver metastases: results of the RTOG dose escalating protocol. *Int J Radiat Oncol Biol Phys* 1993; **27**: 117–123.

27. Yeo SG, Kim DY, Kim TH, *et al.* Whole-liver radiotherapy for end-stage colorectal cancer patients with massive liver metastases and advanced hepatic dysfunction. *Radiat Oncol* 2010; **5**: 97.

28. Pan CC, Kavanagh BD, Dawson LA, *et al.* Radiation-associated liver injury. *Int J Radiat Oncol Biol Phys* 2010; **76**: S94–S100.

29. Dawson LA, McGinn CJ, Normolle D, *et al.* Escalated focal liver radiation and concurrent hepatic artery fluorodeoxyuridine for unresectable intrahepatic malignancies. *J Clin Oncol* 2000; **18**: 2210–2218.

30. Ben-Josef E, Normolle D, Ensminger WD, *et al.* Phase II trial of high-dose conformal radiation therapy with concurrent hepatic artery floxuridine for unresectable intrahepatic malignancies. *J Clin Oncol* 2005; **23**: 8739–8747.

31. Herbsman H, Hassan A, Gardner B, *et al*. Treatment of hepatic metastases with a combination of hepatic artery infusion chemotherapy and external radiotherapy. *Surg Gynecol Obstet* 1978; **147**: 13–17.

32. Friedman M, Cassidy M, Levine M, *et al*. Combined modality therapy of hepatic metastasis. Northern California Oncology Group Pilot Study. *Cancer* 1979; **44**: 906–913.

33. Lokich J, Kinsella T, Perri J, *et al*. Concomitant hepatic radiation and intraarterial fluorinated pyrimidine therapy: correlation of liver scan, liver function tests, and plasma CEA with tumor response. *Cancer* 1981; **48**: 2569–2574.

34. Barone RM, Byfield JE, Goldfarb PB, *et al*. Intra-arterial chemotherapy using an implantable infusion pump and liver irradiation for the treatment of hepatic metastases. *Cancer* 1982; **50**: 850–862.

35. Byfield JE, Barone RM, Frankel SS, *et al*. Treatment with combined intra-arterial 5-FUdR infusion and whole-liver radiation for colon carcinoma metastatic to the liver. Preliminary results. *Am J Clin Oncol* 1984; **7**: 319–325.

36. Rotman M, Kuruvilla AM, Choi K, *et al*. Response of colorectal hepatic metastases to concomitant radiotherapy and intravenous infusion 5 fluorouracil. *Int J Radiat Oncol Biol Phys* 1986; **12**: 2179–2187.

37. Wirtanen GW, Wiley AL, Vermund H, *et al*. Intraarterial iododeoxyuridine infusion combined with irradiation. A pilot study. *Am J Clin Oncol* 1990; **13**: 320–323.

38. Witte RS, Cnaan A, Mansour EG, *et al*. Comparison of 5-fluorouracil alone, 5-fluorouracil with levamisole, and 5-fluorouracil with hepatic irradiation in the treatment of patients with residual, nonmeasurable, intraabdominal metastasis after undergoing resection for colorectal carcinoma. *Cancer* 2001; **91**: 1020–1028.

39. Ricke J, Mohnike K, Pech M, *et al*. Local response and impact on survival after local ablation of liver metastases from colorectal carcinoma by computed tomography-guided high dose- rate brachytherapy. *Int J Radiat Oncol Biol Phys* 2010; **78**: 479–485.

40. Wieners G, Pech M, Hildebrandt B, *et al*. Phase II feasibility study on the combination of two different regional treatment approaches in patients with colorectal "liver-only" metastases: hepatic interstitial brachytherapy plus regional chemotherapy. *Cardiovasc Intervent Radiol* 2009; **32**: 937–945.

41. Wieners G, Mohnike K, Peters N, *et al*. Treatment of hepatic metastases of breast cancer with CT-guided interstitial brachytherapy – a phase II-study. *Radiother Oncol* 2011; **100**: 314–319.

42. Thomas DS, Nauta RJ, Rodgers JE, *et al*. Intraoperative high-dose rate interstitial irradiation of hepatic metastases from colorectal carcinoma. Results of a phase I-II trial. *Cancer* 1993; **71**: 1977–1981.

43. Gray B, Van Hazel G, Hope M, *et al*. Randomised trial of SIR Spheres plus chemotherapy vs. chemotherapy alone for treating patients with liver metastases from primary large bowel cancer. *Ann Oncol* 2001; **12**: 1711–1720.

44. Hendlisz A, Van den Eynde M, Peeters M, *et al*. Phase III trial comparing protracted intravenous fluorouracil infusion alone or with yttrium-90 resin microspheres radioembolization for liver-limited metastatic colorectal cancer refractory to standard chemotherapy. *J Clin Oncol* 2010; **28**: 3687–3694.

45. Cosimelli M, Golfieri R, Cagol PP, *et al*. Multi-centre phase II clinical trial of yttrium-90 resin microspheres alone in unresectable, chemotherapy refractory colorectal liver metastases. *Br J Cancer* 2010; **103**: 324–331.

46. Townsend A, Price T, Karapetis C. Selective internal radiation therapy for liver metastases from colorectal cancer. *Cochrane Database Syst Rev* 2009; (4): CD007045.

47. Sjoquist KM, Goldstein D, Bester L. A serious complication of selected internal radiation therapy: case report and literature review. *Oncologist* 2010; **15**: 830–835.

48. Reddy SK, Barbas AS, Marroquin CE, *et al*. Resection of noncolorectal nonneuroendocrine liver metastases: a comparative analysis. *J Am Coll Surg* 2007; **204**: 372–382.

49. Adam R, Chiche L, Aloia T, *et al*. Hepatic resection for non-colorectal non-endocrine liver metastases: analysis of 1,452 patients and development of a prognostic model. *Ann Surg* 2006; **244**: 524–535.

50. Ruers T, Punt C, Van Coevorden F, *et al*. Radiofrequency ablation combined with systemic treatment versus systemic treatment alone in patients with non-resectable colorectal liver metastases: a randomized EORTC Intergroup phase II study (EORTC 40004). *Ann Oncol* 2012; **23**: 2619–26. doi:10.1093/annonc/mds053 [Epub ahead of print].

51. Wong SL, Mangu PB, Choti MA, *et al*. American Society of Clinical Oncology 2009 clinical evidence review on radiofrequency ablation of hepatic metastases from colorectal cancer. *J Clin Oncol* 2010; **28**: 493–508.

52. Herfarth KK, Debus J, Wannenmacher M. Stereotactic radiation therapy of liver metastases: update of the initial phase-I/II trial. *Front Radiat Ther Oncol* 2004; **38**: 100–105.

53. Mendez-Romero A, Wunderink W, Hussain SM, *et al*. Stereotactic body radiation therapy for primary and metastatic liver tumors: a single institution phase I-II study. *Acta Oncol* 2006; **45**: 831–837.

54. Hoyer M, Roed H, Traberg HA, *et al*. Phase II study on stereotactic body radiotherapy of colorectal metastases. *Acta Oncol* 2006; **45**: 823–830.

55. Rusthoven KE, Kavanagh BD, Cardenes H, *et al*. Multi-institutional phase I/II trial of stereotactic body radiation therapy for liver metastases. *J Clin Oncol* 2009; **27**: 1572–1578.

56. Lee MT, Kim JJ, Dinniwell R, *et al*. Phase I study of individualized stereotactic body radiotherapy of liver metastases. *J Clin Oncol* 2009; **27**: 1585–1591.

57. Ambrosino G, Polistina F, Costantin G, *et al*. Image-guided robotic stereotactic radiosurgery for unresectable liver metastases: preliminary results. *Anticancer Res* 2009; **29**: 3381–3384.

58. Goodman KA, Wiegner EA, Maturen KE, *et al*. Dose-escalation study of single-fraction stereotactic body radiotherapy for liver malignancies. *Int J Radiat Oncol Biol Phys* 2010; **78**: 486–493.

59. Blomgren H, Lax I, Naslund I, Svanstrom R. Stereotactic high dose fraction radiation therapy of extracranial tumors using an accelerator. Clinical experience of the first thirty-one patients. *Acta Oncol* 1995; **34**: 861–870.

60. Wada H, Takai Y, Nemoto K, *et al*. Univariate analysis of factors correlated with tumor control probability of three dimensional conformal hypofractionated high-dose radiotherapy for small pulmonary or hepatic tumors. *Int J Radiat Oncol Biol Phys* 2004; **58**: 1114–1120.

61. Wulf J, Guckenberger M, Haedinger U, *et al*. Stereotactic radiotherapy of primary liver cancer and hepatic metastases. *Acta Oncol* 2006; **45**: 838–847.

62. Katz AW, Carey-Sampson M, Muhs AG, *et al*. Hypofractionated stereotactic body radiation therapy (SBRT) for limited hepatic metastases. *Int J Radiat Oncol Biol Phys* 2007; **67**: 793–798.

63. van der Pool AE, Mendez Romero A, Wunderink W, *et al*. Stereotactic body radiation therapy for colorectal liver metastases. *Br J Surg* 2010; **97**: 377–382.

64. Rule W, Timmerman R, Tong L, *et al*. Phase I dose-escalation study of stereotactic body radiotherapy in patients with hepatic metastases. *Ann Surg Oncol* 2011; **18**: 1081–1087.

65. Chang DT, Swaminath A, Kozak M, *et al*. Stereotactic body radiotherapy for colorectal liver metastases: a pooled analysis. *Cancer* 2011; **117**: 4060–4069.

66. Lock MI, Hoyer M, Bydder SA, *et al*. An international survey on liver metastases radiotherapy. *Acta Oncol* 2012; **51**: 568–574.

CHAPTER 24

Palliative radiotherapy for malignant neuropathic pain, adrenal, choroidal, and skin metastases

Daniel E. Roos[1], Aaron H. Wolfson[2]

[1]Department of Radiation Oncology, Royal Adelaide Hospital; University of Adelaide School of Medicine, Adelaide, Australia

[2]Department of Radiation Oncology, University of Miami Miller School of Medicine, Miami, FL, USA

Malignant neuropathic pain

Clinical circumstance

Neuropathic pain is defined by the Neuropathic Pain Special Interest Group (NeuPSIG) of the International Association for the Study of Pain (IASP) as pain arising as a direct consequence of a lesion or disease affecting the somatosensory part of the nervous system, i.e. afferent, as distinct from efferent motor, or autonomic parts of the nervous system. The confidence with which a diagnosis of neuropathic pain can be made is graded as "possible," "probable," or "definite" based upon an algorithm with four criteria (plausible pain distribution, history suggesting a relevant index lesion or disease, sensory signs confined to the corresponding innervation territory, and confirmatory diagnostic tests) [1].

Neuropathic pain is described by patients using various terms which differ from those commonly used to describe local pain from bone metastases or from soft tissue metastases (Box 24.1). It is experienced in regions innervated by the dermatomes of involved spinal (or cranial) nerves, or portions of these dermatomes innervated by peripheral nerves. Such pain is often described as intractable or opioid resistant and can be very disabling. It needs to be distinguished from "referred pain" from peripheral joints, which is perceived as deep rather than superficial, and is mediated by branches of nerves supplying both the joint and the muscles and bones acting about the joint, for example hip pain radiating towards the knee [2].

Radiation Oncology in Palliative Cancer Care, First Edition. Edited by Stephen Lutz, Edward Chow, and Peter Hoskin.
© 2013 John Wiley & Sons, Ltd. Published 2013 by John Wiley & Sons, Ltd.

Box 24.1 Symptoms typically associated with neuropathic pain

- Characteristics of pain
  - Follows the dermatomal distribution of the affected cranial or spinal nerve
  - Discomfort that differs from common bone metastasis pain, including:
    - Burning
    - Searing
    - Tingling
    - Shooting
    - Stabbing
    - Electric shock
  - Altered sensory function of the affected nerve, including:
    - Paraesthesia
    - Allodynia
    - Hyperalgesia
    - Hyposensitivity

There has recently been increasing interest in the clinical burden caused by neuropathic pain of malignant origin. A systematic review of studies published until 2010 concluded that its prevalence in over 11,000 patients with active cancer and who reported pain is conservatively 19%, but up to 39% if mixed nociceptive/neuropathic pain is included [3]. In a cross-sectional survey, Kerba *et al.* reported that 17% of 98 patients referred to a Canadian comprehensive cancer center for palliation of bone metastases had pain with neuropathic features [4]. Another recent observational study found a 31% prevalence of neuropathic pain amongst 1100 patients with any kind of pain visiting 19 Spanish radiation oncology units. In three-quarters of cases, the neuropathic pain was attributed to tumor and in most of the others to treatment (surgery, radiotherapy (RT), or chemotherapy) [5]. Clearly, malignant neuropathic pain is a significant clinical problem.

When due to malignant tissue in the vicinity of nerves, the question arises as to how effectively neuropathic pain can be palliated by RT directed to the tumor. However, there is debate about whether the pain is due to mechanical pressure on nerves from the adjacent tumor mass, or whether it is instead due to "chemical" irritation of nerves by cytokines elaborated by either the tumor or by host cells acting pathologically in response to the tumor (e.g. osteoclasts), or perhaps due to a combination of both factors. The distinction is of more than academic interest. With the first hypothesis, higher doses of RT might be more effective in relieving neuropathic pain simply via tumor shrinkage, whereas for the latter hypothesis, lower "anti-inflammatory" doses may suffice (as utilized for plantar fasciitis or thyroid eye disease for example) [2].

Radiotherapy treatment

There are very little data in the literature on the use of RT for malignant neuropathic pain to inform the above debate. Only one study has specifically examined RT for this problem. The Trans Tasman Radiation Oncology Group randomized 272 patients with neuropathic pain associated with bone metastases (neuropathic bone pain, NBP) to a single 8 Gy (8/1) vs 20 Gy in 5 fractions (20/5) (TROG 96.05). There were no statistically significant differences between the arms in intention-to-treat overall response rates within 2 months of commencing treatment (53% for 8/1 vs 61% for 20/5, $P = 0.18$), nor in time-to-treatment failure (estimated TTF 2.4 months vs 3.7 months respectively, $P = 0.056$). There were also no statistically significant differences in the rates of re-treatment, cord compression, or pathological fracture at the index site by arm [2].

That the results were very similar for 8/1 and 20/5 argues against the "tumor shrinkage" hypothesis, mirroring the situation with uncomplicated metastatic bone pain where meta-analyses of numerous randomized trials have confirmed equivalent response rates for (low dose) single fractions and (higher dose) fractionated schedules (see Chapter 20). On the other hand, because most outcomes in TROG 96.05 were numerically slightly in favor of 20/5, although not statistically significant, the question remains as to whether higher doses may be more effective. Clearly, further randomized data are needed [6]. Accordingly, at the time of writing, a second NBP trial is under development. Based in Canada, this international project will commence as a randomized Phase II pilot with a mixed control arm of 8/1 *or* 20/5 (pre-specified by center) vs 30/10 as the experimental arm. The diagnosis of NBP will be more stringently specified than in TROG 96.05 using the above new international consensus IASP grading system. Additionally, whereas neither CT planning nor diagnostic MRI to image the index site were routine during the conception and accrual period of TROG 96.05, the proposed study will mandate CT or MRI in order that the anatomical relationship between tumor and involved nerve(s) can be assessed at presentation and follow-up. Subject to viability and results of the pilot study, a subsequent randomized phase III trial may be undertaken aiming to answer the dose question definitively.

Of course, neuropathic pain of malignant etiology does not necessarily have to be associated with *bone* metastases. Examples include painful brachial plexopathy from breast cancer relapsing in supraclavicular nodes, or sacral plexopathy from pre-sacral involvement by rectal cancer. Perineural infiltration from head and neck cutaneous or mucosal primaries can also cause malignant neuropathic pain (trigeminal neuralgia). However, at the time of writing, there appear to have been no randomized trials, nor even any systematic study of RT specifically for neuropathic pain in the extra-osseous setting despite the previously mentioned prevalence of malignant neuropathic pain.

Conclusion

There are very limited data on the role of RT for this common clinical problem. One randomized trial on neuropathic pain due to bone metastases showed similar response rates to those observed for localized bone pain but leaves the question of optimal fractionation open.

Adrenal metastases

Clinical circumstance

Adrenal metastases are common. Up to a quarter of cancer patients are found to have adrenal metastases at autopsy and in patients with a new or prior diagnosis of cancer, more than half of adrenal masses will be malignant. The majority are carcinomas, most commonly adenocarcinoma (56%) [7–9]. Approximately two-thirds are detected synchronously with the primary, the rest with a median latency of about 7 months. They are rarely symptomatic, usually detected incidentally during staging investigations. This has been even more frequently the case since widespread availability of positron emission tomography (PET) [7]. The most common primary is lung where adrenal metastases rank fourth behind brain, lung, and liver, although isolated adrenal metastases after initial treatment are rare (1%) [10]. The other common primaries are breast, melanoma, renal, and gastro-intestinal tract. Median age at diagnosis is typically in the sixth and seventh decades [7–16].

In common with other paired organs (e.g. lungs, kidneys), the adrenals have considerable functional reserve, and accordingly adrenal metastases rarely cause failure of their endocrine function. However, this *can* occur with bilateral involvement, and may be under-diagnosed as the symptoms and electrolyte disturbances can be confused with non-specific effects of dissemination in pre-terminal patients [8]. When symptomatic, the usual presentation is with somatic type back/flank pain and/or visceral type epigastric pain, sometimes associated with nausea or early satiety [11]. However, this can be difficult to distinguish from bone pain, particularly if there is a radiating component, or liver or chest wall involvement by tumor [8].

In the typical clinical setting of disseminated disease, histological confirmation of adrenal metastasis is usually unnecessary. At the other extreme, for example a primary presenting with an apparently solitary adrenal metastasis, or a solitary adrenal lesion appearing after successful treatment of the primary, biopsy would generally be considered appropriate [11].

A number of series report longer survival with metachronous (often defined as >6 months from diagnosis of the primary) compared with synchronous adrenal metastases [12,17]. Median survival in patients treated with conventional external beam radiation therapy (EBRT) is 3–10 months (Table 24.1). However, survival in the stereotactic body radiation therapy (SBRT) series

Table 24.1 Conventional external beam radiation therapy for adrenal metastases.

Series (time frame)	Patients	Primaries	Most common schedule (range) (Gy/number of fractions)	Pain response (assessable patients)	Median survival (range) (months)
Soffen et al. 1990 [11] (1972–1988)	16	lung 15 unknown 1	30/10 – 12 (29/17 – 45/23)	12/16 (75%)	3 (1–11)
Short et al. 1996 [8] (1994–1995)	7	lung 4 others 3	20/5 (20/5 – 45/20)	7/7 (100%)	Not stated[a]
Miyaji et al. 1999 [10] (1994–1996)	3	lung 3	45/25 – 60/30	2/2 (100%)	8 (4–33)
Zeng et al. 2005 [13] (2000–2004)	22	hepatoma 22	50/25 (36/18 – 54/27)	13/14 (93%)	10 (3 36)
Oshiro et al. 2011 [12] (1999–2008)	8	lung 8	39/13 – 54/24[b]	(none symptomatic)	6 (2–22)

[a]4/7 patients still alive at time of reporting
[b]Six different schedules used, none more than twice

(see later) tends to be longer (median 8–21 months), probably reflecting a different mix of primary disease and other prognostic factors. Although it is possible that improved local control for patients with isolated adrenal metastases due to the higher biologically equivalent doses utilized in SBRT may translate to improved survival, randomized evidence is lacking. Of note, for the highly selected subset of resectable lung cancer patients presenting with *operable*, asymptomatic synchronous or metachronous isolated adrenal metastases, a recent systematic review reported median survivals of 12 months and 31 months respectively, although 5-year survival estimates are similar for the two groups (26% and 25% respectively) [17]. As is the case with SBRT, there are no randomized data supporting this aggressive surgical approach. However, for lung cancer, there is a plausible biological rationale for radical treatment in this setting, viz. isolated adrenal metastases *may* reflect direct retroperitoneal lymphatic rather than hematogenous spread, and therefore represent regional extension instead of true systemic involvement [17].

A host of treatment options exist for adrenal metastases including open or laparoscopic surgery, percutaneous ethanol injection, transarterial chemo-embolization, radiofrequency ablation, chemotherapy, and RT (conventional or stereotactic), but there are no randomized comparisons [7,13,15] (Figure 24.1).

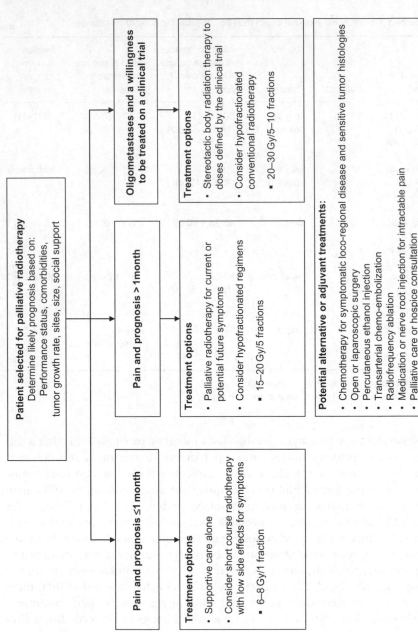

Figure 24.1 Algorithm for use of palliative radiotherapy for patients with adrenal metastases.

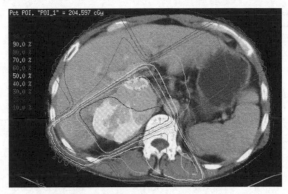

Figure 24.2 Conventional external beam posterior oblique wedged photon pair used to treat a large symptomatic right adrenal metastasis. Representative isodose contours shown. Reproduced from Zeng *et al.* [13], with permission from Oxford University Press.

Radiotherapy treatment

Conventional EBRT has been reported to palliate pain from adrenal metastases since at least the 1970s but the published data are limited and there have been no prospective studies. Fractionation has ranged between 20/5 and 60/30 (Table 24.1). Shorter schedules (e.g. single fractions) could be considered for very poor prognosis patients. When described, beam arrangements have varied from simple opposed anterior-posterior pair [8,11], posterior oblique wedged pair (Figure 24.2) [13], or multi-field [8,12].

Although patient numbers have been small and response definitions variable, pain response has been consistently high (75–100%), sometimes lasting until death (Table 24.1). The unweighted average response rate from the five series is 34/39 = 87%. Radiological response was not usually assessed. Zeng *et al.* reported tumor shrinkage (partial response) in 16/22 patients (73%) with hepatocellular primaries (although this conflicts with tabulated data showing 64% partial response and 36% stable disease). Of note, the doses in this series were higher than typically used for palliation [13].

There are few data on re-treatment of adrenal metastases with EBRT for progression, but second responses have been reported [8,13].

Acute side effects include loss of appetite, mild to moderate nausea, and transient diarrhea [11,13]. Adrenal insufficiency has not been reported, nor has any other late morbidity, reflecting the typically low doses used, the short median survival, and (probably) the absence of prospective studies.

Note that due to widespread disease, many patients in these series (and also those below for SBRT) had sequential or synchronous chemotherapy which likely impacted upon the observed response of their adrenal metastases to radiation, but the relative contributions are unknown in the absence of controlled comparative data.

Table 24.2 Stereotactic body radiation therapy for adrenal metastases.

Series (time frame)	Patients (adrenals irradiated)	Primaries	Most common schedule (range) (Gy/ number of fractions)	Local control (assessable patients)	Pain relief	Median survival (range) (months)
Katoh et al. 2008 [16] (2004–2006)	8 (9)	lung 6 others 2	48/8 (all)	9/9 (100%)	1/1	NS
Chawla et al. 2009 [15] (2001–2007)	30 (35)	lung 20 liver 3 breast 3 others 4	40/10 (16/4 – 50/10)	14/24 (58%)	3/3	11 (0.8–35)
Oshiro et al. 2011 [12] (1999–2008)	11 (11)	lung 11	36/9 – 60/5[a]	8/11 (73%)	NA[b]	12 (0.7–87.8)
Torok et al. 2011 [7] (2002–2009)	7 (9)	lung 5 hepatoma 2	16/1 (10–22/1) and 27/3 (24–36/3)	3/8 (38%)	1/2	8 (NS)
Holy et al. 2011 [14] (2002–2009)	18 (18)	lung 18	40/5 (15/3 – 40/5)	15/18 (78%)	6/8	21 (NS)
Casamassima et al. 2012 [9] (2002–2009)	48 (58)	lung 24 colon 12 others 12	16.5/1 (15–19/1) and 36/3 (30–54/3)	46/48 (96%)	4/4	11[c] (NS)

NS, not stated; NA, not applicable
[a]Seven different schedules used, none more than twice
[b]None symptomatic
[c]Estimated from Casamassima et al., Figure 1 [9]

Newer technologies

During the last few years, there have been several reports on the application of SBRT for the treatment of adrenal metastases (Table 24.2, Figure 24.3). When addressed in these publications, the stated aim is to utilize the highly conformal dose delivery to emulate the long-term disease-free survival (or cure) sometimes observed with surgery, rather than simply to palliate pain. Indeed, most of these patients had asymptomatic lesions [7,9,12,14–16]. Some authors also advocate SBRT to prophylactically palliate bulky adrenal masses [15]. However, SBRT has usually been considered appropriate only in the setting

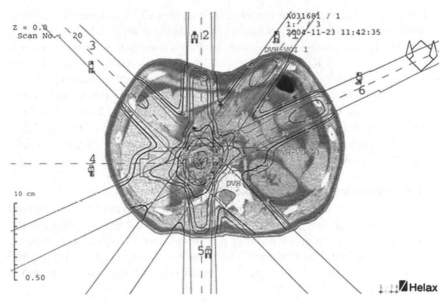

Figure 24.3 Stereotactic body radiotherapy used to treat a small asymptomatic right adrenal metastasis using a 6 static field photon beam technique (see Plate 24.1). Reproduced from Holy *et al.* [14], with permission from Urban und Vogel.

of oligometastases, typically defined as ≤5, conceptualized as a chronic disease state in which widespread metastasis has not evolved [18]. All studies are retrospective.

Table 24.2 shows an enormous range of fractionation schedules ranging from single doses of 10–22 Gy to 15–60 Gy in 3–10 fractions. No one option has yet emerged as dominant. Most series report only *crude* local control rates which range from 38–100% (overall average rate 95/118 = 81%). The largest series (48 patients, 58 lesions) found 90% 1- and 2-year *actuarial* local control [9], whereas corresponding figures from one of the smallest (7 patients, 9 lesions) were 55% and 27% respectively [7].

For the small subset of patients identified with pain in the above series, SBRT appears to be very effective, 15/18 (83%) achieving pain response (Table 24.2).

Acute and late toxicity is reported to be minimal. Mild to moderate nausea [14,15] and fatigue [15] appear to be most common. Gastroduodenal ulceration [12] and adrenal insufficiency [9] have occasionally been observed.

There are very limited data on re-treatment after SBRT. Chawla *et al.* reported successful re-treatment of two adrenal metastases using intensity modulated radiation therapy (IMRT) [15]. Milano *et al.* described 32 (of 121) patients with oligometastases at various sites who underwent one or more repeat courses of SBRT for local failure (9) and/or new lesions (29). Whilst outcomes were promising, none of these patients had an adrenal metastasis re-treated [18].

Data are emerging on the use of newer advanced techniques for adrenal metastases. Several of these, including IMRT, volume modulated arc therapy, and intensity modulated protons, are compared dosimetrically with conventional 3D conformal RT by Scorsetti *et al.* with the conclusion that intensity modulated approaches are superior to the other conformal solutions [19]. Jang *et al.* reported a 60% objective response for "lymph node/adrenal" metastases from helical tomotherapy plus chemotherapy for a subset of 20 (of 42) patients with hepatocellular primaries, but the adrenal results were not described separately. The median dose for the whole series was 51 Gy in 10 fractions (range 30–57.6 Gy) [20].

Special considerations in developing countries

Symptomatic adrenal metastases could be treated most simply with opposed antero-posterior photon beams (including cobalt-60) using conventional simulation and 2D planning if computer planning is unavailable. Diagnostic CT measurements would be transferred onto the simulator film using bony landmarks with at least a 2 cm margin to beam edge. A low cost, convenient fractionation schedule would be 20/5.

Conclusion

Both EBRT and SBRT are effective for palliation of painful adrenal metastases, with response rates of about 85%, although the latter technique is primarily used for local control and disease-free survival benefit. There is no consensus on optimal fractionation schedules, but for EBRT, a 1–2 week course would be reasonable in the majority of patients.

Choroidal metastases

Clinical circumstance

Metastases, usually adenocarcinoma involving the uveal tract, constitute the most common intraocular malignant disease. The prevalence of clinically evident uveal metastases in cancer patients is reported to be 2–9%, and the most common site of involvement is the choroid with <10% involving the iris and <5% the ciliary body [21–24]. Breast cancer dominates ocular metastasis [25], accounting for 40–80% of cases. Hence, choroidal metastases are more common in women overall (70–85%). The median time from diagnosis to development of choroidal metastases from breast is 3–6 years [23,26,27]. The other common primaries are lung and gastrointestinal tract where the time from diagnosis tends to be shorter (median 2.5 months for lung, 11 months for other primaries) [23]. Choroidal metastases are unilateral in about two-thirds of cases, although commonly multi-focal within the eye [24]. Overall, about half are solitary only [22,23]. They are usually sited posterior to the equator (>85%) [21], and there is no predilection for either eye. Simultaneous (15%) or subsequent (15%) brain metastases are common [24]. Median age at diagnosis of choroidal metastases is typically 50–60 years.

Choroidal metastases present with decreased visual acuity/blurred vision (approximately 90%), visual field defect/scotoma (approximately 20%), distorted image, photophobia, and flashes/floaters. Pain and/or redness are rare. The typical fundoscopic appearance is a homogeneous, creamy, plateau lesion often complicated by secondary retinal detachment or hemorrhage. Investigations to confirm the diagnosis may include ultrasound, CT orbits, or fluorescein angiography, but biopsy is rarely needed (unknown primary or no other metastases to biopsy) [23]. However, imaging of the brain (CT or MRI) is justified in view of the risk of synchronous brain metastases and the implications for treatment technique (see later) [28].

Reported median survivals are around 6–12 months (Table 24.3) with breast primaries at the upper end of this range (23 months in one breast only series) [29] and lung primaries at the lower end [23].

Treatment options include observation (if the lesion is inactive, or expected survival is short), RT, chemotherapy/hormonal/biological therapy [25] (the choroid is a vascular structure, not considered to be subject to "sanctuary site" limitations with systemic treatment) [27], laser photocoagulation, photodynamic therapy, transpupillary thermotherapy, local resection and (rarely) enucleation for intractable pain [21,22,27]. There are limited data on the use of brachytherapy (episcleral radioactive plaques) in highly specialized centers [22] and also newer technologies including protons and stereotactic techniques (e.g. CyberKnife), but the following discussion will be limited to conventional EBRT which is regarded as first-line treatment for symptomatic eyes when systemic therapy is either not working or otherwise not indicated. An informative overview of the other treatment options is to be found in Kanthan *et al.* [21].

Radiotherapy treatment

All reported series are retrospective with the exception of a German Cancer Society prospective study [30]. Table 24.3 summarizes data from reports published from 1990 onwards. Visual response was variably reported, most commonly as improvement or stabilization of vision, crude rates for assessable patients being in the range 57–100% (overall average rate 409/551 = 74%). Pre-1990 series are tabulated in Rudoler *et al.* in which the range of visual response was 33–89% [24]. Importantly, even severely affected eyes may improve after RT. In Rudoler *et al.*, 17/47 (36%) initially blind patients (visual acuity ≥20/400) regained useful vision (navigational or excellent) [24]. Most series were too small to analyze prognostic factors for visual outcome, but in the largest, younger age (<55), excellent initial vision (visual acuity ≤20/50), and smaller tumor diameter (<15 mm) were favorable [24]. d'Abbadie *et al.* also found initial vision (≤20/40) to be prognostic, although in their series, tumor progression was used as a surrogate for visual loss [31]. These data argue for earlier intervention. Rosset *et al.* found a dose response for preservation of vision (>35.5 Gy_{10}, where Gy_{10} is the biologically equivalent dose using an alpha/beta ratio of 10 for tumor effects)

Table 24.3 Radiotherapy for choroidal metastases (series published since 1990).

Series (time frame)	Patients (eyes or patients irradiated)	Primaries	Schedules (Gy/number of fractions)	Stable or improved vision (assessable eyes)	Median survival (range) (months)
Burmeister et al. 1990 [32] (approx. 1987–1988)	6 (7)	breast 6	21–27/7–8[a]	5/6 (83%)	5 (NS)[a]
Ratanatharathorn et al. 1991 [27] (1980–1991)	19 (23)	breast 19	26–46/10–25[b]	NS (100%)[b]	6 (1–64)
Nylen et al. 1994 [33] (1985–1992)	17 (21)	breast 14 lung 1 others 2	20–45/5–20	13/16 (81%)	11 (1–54)
Rudoler et al. 1997 [24] (1972–1995)	188 (233)[c]	breast 100 lung 44 others 44	30–40/10–20[d]	89/155 (57%)	9 (NS)
Rosset et al. 1998 [23] (1970–1993)	58 (88)	breast 38 lung 10 others 10	20–53/10–30	48/59 (81%)	11[e] (NS)
Wiegel et al. 2002 [30] (1994–1998)	50 (65)	breast 31 lung 13 others 6	40/20 (all)	58/65 (89%)	7 (1–19)
d'Abbadie et al. 2003 [31] (1966–1992)	123 (97)	breast 88 lung 11 others 24	18–30/3–10[f]	66/97 (68%)[g]	13 (NS)
Demirci et al. 2003 [29] (1974–2001)	254 (129)	breast 254	20–64/8–32	106/129[h] (82%)	23[i] (NS)
Bajcsay et al. 2003 [34] (1994–2002)	17 (24)	breast 11 lung 4 others 2	42–51/NS	24/24 (100%)	12 (1–43)

NS, not stated

[a]This series included 5 other patients with orbital metastases. Fractionation and survival were not separately reported for choroidal metastases

[b]This series included 13 other patients with anterior chamber or orbital metastases. Fractionation and visual outcomes were not separately reported for choroidal metastases. However, all of the 21 (of 32) evaluable patients who completed treatment responded

[c]10 eyes (4%) had ciliary body involvement

[d]72% of patients. The overall dose range was 4–63 Gy at 1.5–4.0 Gy/fraction

[e]Estimated from Rosset et al., Figure 1 [23]

[f]Most common 30/10 followed by 18/3; details of other schedules not provided

[g]Deduced from d'Abbadie et al., Table 5 [31]. Note that tumor response (at 3 months) was reported as a surrogate for visual response

[h]Tumor control (regression or stability) was reported as a surrogate for visual response

[i]Estimated from Demirci et al., Figure 3, for the whole series [29]. Survival was not reported separately for the 129 patients who had radiotherapy for choroid metastases

[23], but no dose response was found in two other series examining this factor [24,31].

Impressive results have been reported for tumor response with regression or stabilization of tumor size in typically ≥85% of patients and improvement in clinically meaningful indices such as freedom from clinically evident recurrence at last follow-up (>90%), and rate of globe preservation (98–100%). Fundoscopic regression is usually evident within 1 month with improvement in visual acuity continuing up to 3 months [23,24,29,33,34].

As noted above for adrenal metastases, many patients in the choroidal series, particularly those with breast primaries, also had chemotherapy and/ or hormonal treatment around the time of the ocular irradiation, the contribution from which is impossible to determine from the available literature.

Most series in which technique is reported advocate use of a lens-sparing (half beam-blocked or angled) lateral photon beam. Alternatives include wedged anterior/lateral pair [27] or direct electrons [24,27]. Bilateral lesions are treated with lens-sparing opposed laterals. Immobilization of the eye is unnecessary for co-operative patients, but eye fixation with vacuum contact lenses has been described [33,34]. There are divergent views as to whether the contralateral eye should be treated prophylactically or instead avoided completely by beam angling. Relapse in the untreated contralateral eye is uncommon, typically <10%, although one author reports the incidence to be 15–20% [30]. Of interest, the prospective German study found that no contralateral choroidal metastases developed using a lens-sparing ipsilateral beam (40 Gy at 2 Gy/fraction) which exited through the fellow eye, delivering 50–70% of the prescribed dose to the contralateral posterior choroid (Figure 24.4(a)) [30]. If synchronous brain metastases are detected, both sites (brain and posterior globes) would ordinarily be treated simultaneously with opposed lateral fields to avoid overlap (Figure 24.4(b)) [28].

Acute side effects may include skin reaction, local alopecia, conjunctivitis, and xerophthalmia, the severity of which are obviously dose and field dependent. Similarly, late side effects including cataract, glaucoma, keratopathy, dry eye syndrome, retinopathy, and optic neuropathy, are a function of technique, dose, and survival time, most rare with low dose palliation.

Special considerations in developing countries

The German technique (see previously) can be easily applied with conventional simulation and 2D planning using the outer canthus as a landmark for the anterior border of a half beam-blocked lateral field (or opposed fields in the case of bilateral involvement) (Figure 24.4). As for adrenal metastases, 20/5 would be a resource favorable fractionation option.

Conclusion

Radiotherapy is a convenient, low toxicity treatment for choroidal metastases with preservation of vision in about 75% of patients. Early referral may lead to improved outcomes.

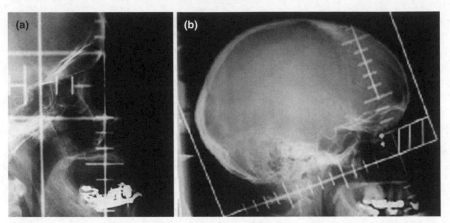

Figure 24.4 (a) Lens-sparing (half beam-blocked) lateral photon field to treat symptomatic right choroidal metastases with exit dose onto the uninvolved left posterior choroid. (b) Opposed lateral photon fields to treat brain and posterior choroidal metastases synchronously. Note position of isocenter and corner shielding to spare lenses. Reproduced from Bottke *et al.* [27], with permission from Urban und Vogel.

Skin metastases (A.H. Wolfson)

Radiotherapy is a proven empirical modality for palliative treatment of symptomatic skin and subcutaneous metastases. Although such involvement is uncommon, the most frequent primary sites are breast, lung, colon, head and neck, kidney, stomach, ovary, and cutaneous malignant melanoma (CMM). Rarely, other primary malignancies spread to the skin, such as gynecologic cancers [35, 36]. Palliative radiotherapy has also been used for locally advanced as well as recurrent primary skin cancers, such as primary cutaneous lymphoma (PCL) [37], Merkel cell carcinoma (MCC) [38], and Kaposi sarcoma [39].

A longstanding palliative regimen in the United States used to treat a variety of metastatic lesions in multiple organ sites, including the skin, has been 10–15 fractions at 2.5–3.0 Gy per fraction over 2–3 weeks using photon and/or electron EBRT. In other countries, hypofractionated treatments to either 20 Gy in 5 fractions or even 8–10 Gy in a single fraction are considered standard. Treatment is usually confined to the discrete site with an accompanying 1–2 cm normal tissue margin and using appropriately constructed bolus material to ensure adequate surface dose. The remainder of this section will focus on primary skin cancers.

Cutaneous recurrence of melanoma occurs in about a third of cases [40]. One therapeutic approach has been to use a hypofractionated regimen of 36/6 delivered twice weekly over 3 weeks to overcome the putative relative radioresistance of this disease [41]. However, some data have suggested that there may not be a therapeutic advantage from employing fraction sizes greater than 3 Gy over more conventional fractionation to palliate metastatic/

recurrent CMM [42]. A randomized trial compared $4 \times 8\,\mathrm{Gy}$ with $20 \times 2.5\,\mathrm{Gy}$ for 126 evaluable patients, about 60% of whom had "soft tissue/skin" melanoma metastases as the index site. There was no difference in response rate between the arms (approximately 60% each) [43]. Although there is still debate about the ideal fractionation to select for subcutaneous or in-transit skin metastases from CMM, there has been a suggestion that both freedom from progression and median survival are improved by delivering a biologically effective total dose greater than $39\,\mathrm{Gy}_{10}$ [44].

Merkel cell carcinoma is considered a highly radiosensitive tumor. In contrast to CMM, radiation therapy has been used as upfront treatment for both inoperable primaries and for locally recurrent lesions. Recommended normal tissue margins on an area of skin recurrence are at least 5 cm, along with electively including the draining lymph node basin [45]. The literature indicates that doses of 40–60 Gy at 2–2.5 Gy per fraction are reasonable to control disease [46]. However, a shorter palliative treatment schedule of 25/5 has been recommended for patients with poor performance status [47]. In addition, one report discussed using high-dose-rate (HDR) brachytherapy to deliver 12/2 to recurrent MCC skin lesions. Not only did this treatment yield long-term complete response but also caused distant untreated lesions to regress. This latter phenomenon is known as the abscopal effect, which has also been described for CMM [48].

Primary cutaneous lymphoma is a spectrum of malignant skin disorders that includes cutaneous T-cell (CTCL) and cutaneous B-cell lymphomas (CBCL). The most common CTCL is mycosis fungoides, which can present as patches, plaques, and tumors. For isolated lesions, optimal total doses of 30–36 Gy at 2 Gy per fraction using superficial electron beam treatment with at least 2 cm normal tissue margin have been recommended [49], although hypofractionated schedules and single doses are also effective in the palliative setting. For advanced forms of mycosis fungoides, including Sezary Syndrome (or erythroderma), the use of total skin electron beam therapy to similar total doses is indicated. For CBCL, local control has been achieved with total doses of at least 36 Gy at 2 Gy per fraction [49]. However, there now exist data to suggest that good palliation of recurrent, persistent lesions of both CTCL and CBCL can be achieved with just 16/2 using electron beam therapy and a normal tissue margin of 2 cm [50].

Special considerations in developing countries

In the absence of electron or brachytherapy options, many skin lesions can be easily treated with orthovoltage X-rays (superficial or deep) using clinical mark-up and brief hypo-fractionated schedules.

Conclusion

EBRT has been used to treat symptomatic cutaneous metastases from a wide variety of carcinomas and for recurrent/metastatic primary skin malignancies including CMM, MCC, and PCL. There are few randomized data to guide choice of fractionation, but 1–2 week courses are often appropriate in the palliative setting.

References

1. Treede RD, Jensen TS, Campbell JN, et al. Neuropathic pain: redefinition and a grading system for clinical and research purposes. *Neurology* 2008; **70**: 1630–1635.
2. Roos DE, Turner SL, O'Brien PC, et al. Randomized trial of 8 Gy in 1 versus 20 Gy in 5 fractions of radiotherapy for neuropathic pain due to bone metastases (Trans-Tasman Radiation Oncology Group, TROG 96.05). *Radiother Oncol* 2005; **75**: 54–63.
3. Bennett MI, Rayment C, Hjermstad M, et al. Prevalence and aetiology of neuropathic pain in cancer patients: a systematic review. *Pain* 2012; **153**: 359–365.
4. Kerba M, Wu JSY, Duan Q, et al. Neuropathic pain features in patients with bone metastases referred for palliative radiotherapy. *J Clin Oncol* 2010; **28**: 4892–4897.
5. Manas A, Monroy JL, Ramos AA, et al. Prevalence of neuropathic pain in radiotherapy oncology units. *Int J Radiat Oncol Biol Phys* 2011; **81**: 511–520.
6. Dennis K, Chow E, Roos D, et al. Should bone metastases causing neuropathic pain be treated with single dose radiotherapy? Editorial. *Clin Oncol (R Coll Radiol)* 2011; **23**: 482–484.
7. Torok J, Wegner RE, Burton SA, Heron DE. Stereotactic body radiation therapy for adrenal metastases: a retrospective review of a non-invasive therapeutic strategy. *Future Oncol* 2011; **7**: 145–151.
8. Short S, Chaturvedi A, Leslie MD. Palliation of symptomatic adrenal gland metastases by radiotherapy. *Clin Oncol* 1996; **8**: 387–399.
9. Casamassima F, Livi L, Masciullo S, et al. Stereotactic radiotherapy for adrenal gland metastases: University of Florence experience. *Int J Radiat Oncol Biol Phys* 2012; **82**: 919–923.
10. Miyaji N, Miki T, Itoh Y, et al. Radiotherapy for adrenal gland metastasis from lung cancer: report of three cases. *Radiat Med* 1999; **17**: 71–75.
11. Soffen EM, Solin LJ, Rubenstein JH, Hanks GE. Palliative radiotherapy for symptomatic adrenal metastases. *Cancer* 1990; **65**: 1318–1320.
12. Oshiro Y, Takeda Y, Hirano S, et al. Role of radiotherapy for local control of asymptomatic adrenal metastases from lung cancer. *Am J Clin Oncol* 2011; **34**: 249–253.
13. Zeng Z-C, Tang Z-Y, Fan J, et al. Radiation therapy for adrenal gland metastases from hepatocellular carcinoma. *Jpn J Clin Oncol* 2005; **35**: 61–67.
14. Holy R, Piroth M, Pinkawa M, Eble MJ. Stereotactic body radiation therapy (SBRT) for treatment of adrenal gland metastases from non-small cell lung cancer. *Strahlenther Onkol* 2011; **187**: 245–251.
15. Chawla S, Chen Y, Katz AW, et al. Stereotactic body radiotherapy for treatment of adrenal metastases. *Int J Radiat Oncol Biol Phys* 2009; **75**: 71–75.
16. Katoh N, Onimaru R, Sakuhara Y, et al. Real-time tumor-tracking radiotherapy for adrenal tumors. *Radiother Oncol* 2008; **87**: 418–424.

17. Tanvetyanon T, Robinson LA, Schell MJ, *et al*. Outcomes of adrenalectomy for isolated synchronous versus metachronous adrenal metastases in non-small cell lung cancer: a systematic review and pooled analysis. *J Clin Oncol* 2008; **26**: 1142–1147.

18. Milano MT, Philip A, Okunieff P. Analysis of patients with oligometastases undergoing two or more curative-intent stereotactic radiotherapy courses. *Int J Radiat Oncol Biol Phys* 2009; **73**: 832–837.

19. Scorsetti M, Mancosu P, Navarria P, *et al*. Stereotactic body radiation therapy (SBRT) for adrenal metastases: a feasibility study of advanced techniques with modulated photons and protons. *Strahlenther Onkol* 2011; **187**: 238–244.

20. Jang JW, Kay CS, You CR, *et al*. Simultaneous multitarget irradiation using helical tomotherapy for advanced hepatocellular carcinoma with multiple extrahepatic metastases. *Int J Radiat Oncol Biol Phys* 2009; **74**: 412–418.

21. Kanthan GL, Jayamohan J, Yip D, Conway RM. Management of metastatic carcinoma of the uveal tract: an evidence-based analysis. *Clin Experiment Ophthalmol* 2007; **35**: 553–565.

22. Shields CL. Plaque radiotherapy for the management of uveal metastasis. *Curr Opin Ophthalmol* 1998; **9**: 31–37.

23. Rosset A, Zografos L, Coucke P, *et al*. Radiotherapy of choroidal metastases. *Radiother Oncol* 1998; **46**: 263–268.

24. Rudoler SB, Shields CL, Corn BW, *et al*. Functional vision is improved in the majority of patients treated with external-beam radiotherapy for choroidal metastases. A multivariate analysis of 188 patients. *J Clin Oncol* 1997; **15**: 1244–1251.

25. Wickremasinghe S, Dansingani KK, Tranos P, *et al*. Ocular presentations of breast cancer. *Acta Ophthalmol Scand* 2007; **85**: 133–142.

26. Chang EL, Lo S. Diagnosis and management of central nervous system metastases from breast cancer. *Oncologist* 2003; **8**: 398–410.

27. Ratanatharathorn V, Powers WE, Grimm J, *et al*. Eye metastasis from carcinoma of the breast: diagnosis, radiation treatment and results. *Cancer Treat Rev* 1991; **18**: 261–276.

28. Bottke D, Wiegel T, Kreusel K-M, *et al*. Is diagnostic CT of the brain indicated in patients with choroidal metastases before radiotherapy? *Strahlenther Onkol* 2005; **181**: 251–254.

29. Demirci H, Shields CL, Chao A-N, Shields JA. Uveal metastasis from breast cancer in 264 patients. *Am J Ophthalmol* 2003; **136**: 264–271.

30. Wiegel T, Bottke D, Kreusel K-M, *et al*. External beam radiotherapy of choroidal metastases – final results of a prospective study of the German Cancer Society (ARO 95-08). *Radiother Oncol* 2002; **64**: 13–18.

31. d'Abbadie I, Arriagada R, Spielmann M, Le MG. Choroid metastases: clinical features and treatments in 123 patients. *Cancer* 2003; **98**: 1232–1238.

32. Burmeister BH, Benjamin CS, Childs WJ. The management of metastases to eye and orbit from carcinoma of the breast. *Aust N Z J Ophthalmol* 1990; **18**: 187–190.

33. Nylen U, Kock E, Lax I, *et al*. Standardized precision radiotherapy in choroidal metastases. *Acta Oncoligica* 1994; **33**: 65–68.

34. Bajcsay A, Kontra G, Recsan Z, *et al*. Lens-sparing external beam radiotherapy of intraocular metastases: our experiences with twenty four eyes. *Neoplasma* 2003; **50**: 459–464.

35. Elit L, Lukka H, Friedman E. Cutaneous metastasis of papillary serous uterine cancer. *Gynecol Oncol* 2001; **82**: 208–211.

36. Marek G, Malgorzata W, Andrzej M. Multiple skin metastases to vulva from carcinoma of the cervical stump. *Ginekol Pol* 2010; **81**: 140–143.

37. De Sanctis V, Osti MF, Berard F, *et al*. Primary cutaneous lymphoma: local control and survival in patients treated with radiotherapy. *Anticancer Res* 2007; **27**: 601–606.

38. Morrison WH, Peters LS, Silva EG, *et al*. The essential role of radiation therapy in securing lococregional control of Merkel cell carcinoma. *Int J Radiat Oncol Biol Phys* 1990; **19**: 583–591.

39. Dogan M, Dogan L, Ozdemir F, *et al*. Fifty-one Kaposi sarcoma patients. *Clin Transl Oncol* 2010; **12**: 629–633.

40. Morris KT, Marquez CM, Holland JM, *et al*. Prevention of local recurrence after surgical debulking of nodal and subcutaneous melanoma deposits by hypofractionated radiation. *Ann Surg Oncol* 2000; **7**: 680–684.

41. Rao NG, Yu H-HM, Trotti A, Sondak VK. The role of radiation therapy in the management of cutaneous melanoma. *Surg Oncol Clin N Am* 2011; **20**: 115–131.

42. Fenig E, Eidelevich E, Njuguna E, *et al*. Role of radiation therapy in the management of cutaneous malignant melanoma. *Am J Clin Oncol* 1999; **22**: 184–186.

43. Sause WT, Cooper JS, Rush MD, *et al*. Fraction size in external beam radiation therapy in the treatment of melanoma. *Int J Radiat Oncol Biol Phys* 1991; **20**: 429–432.

44. Shuff JH, Siker ML, Daly MD, *et al*. Role of radiation therapy in cutaneous melanoma. *Clin Plast Surg* 2010; **37**: 147–160.

45. Decker RH, Wilson LD. Role of radiotherapy in the management of Merkel cell carcinoma of the skin. *J Natl Compr Canc Netw* 2006; **4**: 713–718.

46. Fenig E, Brenner B, Katz A, *et al*. The role of radiation therapy and chemotherapy in the treatment of Merkel cell carcinoma. *Cancer* 1997; **80**: 881–885.

47. Koh CSL, Veness MJ. Role of definitive radiotherapy in treating patients with inoperable Merkel cell carcinoma: the Westmead Hospital experience and a review of the literature. *Australas J Dermatol* 2009; **50**: 249–256.

48. Cotter SE, Dunn GP, Collins KM, *et al*. Abscopal effect in a patient with metastatic Merkel cell carcinoma following radiation therapy: potential role of induced antitumor immunity. *Arch Dermatol* 2011; **147**: 870–872.

49. Smith BD, Wilson LD. Cutaneous lymphomas. *Semin Radiat Oncol* 2007; **17**: 158–168.

50. De Sanctis V, Persechino S, Fanelli A, *et al*. Role of radiation therapy in mycosis fungoides refractory to systemic therapy. *Eur J Dermatol* 2011; **21**: 213–217.

PART 5

Integration of radiation oncology and palliative care

CHAPTER 25

Design challenges in palliative radiation oncology clinical trials

Deborah Watkins Bruner[1], Lawrence B. Berk[2]
[1]Winship Cancer Institute, Emory University, Atlanta, GA, USA
[2]Radiation Oncology at Tampa General Hospital, and University of South Florida, Tampa, FL, USA

Introduction

Medical clinical trials, including palliative care trials, classically use the same paradigm as physical science trials, the objective measurement of an endpoint. For cancer trials, the prototype is to intervene with a pharmaceutical treatment and measure the result. However, the only truly objective endpoint is death. All other endpoints are subjective. Even measuring response requires agreeing on commonly accepted criteria, such as Response Evaluation Criteria In Solid Tumors (RECIST), a set of published rules that define when cancer patients improve ("respond"), stay the same ("stable"), or worsen ("progression") during treatments [1]. The criteria try to precisely define, and control, what is being measured and how it is being measured.

Palliation is treatment without the primary goal of prolongation of survival. Palliation can be a goal for patients receiving curative treatment, by relieving symptoms and improving quality of life [2]. A palliation trial to prevent fractures can be objective: the number of fractures per period of time is measured. However, palliation often cannot be objective in the sense of the physical sciences. A trial to improve quality of life and symptoms can never be objective, because a subjective parameter is being measured. Therefore great care must be taken to use measures that we believe appropriately reflect the parameter we are trying to measure.

Challenges with the validation of palliative metrics

The use of objective measures of outcome in palliative care and symptom management trials can be problematic. A symptom is by definition the subjective patient-reported aspect of a problem. A sign is the observer-reported measurement. Thus skin erythema is a sign of radiation dermatitis, whereas itching and

Radiation Oncology in Palliative Cancer Care, First Edition. Edited by Stephen Lutz, Edward Chow, and Peter Hoskin.
© 2013 John Wiley & Sons, Ltd. Published 2013 by John Wiley & Sons, Ltd.

pain are potential symptoms from radiation dermatitis. Nonetheless, if objective measures are to be used, they must in some way be validated to show they represent a quantitative and reproducible measure of the toxicity. Unfortunately, many objective measures are accepted based solely on reproducibility. In fact many of the "objective" metrics we take for granted as reliable measures have never been validated, such as the National Cancer Institute (NCI) Common Terminology Criteria for Adverse Events (CTCAE) [3].

Symptom management and quality of life endpoints often are not directly measurable, therefore patient perceptions of symptoms or the effect of the symptom on the patient's functioning and quality of life are assessed. Symptom assessments are measured with validated patient-reported outcomes (PROs). The Food and Drug Administration (FDA) in their publication on PRO Guidance for Industry defined a PRO as a measurement of any aspect of a patient's health status that comes directly from the patient, without interpretation of the patient's responses by a clinician or research associate [4]. The FDA Guidance also describes in detail the rigorous process of PRO measure development and validation.

The Functional Assessment of Cancer Therapy (FACT) Fatigue Scale (FACT-F) is just one example of the development and psychometric analysis process required for validation before a measure can be used in a national clinical trial. FACT-F is a subscale that can be added to the general FACT quality of life scale, the 28-item FACT-G, or used alone. This scale was originally developed for use in patients with anemia [5]. Item development began with semi-structured interviews with anemic oncology patients and with medical experts. This phase generated 221 candidate questions. These were then reduced to 39 by eliminating redundant and non-anemia or fatigue specific questions. These 39 questions were then reviewed by a second group of experts and reduced to 20 anemia-related questions, 13 involving fatigue-related areas and 7 non-anemia questions. Thus 13 questions were chosen to comprise the FACT-F. In the validation phase for the FACT-F, the items were given to a separate cohort of cancer patients with anemia.

Other commonly used fatigue scales, the Piper Fatigue Scale (PFS) and the Profile of Mood States (POMS), were co-administered to assess correlations with the new scale. Reliability of the scale was tested by having patients retake the test within 3–7 days. Further, correlations with objective findings such as the hemoglobin levels were assessed. The scale showed good performance in all the areas tested and was therefore considered sufficiently validated for cancer patients at risk of or experiencing anemia. Thus a rigorous process should be used for the validation of measures; however, this process has only evolved over the past few decades.

Evolution of palliative care clinical trials: the Radiation Therapy Oncology Group experience

The quality of the measures used in palliative clinical trials at the Radiation Therapy Oncology Group (RTOG), one of the national clinical trial cooperative groups funded by the NCI since 1968 to increase the survival and improve the quality of life of patients diagnosed with cancer, evolved along with the understanding of the complexities and subtleties of palliation trials. In this chapter, we will use RTOG trials as exemplars of the challenges and progression of metrics in palliative care research. Symptom management during curative treatment and symptom management for patients with incurable disease are both considered as the palliation of symptoms in the trials described below.

Bone metastases

Table 25.1 summarizes the RTOG bone metastases trials. One of the first trials run by the RTOG was RTOG 7402 [6]. This assessed the effect of the number of fractions and the dose of each fraction on the relief of pain among patients with bone metastases. The investigators recognized the need to use a PRO, severity of pain, as part of the primary outcome metric. At the time there was no standard measurement of pain in use; the Brief Pain Inventory, for example, was published 20 years later. They created an ad hoc measurement. The importance of psychometric validation of the measurement, as described above, had not yet emerged. They combined the endpoints by multiplying component scores to generate a new endpoint:

Pain Score = (Pain Severity) × (Pain Frequency)

Narcotic Score = (Medication Type) × (Medication Frequency)

Relief = (Current Pain Score/Original Pain Score) × 100%

This highlights a common problem among subjective trials: ordinal measurements (i.e. numbers assigned to non-quantitative statements) are combined

Table 25.1 Radiation Therapy Oncology Group bone metastases trials.

Trial	Summary	Reference
7402	Phase III comparison of total dose and fraction size	[6]
7810	Phase II trial of hemibody irradiation	[8]
8206	Phase III trial of local irradiation with or without hemibody irradiation	[10]
8822	Phase I/II trial of fractionated hemibody irradiation	[21]
9714	Phase III trial comparing 30 Gy in 10 fractions to 8 Gy in a single fraction	[11]
0517	Phase III trial comparing bisphosphonates to bisphosphonates and systemic radionuclide	M. Seider, et al., in press

and the resultant number is then treated statistically as if it is quantitative. There is no way of quantifying that "mild" pain several times a day (pain score = 2) is worse than "severe" pain occurring less than once a day (=0). Perhaps recognizing this, the authors turned the supposedly quantitative Relief Score back into an ordinal scale by dividing it into Complete Relief (0%), Partial Relief (1–50%), Some Relief (51–99%), No Relief (100%), or progressive pain.

In summary, the original qualitative measure (pain severity) was turned into a quantitative measure (relief as a percent) and then returned to a qualitative measure – complete, partial, some, or no relief. The numeric manipulations were an attempt to describe the data in a clinically meaningful context; however, this creates concerns for validity and reliability of the metrics.

RTOG 7810 was a phase II study of hemi-body irradiation for multiple bone metastases [7]. However, in an attempt to quantify the contribution of the treatment to the patient's quality of life, a new descriptor was added, net pain relief:

$$\text{Net Pain Relief} = 100 \times [(\text{Duration of Pain Relief})/(\text{Survival})]$$

This is an early example of what was later formally developed as the statistical technique Quality Adjusted Time Without Symptoms or Toxicity (Q-TWIST) [8]. Q-TWIST is still a commonly used attempt to quantify the balance of toxicity and benefit of an intervention in the life of a patient [9].

Interestingly, the next RTOG trial of bone metastases, comparing local radiation therapy to local radiation therapy and hemi-body irradiation, RTOG 8206, completely abandoned patient reported outcomes for purely objective outcomes of "skeletal events": time to progression of the target sites based on imaging, time to development of new sites based on imaging, and time to new treatment [10]. This approach shift generates quantitative events that are appropriately analyzed using quantitative statistics. However, by using this approach, the hypothesis changed from "radiation therapy improves pain," a symptom, to "radiation therapy decreases the risk of radiographic progression," a sign. There was no attempt to correlate the sign, skeletal events, with patient suffering.

There was an almost 10-year hiatus before the next randomized RTOG trial on bone metastases. During this decade, the fields of quality of life and symptom measurement matured. Several general health-related quality of life instruments had been developed and validated for cancer patients, including the FACT and European Association for Research and Treatment of Cancer (EORTC) QLQ30. Both of these measures have validated subscales for specific disease sites (e.g. for lung cancer, breast cancer) and for specific symptoms (e.g. bone pain, fatigue). The next trial, RTOG 9714, was designed to be a pivotal trial to define the treatment of bone metastases, a large trial comparing 8 Gy in a single fraction to 30 Gy in 10 fractions. There was vigorous debate within the RTOG Symptom Management Committee about the appropriate endpoint. The Brief Pain Inventory (BPI) was the initial primary endpoint. The BPI is a validated and widely used patient-oriented measure for pain but has limitations: in particular it does not account for the type and amount of pain medication being used. It was decided to use a strict but rigorous primary endpoint, complete relief, defined as pain score of 0 for two consecutive analysis periods with no use of narcotics. Further discussion centered on whether there should have to be no pain at all or only no pain at the site treated. Concerns were raised that pain at another site could mask the response at the primary site, and the philosophical question was raised as to whether the patient had benefit from treatment at one site if they still had pain at other sites. The final decision was that the primary endpoint would be no pain at any site and no narcotic use. We were aware that this would tend to make radiation therapy appear less efficacious for treating bone metastases than it clinically might be, but it was felt to be the most reproducible endpoint.

The BPI, FACT-G, and Health Utilities Index, and the measures used in RTOG 7402 (to allow direct comparisons and continuity within the trials) were included as secondary measures. This trial was completed successfully, and the collection of multiple endpoints and extensive clinical data has allowed multiple secondary analyses to be published. Results demonstrated a non-significant difference in complete response rate of 15% and a partial response rate of 50% in the 8-Gy arm compared with 18% and 48% respectively in the 30-Gy arm. Both arms demonstrated good pain relief with 33% of all patients no longer requiring narcotic medications at 3 months follow-up [11]. The incidences of subsequent pathologic fractures were equivalent at 5% for the 8-Gy arm and 4% for the 30-Gy arm. The retreatment rate was statistically significantly higher in the 8-Gy arm (18%) than in the 30-Gy arm (9%); however, retreatment was based on clinician discretion and not protocol driven criteria. The findings have been subsequently used as the foundation for the recent publication: American Society for Radiation Oncology (ASTRO) Palliative radiotherapy for bone metastases: an ASTRO evidence-based guideline [12].

The most recent RTOG trial for bone metastases was RTOG 0517, a randomized trial of zoledronic acid with or without systemic bone-seeking radionuclides (either strontium-89 or samarium-153 lexidronam) for patients with asymptomatic bone metastases. The primary objective was to determine whether the addition of a radionuclide delayed the time to development of malignant skeletal-related events, defined as a pathologic bone fracture, spinal cord compression, surgery to bone, or radiation to bone. This endpoint was the same as that used for RTOG 8206, the hemi-body irradiation trial. Secondary endpoints included the effect of treatment on quality of life (measured with FACT-G) and pain control (measured with the BPI). Because the patients eligible for this trial did not have pain, the need for treatment from bone metastases, rather than the level of pain from bone metastases, was chosen as the most relevant primary endpoint.

Table 25.2 Radiation Therapy Oncology Group brain metastases trials.

Trial	Summary	Reference
1 and 2	Phase III trials comparing total dose and fractionation	[13]
7916	Phase III trial of radiation therapy with or without misonidazole	[14]
8528	Phase I/II trial of accelerated hyperfractionation	[15]
9104	Phase III trial comparing 30 Gy in 10 fractions to 54.4 Gy in 34 fractions of 1.6 Gy BID	[16]
9508	Phase III trial of whole brain vs whole brain with a stereotactic boost for 1 to 3 metastases	[22]
BR0018	Phase II trial of collecting neurocognitive data	[19]
0118	Phase III trial of thalidomide and radiation therapy	[23]
0119	Randomized Phase II trial of am vs pm melatonin and radiation therapy	[24]
0614	Phase III trial of memantine in conjunction with radiation therapy	Completed [25]
0933	Phase II trial of hippocampal sparing during radiation therapy	Completed, publication pending

Brain metastases

The RTOG has studied both palliation of brain metastases and palliation of the effect of brain radiation on the patient. Table 25.2 summarizes the RTOG brain metastases trials.

The very first RTOG trials, RTOG Trials 1 and 2, explored the treatment of brain metastases with whole brain radiation therapy [13]. The studies, similar to the bone metastases studies, looked at the effect of different daily fraction size and total dose on treatment efficacy. The endpoint was a clinician graded, non-validated measure created specifically for the protocols called the Neurological Function Class (NFC), a four-point scale from "able to work, neurologic findings minor or absent" to "requires hospitalization and in serious physical or neurologic state, including coma." The study measured the median duration of improvement and the time to progression of the NFC.

The next trial, RTOG 7916, was a Phase III trial of whole brain radiation therapy with or without the radiosensitizer, misonidazole, and a co-randomization of 30 Gy in 10 fractions vs 30 Gy in 6 fractions [14]. The primary endpoint was survival, and the change in the NFC was a secondary endpoint, as was the Karnofsky Performance Status (KPS). As an attempt to determine whether any improvement in NFC was of significance to the patient, the percentage of total survival time before deteriorating KPS or NFC was also calculated.

Two RTOG studies looked at twice daily (BID) radiation for brain metastases. The first trial, RTOG 8528 was a Phase I/II trial of BID radiation therapy at doses increasing from 48 Gy to 70.4 Gy in 1.6 Gy fractions. The primary endpoint was the improvement in either the patient (as defined by the NFC) or the patient's CT scan [15].

This led to a randomized trial, RTOG 9104, comparing 30 Gy in 10 fractions vs 54.4 Gy in 34 fractions of 1.6 Gy BID. The primary outcome of the trial was survival. This trial is significant because it introduced the first attempt to measure neurocognitive functioning with a standardized metric, the Mini Mental Status Exam (MMSE) [16]. A secondary analysis showed that a decline in the MMSE score correlated strongly with poorer survival [17,18].

RTOG BR0018 was a trial specifically designed to test the feasibility of doing comprehensive neurocognitive testing among patients with brain metastases. The battery included the Mini Mental Status Exam, the Hopkins Verbal Learning Test, the Verbal Fluency/Controlled Word Association Test, and the Ruff 2 and 7. The pre-treatment compliance for testing was >90%, the treatment at the end of radiation therapy was 84%, and the one month follow-up compliance was 70–78%. This study showed that extensive neurocognitive testing is feasible in large cooperative group trials [19].

Because BR0018 showed the feasibility of doing neurocognitive testing in patients with brain metastases, a trial was instituted specifically to try to prevent the neurocognitive deterioration caused by whole brain radiation therapy. RTOG 0614 was a phase III trial evaluating memantine as a neurocognitive protective agent. The primary endpoint was the decline in neurocognitive function from baseline to 24 weeks as measured by the Hopkins Verbal Learning Test (HVLT-Revised). At the completion of this trial, RTOG 0933, a Phase II trial was started of hippocampal sparing to reduce the neurocognitive damage associated with radiotherapy, and the primary endpoint is the HVLT-Revised at 4 months after radiation therapy.

International research efforts

Many of the same goals and efforts of the RTOG are shared by international radiotherapy research collaborative groups such as the Trans Tasman Radiation Oncology Group (TROG), the Canadian Cancer Society Research Interest Group (CCSRI), and the European Organisation for Research and Treatment of Cancer (EORTC). The EORTC has devoted significant energy towards the development of validated instruments to measure quality of life in cancer patients. The previously-mentioned EORTC QLQ-30 instrument is one of the most widely used health-related QOL questionnaires in palliative oncology research trials, measuring patient-reported answers to 30 questions about their physical, psychologic, and social functioning status [20]. Because of concerns about burdening patients with lengthy questionnaires at the end of life, the EORTC has also developed the shorter QLQ-15 instrument to serve as a "core questionnaire" for palliative oncology [21]. The EORTC QLQ-BM22 module has been created to help measure the health-related quality of life for patients with symptomatic bone metastases [22]. All future clinical trials involving these patient groups should use the EORTC or FACT questionnaires, or similarly validated instruments.

Conclusion

In summary, this chapter describes some of the design issues related to choosing appropriate and validated metrics for palliative trials. Substantial areas for future research in palliative care remain, especially in the need for a common set of palliative metrics and time points for measurement that can be used in future clinical trials. For example, there is some research to suggest that consistent assessments may be valuable tools for selecting patients for palliative radiotherapy trials [24].

Such consistency would better inform outcomes of these trials for cross-study comparisons and meta-analyses. This in turn would inform the ability to synthesize research for use in guidelines and inform symptom/toxicity intervention research. For example, a NCI-sponsored clinical trials planning meeting on the "Identification of Core Symptoms and Health-Related Quality of Life Domains for use in Cancer Research," was held in September 2011 to address similar issues across disease sites during acute treatment. An extensive process of literature and source data review identified a lengthy list of symptoms ranked by prevalence. A panel of experts narrowed the list to a core set of symptoms that may serve as a guide to common reporting across all acute phase cancer clinical trials. If adopted, this core set of PROs could facilitate comparison and combination of data across cancer clinical trials around the world. The publications from this meeting are in development. Palliative care research would benefit from a similar process.

References

1. Therasse P, Arbuck SG, Eisenhauer EA, *et al.* New guidelines to evaluate the response to treatment in solid tumors. european organization for research and treatment of cancer, national cancer institute of the united states, national cancer institute of Canada. *J Natl Cancer Inst* 2000; **92**: 205–216.
2. World Health Organization. WHO definition of palliative care. http://www.who.int/cancer/palliative/definition/en/. Updated 2012. (accessed November 19, 2012).
3. Bruner DW. Should patient-reported outcomes be mandatory for toxicity reporting in cancer clinical trials? *J Clin Oncol* 2007; **25**: 5345–5347.
4. U.S. Food and Drug Administration. Guidance for industry: Patient-reported outcome measures: Use in medical product development to support labeling claims. Available at: http://www.fda.gov/downloads/Drugs/GuidanceComplianceRegulatory

Information/Guidances/UCM193282.pdf. Updated 2009. (accessed November 16, 2012).

5. Yellen SB, Cella DF, Webster K, *et al.* Measuring fatigue and other anemia-related symptoms with the functional assessment of cancer therapy (FACT) measurement system. *J Pain Symptom Manage* 1997; **13**: 63–74.

6. Tong D, Gillick L, Hendrickson FR. The palliation of symptomatic osseous metastases: final results of the study by the radiation therapy oncology group. *Cancer* 1982; **50**: 893–899.

7. Salazar OM, Rubin P, Hendrickson FR, *et al.* Single-dose half-body irradiation for palliation of multiple bone metastases from solid tumors. Final radiation therapy oncology group report. *Cancer* 1986; **58**: 29–36.

8. Gelber RD, Goldhirsch A, Cole BF. Evaluation of effectiveness: Q-TWiST. the international breast cancer study group. *Cancer Treat Rev* 1993; **19**(Suppl A): 73–84.

9. Corey-Lisle PK, Peck R, Mukhopadhyay P, *et al.* Q-TWiST analysis of ixabepilone in combination with capecitabine on quality of life in patients with metastatic breast cancer. *Cancer* 2012; **118**: 461–468.

10. Poulter CA, Cosmatos D, Rubin P, *et al.* A report of RTOG 8206: a phase III study of whether the addition of single dose hemibody irradiation to standard fractionated local field irradiation is more effective than local field irradiation alone in the treatment of symptomatic osseous metastases. *Int J Radiat Oncol Biol Phys* 1992; **23**: 207–214.

11. Hartsell WF, Scott CB, Bruner DW, *et al.* Randomized trial of short- versus long-course radiotherapy for palliation of painful bone metastases. *J Natl Cancer Inst* 2005; **97**: 798–804.

12. Lutz S, Berk L, Chang E, *et al.* Palliative radiotherapy for bone metastases: an ASTRO evidence-based guideline. *Int J Radiat Oncol Biol Phys* 2011; **79**: 965–976.

13. Borgelt B, Gelber R, Larson M, *et al.* Ultra-rapid high dose irradiation schedules for the palliation of brain metastases: final results of the first two studies by the radiation therapy oncology group. *Int J Radiat Oncol Biol Phys* 1981; **7**: 1633–1638.

14. Komarnicky LT, Phillips TL, Martz K, *et al.* A randomized phase III protocol for the evaluation of misonidazole combined with radiation in the treatment of patients with brain metastases (RTOG-7916). *Int J Radiat Oncol Biol Phys* 1991; **20**: 53–58.

15. Epstein BE, Scott CB, Sause WT, *et al.* Improved survival duration in patients with unresected solitary brain metastasis using accelerated hyperfractionated radiation therapy at total doses of 54.4 gray and greater. results of radiation therapy oncology group 85-28. *Cancer* 1993; **71**: 1362–1367.

16. Murray KJ, Scott C, Greenberg HM, *et al.* A randomized phase III study of accelerated hyperfractionation versus standard in patients with unresected brain metastases: a report of the radiation therapy oncology group (RTOG) 9104. *Int J Radiat Oncol Biol Phys* 1997; **39**: 571–574.

17. Murray KJ, Scott C, Zachariah B, *et al.* Importance of the mini-mental status examination in the treatment of patients with brain metastases: a report from the radiation therapy oncology group protocol 91-04. *Int J Radiat Oncol Biol Phys* 2000; **48**: 59–64.

18. Regine WF, Scott C, Murray K, *et al.* Neurocognitive outcome in brain metastases patients treated with accelerated-fractionation vs. accelerated-hyperfractionated radiotherapy: an analysis from radiation therapy oncology group study 91-04. *Int J Radiat Oncol Biol Phys* 2001; **51**: 711–717.

19. Regine WF, Schmitt FA, Scott CB, *et al.* Feasibility of neurocognitive outcome evaluations in patients with brain metastases in a multi-institutional cooperative group setting:

results of radiation therapy oncology group trial BR-0018. *Int J Radiat Oncol Biol Phys* 2004; **58**: 1346–1352.

20. Kyriaki M, Eleni T, Efi P, *et al.* The EORTC core quality of life questionnaire (QLQ-C30, version 3.0) in terminally ill cancer patients under palliative care: validity and reliability in a Hellenic sample. *Int J Cancer* 2001; **94**: 135–139.

21. Groenvold M, Petersen MA, Aaron NK, *et al.* The development of the EORTC QLQ-C15-PAL: a shortened questionnaire for cancer patients in cancer care. *Eur J Cancer* 2006; **42**: 55–64.

22. Chow E, Nguyen J, Zhang L, *et al.* International field testing of the reliability and validity of the EORTC QLQ-BM22 module to assess health-related quality of life in patients with bone metastases. *Cancer* 2012; **118**: 1457–1465.

23. Knisely JP, Berkey B, Chakravarti A, *et al.* A phase III study of conventional radiation therapy plus thalidomide versus conventional radiation therapy for multiple brain metastases (RTOG 0118). *Int J Radiat Oncol Biol Phys* 2008; **71**: 79–86.

24. Berk L, Berkey B, Rich T, *et al.* Randomized phase II trial of high-dose melatonin and radiation therapy for RPA class 2 patients with brain metastases (RTOG 0119). *Int J Radiat Oncol Biol Phys* 2007; **68**: 852–857.

25. Laack N, *et al.* Memantine for the Prevention of Cognitive Dysfunction in Patients Receiving Whole-brain Radiation Therapy (WBRT): First Report of RTOG 0614, a Placebo-controlled, Double-blind, Randomized Trial. ASTRO's 54th Annual Meeting, Boston, MA 2012.

CHAPTER 26

Radiation oncology cost-effectiveness

Andre Konski
Department of Radiation Oncology, Wayne State School of Medicine, Barbara Ann
Karmanos Cancer Center, Detroit, MI, USA

Introduction

The previous chapters in this text have highlighted radiation's efficacy in the
treatment and palliation of symptoms from locally advanced and metastatic
cancer. The technical aspects of radiotherapy have advanced from relatively
"crude" linear accelerators, by today's standards, with limited imaging capabilities to highly sophisticated machines capable of generating high dose rates
of radiation guided by on-board imaging including megavoltage and cone
beam computed tomography. This highly sophisticated delivery equipment
has increased the cost of care leading to a number of articles in the lay press
evaluating radiotherapy's place in cancer therapy.

The underuse of radiotherapy in the palliative management of patients has
been documented. In one of the first studies published investigating the use
of a modality as compared to an accepted standard, a 12-week survey of
radiotherapy practices in Sweden reported on the frequency of use of radiotherapy in the management of patients with bone and brain metastases,
among other sites. The researchers found an underutilization of radiotherapy
in the treatment of bone metastasis with only 1 of 10 eligible patients receiving
radiotherapy while only 1 in 100 received radiotherapy for brain metastasis
[1]. An etiology for the underuse was not given.

Two contemporary studies performed in the United States confirmed the
Swedish findings. An underutilization of radiotherapy services was found in
480 respondents out of over 1800 National Hospice and Palliative Care Organizations (NHPCO) surveyed. Less than 3% on average of hospice patients
received radiotherapy in 2002 [2]. Barriers to receipt of radiotherapy included
cost of radiotherapy, transportation difficulties, short life expectancy, and
educational deficiencies between the specialities. Radiotherapy cost was cited
by 64.1% of respondents as the reason for lack of referral. Transportation
issues were cited by 59.6% of respondents which is of interest given that 76.1%

Radiation Oncology in Palliative Cancer Care, First Edition. Edited by Stephen Lutz,
Edward Chow, and Peter Hoskin.

of respondents felt that radiotherapists were reluctant to prescribe a single radiotherapy fraction. McCloskey *et al.* found similar results in a latter survey of physician members of the American Society for Radiation Oncology (ASTRO), the American Academy of Hospice and Palliative Medicine (AAHPM), and a random sample American Society of Clinical Oncology (ASCO). With a 27%, 26%, and 14% response rate respectively, most agreed radiation oncologists should be more involved in palliative care but found referrals for such therapy were declining. Once again, barriers included the cost of radiotherapy or poor reimbursement, emotional burden of care, insufficient training/knowledge, and the sense of unwillingness of others to share delivery of such services [3].

Barriers to the appropriate utilization of radiotherapy in the palliation of symptoms will increase as cost of radiotherapy services increases with the adoption of newer technology. The majority of studies published to date evaluating the economic aspect of palliative care have been performed in an era without the widespread adoption of focused radiotherapy techniques such as stereotactic radiosurgery (SRS) and stereotactic body radiation therapy (SBRT). Fixed hospice per diem rates may not be able to cover the cost of these new and potentially expense technologies, further limiting radiotherapy utilization.

Cost-effectiveness

Radiotherapy has been shown in a number of studies to provide cost-effective care in the palliation of cancer symptoms, most notably bone metastasis. Macklis and colleagues compared radiotherapy to narcotic analgesics in a group of outpatient oncology patients with a Karnofsky performance status (KPS) score of 70 and above. Radiotherapy costs were estimated from Medicare-allowable charges with narcotic costs estimated from published values. The authors found a statistically significant decrease in pain scores after radiotherapy. The estimated cost per patient ranged from $1,200–$2,500 for radiotherapy as compared to $9,000–$36,000 for narcotic use [4]. Similar results were found in an analysis of palliative treatment for patients with bone metastasis from prostate cancer using a Markov model [5]. A Markov model is a modeling technique derived from matrix algebra that constructs a finite set of mutually exclusive possible health states. Transitions are allowed between these health states and the health states are efficiently represented recursive events that occur over time. The time that these events can occur over, however, is uncertain. The available options for treatment in this study of men with hormone refractory prostate cancer were pain medication, single fraction of external beam radiation therapy (EBRT), multi-fraction radiotherapy, and chemotherapy. Radiotherapy costs, like the last study, were modeled from Medicare data, with drug and other costs obtained from the literature. Both single and multi-fraction courses of EBRT were found to be cost-effective if the ceiling of cost-effectiveness is assumed to be $50,000/Quality-adjusted life year (QALY). Single fraction radiotherapy had a cost-effective ratio of $6,857/QALY as compared to the use of pain medication, while multi-fraction radiotherapy had a cost-effective ratio of $36,000/QALY [5]. Chemotherapy was both more costly and provided lower quality-adjusted life months as compared to the use of narcotic medication.

Economic analyses have been performed on two of the largest bone metastases trials. Konski *et al.* performed an economic analysis of Radiation Therapy Oncology Group (RTOG) 97-14 using both modeled costs from Medicare data and resource utilization data from a select group of centers participating in the trial [6]. RTOG 97-14 compared the effectiveness of a single 8 Gy fraction to 30 Gy in 10 fractions in palliating pain from prostate and breast cancer bone metastasis. The modeled cost and actual trial results were used to inform a Markov model similar to the one used to model radiotherapy costs to treat bone metastases previously mentioned. The use of 8 Gy in a single fraction resulted in an expected mean cost of $998 for 7.26 quality-adjusted life months of survival as compared to an expected mean cost of $2,316 for 9.53 quality-adjusted life months of survival [6]. This results in an incremental cost-effectiveness ratio (ICER) of $6,973, far below the commonly accepted threshold of $50,000/QALY. In a separate analysis, the authors found the cost to avoid retreatment by using 30 Gy in 10 fractions instead of 8 Gy in 1 fraction to be only $131. The difference in cost is so small between the two regimens it can be argued that 8 Gy in 1 fraction should be the standard of care even though the ICER is well below the commonly accepted standard of $50,000/QALY.

The studies reported so far used a payer's perspective for the economic analysis, meaning they only considered costs paid by an insurance company or government health-care provider such as Medicare. Van den Hout *et al.* published an economic analysis of the Dutch Bone Metastases trial from a societal perspective [7]. The Dutch Bone Metastases trial compared 8 Gy in a single fraction to 4 Gy in 6 fractions for a wide variety of tumor types. From a societal perspective, all costs borne by society are included in the analysis. Costs such as transportation costs, which are important for patients with a short life expectancy and in pain, and costs to build and equip the centers are included in the analysis. In addition, non-medical costs such as out-of-pocket expenses, cost of domestic help during the treatment, and paid and unpaid labor costs, all of which are not included in an analysis from a payer's perspective, were included in the analysis. For a willingness-to-pay between $5,000 and $40,000/QALY, the single fraction schedule was statistically significantly more cost-effective when compared to the multiple-fraction radiotherapy schedule [7].

A health economic study was performed on a randomized trial evaluating the use of stents or three endoluminal brachytherapy insertions in the treatment of dysphagia from esophageal cancer [8]. Thirty patients were randomly assigned to either a self-expanding metal stent or 3×7 Gy brachytherapy insertions. Hospital debits were used to calculate costs in this Swedish study.

An overall survival or complication rate did not occur between the two groups but the group receiving the stents had a significant difference in change of dysphagia scores between the time of inclusion and the one-month follow-up visit. The group receiving brachytherapy had a statistically significant higher lifetime medical costs as compared to the groups receiving the stents, mostly as a result of the higher cost of the initial treatment. In a sensitivity analysis, a reduction in the brachytherapy charges was necessary for brachytherapy to be cost-competitive [8]. The opposite was found, however, in a study from nine hospitals in the Netherlands [9]. 209 patients with dysphagia from either esophageal or gastroesophageal cancer were randomly assigned to either stent placement, n=108, or a single dose of 12 Gy endoluminal brachytherapy, n=101. Dysphagia was found to rapidly improve with stent placement but long-term dysphagia relief was better with the brachytherapy. The quality of life was better in the group receiving brachytherapy compared to stenting. A formal economic analysis was performed and published separately [10]. Although initial costs were higher in the group receiving the stents, total medical costs were similar between the two, most likely as a result of higher total hospital stays in the group receiving the brachytherapy. It is difficult to determine how this would translate to an American population since these procedures are usually performed as an outpatient and do not usually incur hospital stays in the uncomplicated case.

Newer technologies

In an analysis of some of the newer radiotherapy technologies, Haley *et al.* performed a matched-pair analysis investigating the efficacy and cost-effectiveness of EBRT and SBRT in the treatment of spine metastases [11]. The authors compared 30 Gy in 10 fractions with a 3-dimensional (3D) radiotherapy plan, to 20 Gy in 5 fractions with a 3D plan, to 30 Gy in 10 fractions with a 2D plan, and 20 Gy in 5 fractions with a 2D plan. The authors used 2010 Medicare hospital fee schedule reimbursement for both the technical and professional fees. The authors ascribed a cost of $7,729 for the SBRT cost which was delivered in a single fraction [11]. Unfortunately the authors did not include retreatment costs in the analysis. 30 Gy in 10 fractions was 80% of the SBRT cost, while 20 Gy in 5 fractions was 59% of the SBRT costs. Only 9% of the patients receiving SBRT required retreatment, while 23% of patients receiving EBRT required retreatment. Had the retreatment costs been included in the analysis the difference between SBRT and non-SBRT would have been less. In addition, the SBRT was given in a single fraction, so the differences between the two groups would have been different had the analysis been performed from a societal perspective where transportation costs would have been higher in the multi-fraction treatment regimens. The use of single dose SBRT will be important to alleviate one of the barriers to the use of radiotherapy in the palliation of pain since it will require only a few visits as compared to up to 10 or more visits.

Using a Markov analysis, Papatheofanis *et al.* performed a cost-utility analysis of another modern radiotherapy technology, the CyberKnife, in the treatment of metastatic spinal tumors [12]. The authors also used published results in the literature and Medicare reimbursement data to inform the model. The authors reported a net health benefit of 0.08 QALY with a net cost increase of $1,933 resulting in a ICER of $41,500/QALY meeting the usually accepted ceiling for adopting a new treatment [12]. The results may have been different if a societal perspective was taken given the high acquisition cost of a Cyber-Knife linear accelerator.

Adoption of new technology can be difficult to impossible in low to middle income countries. These countries have tremendous competing needs for limited resources making adoption of the new technology and treatment techniques close to impossible. In one of the few economic analyses performed from a societal viewpoint, Vuong *et al.* compared SRS to surgical resection in the treatment of brain metastasis in Vietnam [13]. 111 patients, 64 treated with surgery and 47 with SRS, were retrospectively reviewed. A statistically significant difference in survival was not apparent between the two groups at 18 months. The mean number of hospital days was statistically significantly longer in patients undergoing resection compared to patients receiving SRS, but the direct costs of resection were significantly lower in patients undergoing resection compared to SRS. On the other hand, indirect medical costs were higher in patients undergoing resection compared to SRS, with a resultant higher cost of life-year gained for patients undergoing resection compared to SRS. The authors concluded from a patient's perspective that SRS was more cost-effective but lower direct medical costs charged by the hospital may prevent poorer and older patients in this low to middle income country from choosing SRS [13].

Conclusion

Radiotherapy is an integral part of palliative care for patients with cancer. Perceived barriers to the incorporation of radiotherapy, including cost and access, can be overcome by the use of hypofractionated treatment regimens. The adoption of newer technology such as SRS and SBRT has been shown to be cost-effective in a few of the early studies published to date. More studies are needed to confirm these findings.

References

1. A prospective survey of radiotherapy in Sweden. *Acta Oncol* 1996; **35**(Suppl 6): 47–56.
2. Lutz S, Spence C, Chow E, *et al.* Survey on use of palliative radiotherapy in hospice care. *J Clin Oncol* 2004; **22**: 3581–3586.
3. McCloskey SA, Tao ML, Rose CM, *et al.* National survey of perspectives of palliative radiation therapy: role, barriers, and needs. *Cancer J* 2007; **13**: 130–137.

4. Macklis RM, Cornelli H, Lasher J. Brief courses of palliative radiotherapy for metastatic bone pain: a pilot cost-minimization comparison with narcotic analgesics. *Am J Clin Oncol* 1998; **21**: 617–622.
5. Konski A. Radiotherapy is a cost-effective palliative treatment for patients with bone metastasis from prostate cancer. *Int J Radiat Oncol Biol Phys* 2004; **60**: 1373–1378.
6. Konski A, James J, Hartsell W, *et al.* Economic analysis of radiation therapy oncology group 97-14: multiple versus single fraction radiation treatment of patients with bone metastases. *Am J Clin Oncol* 2009; **32**: 423–428.
7. van den Hout WB, Tijhuis GJ, Hazes JM, *et al.* Cost effectiveness and cost utility analysis of multidisciplinary care in patients with rheumatoid arthritis: a randomised comparison of clinical nurse specialist care, inpatient team care, and day patient team care. *Ann Rheum Dis* 2003; **62**: 308–315.
8. Wenger U, Johnsson E, Bergquist H, *et al.* Health economic evaluation of stent or endo-luminal brachytherapy as a palliative strategy in patients with incurable cancer of the oesophagus or gastro-oesophageal junction: results of a randomized clinical trial. *Eur J Gastroenterol Hepatol* 2005; **17**: 1369–1377.
9. Homs MY, Steyerberg EW, Eijkenboom WM, *et al.* Single-dose brachytherapy versus metal stent placement for the palliation of dysphagia from oesophageal cancer: multi-centre randomised trial. *Lancet* 2004; **364**: 1497–1504.
10. Polinder S, Homs MY, Siersema PD, *et al.* Cost study of metal stent placement vs single-dose brachytherapy in the palliative treatment of oesophageal cancer. *Br J Cancer* 2004; **90**: 2067–2072.
11. Haley ML, Gerszten PC, Heron DE, *et al.* Efficacy and cost-effectiveness analysis of external beam and stereotactic body radiation therapy in the treatment of spine metas-tases: a matched-pair analysis. *J Neurosurg Spine* 2011; **14**: 537–542.
12. Papatheofanis FJ, Williams E, Chang SD. Cost-utility analysis of the cyberknife system for metastatic spinal tumors. *Neurosurgery* 2009; **64**(2 Suppl): A73–A83.
13. Vuong DA, Rades D, Le AN, *et al.* The cost-effectiveness of stereotactic radiosurgery versus surgical resection in the treatment of brain metastasis in Vietnam from the per-spective of patients and families. *World Neurosurg* 2012; **77**: 321–328.

CHAPTER 27

Quality measures and palliative radiotherapy

James A. Hayman[1], Rinaa S. Punglia[2], and Anushree M. Vichare[3]

[1]Department of Radiation Oncology, University of Michigan, Ann Arbor, MI, USA
[2]Department of Radiation Oncology, Dana-Farber Cancer Institute and the Brigham and Women's Hospital, Harvard Medical School, Boston, MA, USA
[3]American Society for Radiation Oncology, Fairfax, VA, USA

Introduction

Due to the rising cost of health care, there is increasing interest in value, which is defined as quality divided by cost. Accordingly, one can increase value by increasing the quality of medical care and/or decreasing its cost. In the context of health care, the Institute of Medicine has defined quality as "the degree to which health care services for individuals and populations increase the likelihood of desired outcomes and are consistent with current professional knowledge" [1], later adding that it should be safe, effective, patient-centered, timely, efficient, and equitable [2]. The Agency for Healthcare Research and Quality (AHRQ) defines quality as "doing the right thing, at the right time, in the right way, for the right person – and having the best possible result" [3].

As health-care providers interested in palliative care, specifically the use of palliative radiotherapy, these definitions appear eminently reasonable and easily achievable. However, there are examples in the radiation oncology literature where there is evidence of variation in how patients are treated with palliative radiation that far exceeds what would be expected based on the medical evidence, clinical grounds, and/or patient preference [4]. This variability suggests that the National Cancer Policy Board statement that "for many patients with cancer there is a wide gulf between what could be construed as the ideal and the reality of their experience with cancer care" unfortunately applies to palliative radiation too [5].

In order to improve something first you have to be able to measure it, hence the current interest in quality measures. Quality measures provide a

Radiation Oncology in Palliative Cancer Care, First Edition. Edited by Stephen Lutz, Edward Chow, and Peter Hoskin.
© 2013 John Wiley & Sons, Ltd. Published 2013 by John Wiley & Sons, Ltd.

mechanism for assessing health care against standards based on established clinical evidence. The goal of this chapter is to introduce the principle concepts of quality measurement in the context of palliative radiation. We will begin by introducing the characteristics of quality measures and discussing how measures are created. We will then review how they are presently being used to improve quality of care and conclude with how they might be used even more effectively in future quality improvement initiatives.

Quality measures: characteristics

Quality measures have historically been categorized as structural, process, or outcomes measures [6]. Other types of measures include access, care-coordination, resource-use, patient experience, and composite measures. Structural measures assess the characteristics of the setting or system in which health care is provided. They can include facility characteristics such as staffing levels, use of an electronic medical record, or the number of treatment courses delivered yearly or provider characteristics such as years in practice or board certification. Structural measures are appealing because they are relatively easy to assess and can impact multiple outcomes such as quality of life and patient satisfaction due to their cross-cutting nature. However, because their presence does not ensure that high quality care will be delivered, their link with improved patient outcomes is often implied.

Process measures are currently the most common type of quality measure in use. They measure whether steps known to benefit patients are followed correctly and completely. While they often focus on technical aspects of medical care, they can also deal with how providers and patients interact (e.g. shared decision-making). Given the technical nature of radiation oncology, the question of not just if something was done but whether it was done correctly is also highly relevant. Current examples of process measures relevant to palliative radiation include a pair of measures focused on reporting a quantified pain score for those patients receiving external beam radiation and the creation of a care plan for those patients in pain [7,8], and another measure focusing on fractionation schedules for external beam radiation treatment of painful bone metastases [9]. Because they are often derived from clinical trials' data or expert consensus and focus on what we have done rather than who we are or where we work, process measures have greater physician acceptance than structural measures. However, it is much more difficult to collect the data needed for process measures than structural measures, and their linkage with outcomes is also often implied rather than proven.

Process measures can be further subcategorized into overuse, underuse, and misuse measures [10]. Overuse occurs when there is too much care and the drawbacks outweigh the benefits, such as the use of prolonged fractionation in patients with limited life expectancies. For example, one study of patients referred for palliative radiation found that over one-quarter were undergoing treatment for 81–100% of their remaining lifespan [11]. Underuse occurs when an effective treatment is not provided that would have been beneficial, such as the lack of use of radiation in hospice. Lastly, misuse occurs when appropriate care is delivered but the patient does not experience its full benefit due to an error in how it is delivered.

Outcomes measures are the most relevant type of measure because they directly assess the impact of care on patients' health. For palliative radiation, potential outcomes include symptom relief, quality of life, and patient and/ or caregiver satisfaction. Outcomes measures can be difficult to interpret when there is a long delay between a particular intervention and the outcome (e.g. radiation for low-risk prostate cancer and overall survival). While this could be less of an issue for palliative radiation due to patients' limited life expectancy, there are still potential confounding factors such as concurrent therapies including narcotics and steroids and/or differences in baseline patient characteristics which can be difficult to adjust for. In addition, even though palliative radiation is utilized relatively commonly, there still may not be enough cases or adverse events to ensure that differences from a benchmark represent true differences and are not just a result of random variation. For all these reasons, outcomes measures have typically not been used in radiation oncology.

Quality measures can also be categorized based on the aspect of care that they are trying to improve. Using the framework mentioned above by the Institute of Medicine in their report "Crossing the Quality Chasm" [2], the six aims of quality improvement include safety, effectiveness, patient-centeredness, timeliness, efficiency, and equity. Care that is safe avoids injury. Effective care is based on scientific knowledge of who is most and least likely to benefit thereby avoiding underuse and overuse, respectively. Patient-centered care is responsive to individual patient preferences, needs, and values and ensures that the patient's values drive clinical decision-making. Timely care reduces waits and minimizes potentially harmful delays. Efficient care does not waste resources and, lastly, equitable care does not vary based on personal characteristics such as gender, ethnicity, geography, or socioeconomic status. The aim of most oncology quality measures to date has been effectiveness, followed by safety.

There are also several other factors that can be used to categorize quality measures. Measures can be subdivided based on their intended use: research, quality improvement, and/or accountability. Measures can either be general measures applicable to all cancer patients or they can be site-specific and, for example, only apply to breast cancer. Measures can focus on a specific point along the cancer continuum such as measures related to prevention, screening, diagnosis, staging, primary treatment, adjuvant treatment, and survivorship or, most relevant to this book, palliative care and end-of-life care. Measures can address care provided in certain settings such as during hospitalization, in hospice, or in a hospital-based or freestanding radiation treatment facility. Measures can vary based on level of provider (e.g. individual, practice, institution, health system, health plan, geographic region) and type

Table 27.1 Example of measure characteristics: external beam radiotherapy for bone metastases measure.

Characteristic	Example
Type	Process/Overuse
Aim	Effectiveness
Intended use	Quality improvement
Disease type	All cancers
Care continuum	Palliative/end-of-life care
Care setting	Hospital, freestanding facility
Care level	Individual physician, physician practice, facility, health plan
Data sources	Electronic health records, paper records
Purpose	Public reporting, payment program, quality improvement

of provider (e.g. physician, medical physicist, radiation therapist). Lastly they can also be classified based on the type of data used to report the measure, such as billing claims, electronic medical record, paper record, or patient survey. As an example, the defining characteristics of ASTRO's external beam radiotherapy for bone metastases quality measure are listed in Table 27.1.

Developing quality measures

Use of a quality measure can be defined as the quantification of the degree of adherence to an evidence- or consensus-based indicator of quality care [12]. Accordingly, quality measure development ideally starts with an evidence- or formal consensus-based guideline recommendation but in reality often arises from informal expert consensus. For example, ASTRO's recently developed bone metastasis quality measure, External Beam Radiotherapy for Bone Metastases [9], arose from a recommendation from ASTRO's evidence-based guideline on the same subject (see Table 27.2) [13]. Based on the recommendation, one next develops a quality indicator. In the case of the ASTRO bone metastasis measure, the indicator is that the fractionation for external beam treatment of a previously untreated painful bony metastasis should consist of 30 Gy in 10, 24 Gy in 6, 20 Gy in 5, or 8 Gy in 1 fraction(s), whereas the quality measure is the percentage of patients receiving external beam treatment of a previously untreated painful bony metastasis who receive one of these fractionation schedules.

Specification of the quality measure from the indicator requires defining the specific aspect of care being measured as well as relevant data elements such as patient population, provider type, care setting, and measurement or reporting time period. Since most process and outcomes measures are typically reported as percentages, this requires defining the numerator, the aspect of care under investigation, and the denominator, the eligible patients, including reasons for excluding patients from the denominator (e.g. medical, patient, health system). Also included are the potential sources of data to be used in the measure and, if appropriate, any risk-adjustment methods. As an example, the measure specifications for the ASTRO bone metastases measure are listed in Table 27.2.

Table 27.2 Example of measure specifications: external beam radiotherapy for bone metastases measure

Guideline	Palliative radiotherapy for bone metastases: an ASTRO evidence-based guideline
Guideline recommendation	Multiple prospective randomized trials have shown pain relief equivalency for dosing schema, including 30 Gy in 10 fractions, 24 Gy in 6 fractions, 20 Gy in 5 fractions, and a single 8-Gy fraction for patients with previously unirradiated painful bone metastases. Fractionated RT courses have been associated with an 8% repeat treatment rate to the same anatomic site because of recurrent pain vs 20% after a single fraction; however, the single fraction treatment approach optimizes patient and caregiver convenience.
Quality indicator	Fractionation for external beam treatment of a previously untreated painful bony metastasis should consist of 30 Gy in 10, 24 Gy in 6, 20 Gy in 5, or 8 Gy in 1 fraction(s)
Quality measure	Percentage of patients, regardless of age, with a diagnosis of painful bone metastases and no history of previous radiation who receive external beam radiation therapy (EBRT) with an acceptable fractionation scheme as defined by the guideline.
Numerator	All patients, regardless of age, with painful bone metastases, and no previous radiation to the same anatomic site who receive EBRT with any of the following recommended fractionation schemes: 30 Gy/10fxns, 24 Gy/6fxns, 20 Gy/5fxns, 8 Gy/1fxn.
Denominator	All patients with painful bone metastases and no previous radiation to the same anatomic site who receive EBRT
Denominator exclusions	Medical reasons: • Previous radiation treatment to the same anatomic site • Patients with femoral axis cortical involvement greater than 3 cm in length • Patients who have undergone a surgical stabilization procedure • Patients with spinal cord compression, cauda equina compression, or radicular pain
Risk adjustment	Not required for this measure

Fxn, fraction.

Desirable attributes of quality measures

Once a measure has been specified, the next step is pilot testing with the ultimate goal of seeking endorsement. To achieve endorsement, it is required that measures have certain key attributes. The most critical attributes are importance and scientific acceptability. To be "important" a quality measure must focus on an aspect of care that affects large numbers of patients with significant disease burden, where there is evidence of opportunity for improvement due to identified unexplainable variation or gaps in care, and where the body of evidence that supports the measure is of sufficient size, quality, and consistency. Scientific acceptability of a measure is assessed on the basis of its validity and reliability. A valid quality measure measures what it intends to measure. This is typically assessed by face validity based on expert opinion or convergent validity based on similar results from another measure focused on the same issue. Reliability is the degree to which the results of a measure are consistent across users and settings, which is typically related to how clearly the measure was specified. Other important measure attributes include usability, the extent to which the end-users of the measure (e.g. patients, payers, policy makers) understand the results of the measure and find them useful for decision-making, and feasibility, the extent to which the data required for a measure can be obtained without excessive burden. Ideally the data necessary for the measure can be collected as part of routine workflow.

Uses of quality measures

Quality measures have three main uses: research, quality improvement, and accountability. Quality measures often are first developed as part of observational research focused on identifying unexplainable variations in care. When a gap in care is identified that is worthy of being closed, the measure can be used for quality improvement. Typically, the measure is first used to assess baseline performance, then a quality improvement intervention is undertaken, next performance is reassessed by re-measurement and then the plan-do-check-act cycle continues. This can be as part of an internal quality improvement program with comparisons made within the same organization and/or as part of a broader quality improvement program with benchmarking of results relative to other providers or organizations. Often operated by professional societies, these programs coordinate regularly repeated cycles of performance measurement followed by reporting of comparative data, hopefully stimulating providers or practices to address their quality shortcomings. Ideally such programs also include tools for quality improvement. Participation in such programs is usually voluntary and data are typically not reportedly publicly. When used for accountability, measures can be used for public reporting (e.g. report cards), as part of practice accreditation, for payment programs (e.g. pay for reporting or performance), or for the selection of preferred facilities or providers such as centers of excellence programs. As measures progress from being used for research to quality improvement and then accountability, the potential impact of their use increases and, therefore, the need for evidence of measures' importance, scientific acceptability, usability, and feasibility increases as well.

Current uses of quality measures in radiation oncology

In the United States there is a long history of using quality measures to improve quality of care in radiation oncology through the Patterns of Care Studies (PCS). Starting in 1973, facilities were surveyed regarding cancer-specific processes of care which were retrospectively assessed by comparison to standards developed by expert consensus [14,15]. In later years, data on outcomes such as overall survival, disease-free survival, and complication rates were also collected. Only once – in 1984–1985 – did PCS focus on the use of palliative radiation [16]. More recently, PCS renamed itself Quality Research in Radiation Oncology (QRRO) and it has focused on cancers in which radiation oncology plays a major role and on emerging technologies in radiation oncology [17]. Part of this initiative was the development of quality measures for all cancers as well as those specific to breast, cervix, gastric, lung, and prostate cancer, but none focus specifically on palliative radiotherapy [18].

In addition to PCS/QRRO, quality measures for radiation oncology have also been developed for, and used in, national payment and physician practice improvement programs. In 2006, Congress created the Physician Quality Reporting Initiative (PQRI) through which physicians were incentivized by a small increase in their professional reimbursement from Medicare to voluntarily report performance on a limited number of quality measures for a certain percentage or number of their Medicare beneficiaries (e.g. pay-for-reporting). Now known as the Physician Quality Reporting System (PQRS), over time the program's incentive has declined and will eventually transition to a penalty in 2015. Currently, the names of PQRS participants who successfully report are made public; however, information on performance along with national averages is reported only to participants. Since its inception, the ease with which physicians can successfully report has improved slightly and the number of measures available for reporting has slowly increased.

Unfortunately, for oncology in general, radiation oncology in particular, and palliative radiotherapy specifically, the number of relevant quality measures is quite limited. Of the measures that are specific to oncology that radiation oncologists can report on, most were developed by ASTRO in partnership with other medical specialty organizations and the American Medical Association's Physician Consortium for Performance Improvement (AMA-PCPI). Due to the lack of clinical practice guidelines related to radiation oncology, many of the measures for radiation oncology have been process measures developed through informal expert consensus. Most measures included in

PQRS have been endorsed by the National Quality Forum (NQF). Measures submitted for NQF endorsement are carefully reviewed and assessed for the attributes described above with input from a variety of experts and stakeholders. The process is intended to identify "best in class" measures that warrant endorsement. It is beyond the scope of this article to describe all oncology quality measures.

However, it should be noted, that while some measures can be reported on for all cancers, others are specific to certain cancers such as breast, prostate, colorectal, lung, and pancreas. Just because a measure addresses a radiotherapy issue does not mean it is appropriate for radiation oncologists to report on it (e.g. the percentage of patients undergoing breast-conserving surgery for breast cancer who receive radiation), and only three oncology measures are directly related to palliative radiotherapy. Although not specific to radiation oncology, there are also end-of-life cancer-related quality measures addressing the issues of chemotherapy use, ER visits, hospitalization, ICU admission, and hospice use in the last days of life [19], developed by the American Society of Clinical Oncology (ASCO), along with a series of symptom management and end-of-life measures for patients with advanced cancer, that were developed by the RAND Corporation [20].

Professional organizations also use quality measures in quality improvement and practice accreditation programs. In response to the need of its physician members to fulfill the Part IV: Practice Improvement component of the American Board of Radiology's (ABR) Maintenance of Certification (MOC) program, ASTRO has created Performance Assessment for the Advancement of Radiation Oncology Treatment (PAAROT), a quality improvement program for individual radiation oncologists [21]. PAAROT assesses quality of care at the physician-level by requiring radiation oncologists to report data from 10 consecutive cases on mostly consensus-derived process measures via a secure website. Physicians are provided with feedback on their performance relative to other participants. To meet the MOC practice improvement requirement they must then identify one measure to improve upon, implement a change in their practice, and reassess their performance by reporting on another 10 cases after 3 months and whether the desired level of improvement was achieved. Structure and process quality measures also play a part in the ASTRO-American College of Radiology (ACR) Radiation Oncology Practice Accreditation (ROPA) Program [22]. Based on the ACR Technical Standards and Guidelines, and the ASTRO Guidelines and White Papers, structure and process measure data are collected as part of an online application and onsite visit involving the review of at least 10 cases and are used in determining whether to grant accreditation.

International quality measures in radiation oncology

Several countries around the world employ radiotherapy quality measures that exist in various stages of development. In England, the National Institute for Health and Clinical Excellence (NICE) uses an evidence-based approach to define which medical interventions offer the best quality and value for patient care [23]. NICE quality measures address three dimensions including clinical effectiveness, patient safety, and patient experience. Their guidelines are made available in formats appropriate both for health-care providers and for patients, with guidance offered for all of the most common cancer diagnoses.

In Canada, the Canadian Partnership for Quality Radiotherapy (CPQR) has published guidelines to optimize safe delivery of radiation therapy and to increase the ability to evaluate and report on quality care measures [24]. The CPQR involves collaboration between the Canadian Association of Radiation Oncologists, the Canadian Association of Medical Radiation Technologists, and the Canadian Organization of Medical Physicists to measure system performance and advance the implementation of evidence-based quality initiatives. Ongoing initiatives include development of a more sophisticated instrument to measure concordance with treatment guidelines and quality measures.

The Australian Council on Healthcare Standards (ACHS) was established in 1974 and provides measurement and implementation of quality improvement systems for more than 1400 Australian health-care organizations. The ACHS includes representatives from health-care, governmental, and consumer organizations. In 1996 the ACHS launched an Evaluation and Quality Improvement Program (EQuIP) to allow for systematic external peer review of the continuum of care. The most recent quality measures for radiotherapy are included in *The Australian Council on Healthcare Standards' Australasian Clinical Indicator Report: 2003–2010* [25]. Of note, while NICE has developed quality standards for end-of-life care, none of these international quality measures programs currently include measures focused on palliative radiation therapy.

Conclusion

Having reviewed the characteristics of quality measures and their current uses, we would like to conclude with our thoughts on how their use will drive future quality improvement in radiation oncology in the United States and internationally. Currently, data on variation and gaps in care in radiation oncology are limited and when available are neither comprehensive, representative, nor timely. Hopefully, the on-going development of large-scale longitudinal registries such as the National Radiation Oncology Registry (NROR) will identify where quality improvement is needed. Some of these care gaps will be specific to the United States while others might be worldwide. With this knowledge, guidelines can then be developed that address these gaps in care and their recommendations can be used to develop the next generation of quality measures, thereby reducing reliance on measures based on informal expert consensus. In fact, recently palliative radiotherapy guidelines for the treatment of bone metastases, brain metastases, and the use of thoracic radiation have been developed by ASTRO through international collaboration [13,26,27] and one of the recommendations from the bone metastases guideline has been developed into the palliative quality measure as described previously. However, to assess quality of care more comprehensively, a much larger measure set will need to be developed in the future that includes common cancers, common indications for treatment, such as palliation, existing and emerging technologies, and relevant care settings. There is also interest in developing more cross-cutting measures and measures related to the recently announced three aims of the National Quality Strategy: "Better Care," "Healthy People and Communities," and "Affordable Care" [28]. Because of the weak relationship between most structural measures and outcomes and the challenges associated with outcomes measures described above (e.g. confounding factors, delay between treatment and outcome, difficulty of risk-adjustment, small sample size), most quality measures will likely be process measures, although for palliative measures some of these issues are less problematic. As more measures become available it is also likely that the focus will shift from quality measurement to quality improvement, leading to increased development of quality improvement tools. With better measures and tools, physician- and practice-level quality improvement programs will hopefully lead to greater gains in quality. However, it is also inevitable that performance data will be publicly reported and doing so will likely lead to additional efforts to improve quality. Although it may take years for all of these components to fall into place, eventually we will have a system based on quality measures that supports continuous quality improvement for all cancer patients including those receiving palliative radiotherapy.

References

1. Lohr KN (ed.) *Medicare: A Strategy for Quality Assurance*. Washington, DC: National Academy Press, 1990.
2. Committee on Quality of Health Care in America, Institute of Medicine. *Crossing the Quality Chasm: A New Health System for the 21st Century*. Washington, DC: National Academy Press, 2001.
3. Agency for Healthcare Research and Quality. Your guide to choosing quality care. Available at: http://archive.ahrq.gov/consumer/qnt/qntqlook.htm (accessed April 27, 2012).
4. Fairchild A, Barnes E, Ghosh S, *et al.* International patterns of practice in palliative radiotherapy for painful bone metastases: evidence-based practice? *Int J Radiat Oncol Biol Phys* 2009; **75**: 1501–1510.
5. Hewitt M, Simone JV (eds) *Ensuring Quality Cancer Care*. Washington, DC: National Academy Press, 1999.
6. Donabedian A. The quality of care. How can it be assessed? *JAMA* 1988; **260**: 1743–1748.
7. National Quality Measures Clearinghouse. Oncology: percentage of visits for patients, regardless of age, with a diagnosis of cancer currently receiving chemotherapy or

radiation therapy in which pain intensity is quantified. Available at: http://www.qualitymeasures.ahrq.gov/content.aspx?id=27999 (accessed April 27, 2012).

8. National Quality Measures Clearinghouse. Oncology: percentage of visits for patients, regardless of age, with a diagnosis of cancer currently receiving chemotherapy or radiation therapy who report having pain with a documented plan of care to address pain. Available at: http://www.qualitymeasures.ahrq.gov/content.aspx?id=28000 (accessed April 27, 2012).

9. American Society for Radiation Oncology. External beam radiotherapy for bone metastases. Available at: http://www.qualityforum.org/QPS/1822 (accessed November 25, 2012).

10. Donaldson MS (ed.) *Measuring Quality of Care: A Statement by the National Roundtable on Health Care Quality*. Washington, DC: National Academy Press, 1999.

11. Gripp S, Mjartan S, Boelke E, Willers R. Palliative radiotherapy tailored to life expectancy in end-stage cancer patients: reality or myth? *Cancer* 2010; **116**: 3251–3256.

12. Schachter HM, Mamaladze V, Lewin G, *et al*. *Measuring the Quality of Breast Cancer Care in Women*, Evidence report/technology assessment no. 105. Rockville, MD: Agency for Healthcare Research and Quality, 2004.

13. Lutz S, Berk L, Chang E, *et al*. Palliative radiotherapy for bone metastases: an ASTRO evidence-based guideline. *Int J Radiat Oncol Biol Phys* 2011; **79**: 965–976.

14. Hanks GE, Coia LR, Curry J. Patterns of care studies: past, present, and future. *Semin Radiat Oncol* 1997; **7**: 97–100.

15. Owen JB, Sedransk J, Pajak TF. National Averages for process and outcome in radiation oncology: methodology of the patterns of care study. *Semin Radiat Oncol* 1997; **7**: 101–107.

16. Coia LR, Hanks GE, Martz K, *et al*. Practice patterns of palliative care for the United States 1984–1985. *Int J Radiat Oncol Biol Phys* 1988; **14**: 1261–1269.

17. Crozier C, Erickson-Wittmann B, Movsas B, *et al*. Shifting the focus to practice quality improvement in radiation oncology. *J Healthc Qual* 2011; doi doi: 10.1111/j.1945-1474.2010.00119.x. [Epub ahead of print].

18. Quality Research in Radiation Oncology. Quality research in radiation oncology. Clinical performance measures. Available at: http://www.qrro.org/intro_to_QIs.html (accessed April 27, 2012).

19. Earle CC, Neville BA, Landrum MB, *et al*. Trends in the aggressiveness of cancer care near the end of life. *J Clin Oncol* 2004; **22**: 315–321.

20. National Quality Measures Clearinghouse. Cancer Quality-ASSIST Project Quality Indicators. Available at: http://www.qualitymeasures.ahrq.gov/browse/by-organization-indiv.aspx?orgid=2198 (accessed April 27, 2012).

21. American Society for Radiation Oncology. Performance Assessment for the Advancement of Radiation Oncology Treatment (PAAROT). Available at: https://www.astro.org/Educational-Resources/PAAROT/Index.aspx (accessed April 27, 2012).

22. American Society for Radiation Oncology. ACR-ASTRO Radiation Oncology Practice Accrediation Program. Available at: https://www.astro.org/Practice-Management/Practice-Accreditation/Index.aspx (accessed April 27, 2012).

23. National Institute for Health and Clinical Evidence: Who we are. Available at: http://www.nice.org.uk/aboutnice/whoweare/who_we_are.jsp (accessed July 24, 2012).

24. Canadian Partnership Against Cancer: Canadian Partnership for Quality Radiotherapy. Available at: http://www.partnershipagainstcancer.ca/priorities/quality-standards/strategic-initiatives/canadian-partnership-for-quality-radiotherapy/ (accessed July 24, 2012).

25. Australian Council on Healthcare Standards (ACHS). Australasian Clinical Indicator Report: 2003–2010: 12th Edition. Sydney NSW: ACHS,2011; 95–96.

26. Rodrigues G, Videtic GMM, Sur R, *et al*. Palliative thoracic radiotherapy in lung cancer: an American Society for Radiation Oncology evidence-based clinical practice guideline. *Pract Radiat Oncol* 2011; **1**: 60–71.

27. Tsao MN, Rades D, Wirth A, *et al*. Radiotherapeutic and surgical management for newly diagnosed brain metastasis(es): an American Society for Radiation Oncology evidence-based guideline. *Pract Radiat Oncol* 2012; **2**: 210–225. Available at: http://www.sciencedirect.com/science/article/pii/S1879850011003808 (accessed November 16, 2012).

28. Agency for Healthcare Research and Quality. About the National Quality Strategy. Available at: http://www.ahrq.gov/workingforquality/about.htm (accessed November 25, 2012).

CHAPTER 28

Use of technologically advanced radiation oncology techniques for palliative patients

Simon S. Lo[1], Bin S. Teh[2], Samuel T. Chao[3], Arjun Sahgal[4], Nina A. Mayr[5], and Eric L. Chang[6]

[1]University Hospitals Seidman Cancer Center, Case Comprehensive Cancer Center, Case Western Reserve University, Cleveland, OH, USA
[2]The Methodist Hospital, Cancer Center and Research Institute, Weill Cornell Medical College, Houston, TX, USA
[3]Cleveland Clinic Lerner College of Medicine, Cleveland, OH, USA
[4]Princess Margaret Hospital and the Sunnybrook Health Sciences Center, University of Toronto, Toronto, Ontario, Canada
[5]Arthur G. James Cancer Hospital, The Ohio State University, Columbus, OH, USA
[6]Keck School of Medicine at University of Southern California, Los Angeles, CA, USA

Introduction

There has been a rapid development in advanced technology for radiation therapy in the last 20 years. In the past, virtually all patients treated with palliative intent were treated with conventional radiation therapy techniques. With the availability of newer technologies, more patients are increasingly treated with palliative radiation therapy using advanced techniques because of the perceived advantage of better symptom control and normal tissue sparing. This chapter will provide an overview of clinical applications of technologically advanced radiation therapy in the palliative setting.

Overview of technologically advanced radiotherapy techniques

With the emergence of advanced technologies, there are several commercially available treatment devices that can be used for technologically advanced radiation therapy [1–3]. One common feature of these devices is the capability

Radiation Oncology in Palliative Cancer Care, First Edition. Edited by Stephen Lutz, Edward Chow, and Peter Hoskin.
© 2013 John Wiley & Sons, Ltd. Published 2013 by John Wiley & Sons, Ltd.

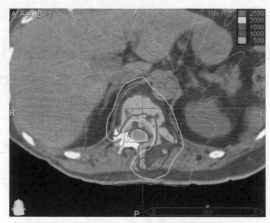

Figure 28.1 Stereotactic body radiotherapy for re-irradiation of breast cancer spinal metastasis at T12 which had prior external beam radiotherapy to 37.5 Gy in 15 fractions; a dose of 25 Gy in 5 fractions was prescribed to 78%, while limiting the spinal cord maximum point dose to 10 Gy in 5 fractions; the beams were manipulated by the computer such that the radiation dose was steered away from the spinal cord; the patient obtained prompt pain relief after the treatment (pain decreased from 6 to 1 on an 11-point scale) (see Plate 28.1).

to produce a highly conformal radiation isodose distribution, and therefore the collateral damage to normal tissue or organs-at-risk (OARs) can be minimized (Figure 28.1). The earliest prototype of highly conformal radiation therapy is Gamma Knife-based stereotactic radiosurgery (SRS), which involves the precise and focused delivery of a single, high dose of radiation to an intracranial target volume in a single session. The Gamma Knife device utilizes 192 cobalt-60 sources (previously 201) to deliver gamma rays converging at a target volume [2]. Subsequently, alternative devices such as adapted or specialized linear accelerators and proton-generating cyclotron or synchrotron machines have been used to deliver SRS with similar outcomes [3–7]. Using these alternative devices, stereotactic radiation delivery to intracranial targets can be fractionated by using relocatable immobilization devices such as a Gill-Thomas-Cosman head frame or aquaplast mask, therefore coming to be known as stereotactic radiation therapy (SRT) [8].

Building upon the experience of intracranial SRS, investigators from Karolinska Institute of Stockholm, Sweden and the National Defense Medical College of Japan developed methods to account for respiratory motion and provide robust immobilization. They pioneered the extension of stereotactic radiation delivery for use in extracranial tumors, leading to an approach named stereotactic body radiation therapy (SBRT) or more recently, stereotactic ablative radiation therapy (SABR) [1,9]. SBRT has been used to treat various primary and metastatic tumors for curative and palliative intent [1]. There are several linear accelerator systems on the market, such as the Novalis system, TomoTherapy system, CyberKnife system, Varian TrueBeam, and Elekta

Synergy-S and Axesse, which are equipped to deliver SBRT [1]. The common feature of these machines is the image guidance capability. The CyberKnife system consists of a lightweight linear accelerator mounted on a robotic arm, and the treatment planning system is different from those of other linear accelerator systems [6]. Regardless of the system used, the key to delivery of high quality treatment is the seamless collaboration of treatment team and rigorous quality assurance process.

Other advanced radiation therapy techniques include intensity modulated radiation therapy (IMRT), image-guided radiation therapy (IGRT), and proton beam therapy [3,10,11]. IMRT involves an inverse planning process with dose constraints set for each OAR, and it can be delivered using most modern machines. IGRT refers to conventionally fractionated radiation therapy delivered with the use of image guidance prior to each treatment. Most machines that are equipped to deliver SBRT can also deliver IGRT [10]. IGRT is used to treat primary cancer with curative intent in most circumstances. Proton beam therapy has traditionally been used to treat skull base tumors, such as chordoma and chondosarcoma, pediatric tumors, and ocular tumors, but its use has recently been extended to prostate cancer [3].

Clinical applications reported in the literature

Most of the data from literature on the use of advanced radiation therapy techniques for palliation of symptoms pertain to IMRT, SRS, SRT, and SBRT for brain, spinal, and bone metastases [12–15]. SBRT for liver and lung oligometastases is usually given with a curative intent and is therefore beyond the context of this chapter.

Brain metastasis

Brain metastasis is a common occurrence in patients with solid tumors. The most common primary tumors that metastasize to brain are lung cancer, breast cancer, melanoma, renal cell carcinoma, and colorectal cancer. Although the main aim of treatment is palliation, survival is frequently prolonged in patients with good performance status. Advanced radiation therapy techniques have been used in patients with brain metastases in an aim to escalate the radiation dose to the metastatic lesions or to spare normal brain parenchyma or other OARs.

Stereotactic radiosurgery

In the past two decades, SRS has been used extensively to treat brain metastasis. There have been prospective trials, including phase III randomized trials, investigating the role of SRS in the management of brain metastasis [16–19]. In a Radiation Therapy Oncology Group (RTOG) phase III randomized trial comparing whole brain radiation therapy (WBRT) alone and

WBRT combined with SRS for patients with one to three brain metastases, it was observed that addition of SRS had led to improvement of survival in patients with one brain metastasis and improvement of Karnofsky Performance Status (KPS) at 6 months' follow-up [16].

There have been three trials comparing SRS alone to SRS combined with WBRT for patients with one to three or four metastases (Table 28.1). Increased

Table 28.1 Summary of phase III trials of stereotactic radiosurgery for brain metastasis.

Study	Number of patients	Number of metastasis	Treatment arms	Outcomes
Radiation Therapy Oncology Group [16]	331	1–3	WBRT vs WBRT + SRS	WBRT vs WBRT + SRS
				Median OS: 5.7 vs 6.5 mos ($P = 0.14$); 4.9 vs 6.5 mos for 1 metastasis ($P = 0.04$)
				Overall time to intracranial tumor progression or neurologic death rates: No difference
				Stable or improved KPS at 6 months' follow-up: 27% vs 43% ($P = 0.03$)
Japanese Radiation Oncology Study Group [18]	132	1–4	SRS vs SRS + WBRT	SRS vs SRS + WBRT
				1 year OS: 28.4% vs 38.5% (P = NS)
				Median OS: 8 vs 7.5 mos (P = NS)
				1 year brain tumor recurrence rate: 76.4% vs 46.8% ($p < 0.001$)
				Death attributed to neurologic causes: 19.3% vs 22.8% (P = NS)
M.D. Anderson Cancer Center [17]	58	1–3	SRS vs SRS + WBRT	SRS vs SRS + WBRT
				Mean posterior probability of decline in learning and memory function: 24% vs 52%
European Organisation for Research and Treatment of Cancer [19]	359	1–3	Surgery or SRS vs Surgery or SRS combined with WBRT	Intracranial progression caused death in 44% of patients in the surgery or SRS arm and in 28% of patients in the WBRT arm.
				WBRT did not improve duration of functional independence or OS

WBRT, whole brain radiation therapy; SRS, stereotactic radiosurgery; OS, overall survival; KPS, Karnofsky performance status; mos, months; NS, not significant risk of intracranial recurrence was observed with the omission of WBRT in all three trials, but there was no negative impact on survival [17–19]. In the phase III trial from M.D. Anderson Cancer Center, omission of WBRT resulted in better preservation of neurocognitive function despite higher incidence of intracranial failure [17]. Recently, the American Society for Radiation Oncology (ASTRO) has published guidelines on the use of SRS for newly diagnosed brain metastasis, and SRS alone is regarded as one of the primary treatment options for patients with up to four lesions [20].

SRS has also been used in a recurrent and progressive setting with good local control based on radiographic response [21]. However, there is insufficient evidence as to the clinical benefit and risks of its use in the setting of recurrence when compared to other competing management options.

Scalp-sparing whole brain radiation therapy

Alopecia is one of the most noticeable side effects of whole brain radiation therapy, causing significant psychologic distress in some patients. With the use of IMRT it is possible to reduce the radiation dose given to the superficial scalp, therefore decreasing the extent of alopecia. Data from the literature on the use of this strategy are, however, very limited [22,23]. In one study from the University of Wisconsin, 10 patients treated with scalp-sparing whole brain IMRT had subjectively less alopecia than historical norms, thereby raising the possibility that this type of approach might positively influence quality of life in this patient group [23].

Hippocampus-sparing whole brain radiation therapy

Radiation-induced damage of the hippocampi has been implicated in neuro-cognitive decline after WBRT. It has been speculated that the hippocampus is a source of stem cells responsible for neuro-regeneration. Significant short-term memory impairment was observed in rodents even after exposure of the hippocampi to a low dose of radiation ($\leq 2\,Gy$). Investigators from University of Wisconsin and Rush University have observed that the prevalence of brain metastases within 5mm of the hippocampus is very low, and they have determined that it is safe to spare the hippocampi using TomoTherapy- or linear accelerator-based whole brain IMRT [24–27]. A phase II RTOG trial was written and has been accruing patients to measure the value of hippocampus-sparing whole brain IMRT for brain metastasis (www.rtog.org).

Stereotactic radiation therapy

For patients not eligible for SRS due to size (>4 cm) or location (close to the optic apparatus), SRT has been used as the primary or post-operative in patients who have 1–3 brain metastases. However, the data in the literature regarding this approach are limited. Overall, the results are thought to be similar to those achieved with SRS [28,29].

Spinal metastasis

SBRT has been used in an attempt to deliver highly focal radiation doses to spinal metastatic lesions, aiming to improve tumor control and hence pain relief. There have been abundant data from prospective trials and retrospective studies in the literature on the use of SBRT for spinal metastasis in various settings [1,13–15]. Pertaining to pain control, the most relevant scenarios are primary treatment for spinal metastasis and re-irradiation of recurrent spinal metastasis.

One of the largest studies included 393 patients with 500 spinal metastases treated with single fraction SBRT treated at University of Pittsburgh Medical Center. In that patient group, long-term pain improvement based on a 10-point visual analog scale was achieved in 290 out of 336 evaluable cases [30]. In a study from University of California San Francisco, 38 patients with 60 spinal metastases were treated with CyberKnife-based SBRT using 1–5 fractions, and 31 of 46 painful sites achieved pain improvement [31].

In a phase I/II trial from M.D. Anderson Cancer Center, 149 patients with 166 uncomplicated spinal metastases were treated with SBRT to either 30 Gy in 5 fractions or 27 Gy in 3 fractions. Patients' symptoms were measured with both the Brief Pain Inventory (BPI) and the M.D. Anderson Symptom Inventory (MDASI) before treatment and at several time points up to 6 months after treatment. Frequency and duration of complete pain relief were the primary endpoints of this study. At a median follow-up time of 15.9 months, the number of patients reporting no pain from bone metastases, based on BPI, increased from 26% to 54% 6 months after SBRT [32]. BPI-based pain reduction from baseline to 4 weeks after SBRT was clinically meaningful. Opioid use was reduced from 28.9% to 20% during the first 6 months after SBRT. Patients also reported significant pain reduction according to the MDASI during the first 6 months after SBRT as well as significant reductions in a composite score of the six MDASI symptom interference with daily life items [32]. In another phase I/ II trial of single fraction SBRT for previously unirradiated spinal metastasis, 61 patients with 63 non-cervical spinal or paraspinal metastases were treated to a dose of 16–24 Gy in one fraction. More patients were pain free at 3 and 6 months than at baseline, and the pain levels were lower at 3 and 6 months compared with those at baseline. It was also observed that pain level correlated with local control [33]. Table 28.2 summarizes selected studies of SBRT for spinal metastasis with symptomatic endpoints.

Spinal cord compression

The standard treatment for spinal cord compression, except for radiosensitive tumors such as plasma cell tumors, lymphoma, small cell carcinoma, and

Table 28.2 Selected studies of stereotactic body radiation therapy for spinal metastases or spinal cord compression with symptomatic endpoints.

Series/type	No. of patients/ Tumors/ No. of tumors with prior EBRT	Patient type	Dose (Gy)	Follow-up	Pain control or improvement of neurologic symptoms	Radiation myelopathy
Gerszten [30]/ Retrospective	393/ 500/ 344	Mixed	20 in 1 fxn (range, 12.5–25)	21 months	86%	0
Gibbs [47]/ Retrospective	74/ 102/ 50	Mixed	14–25 in 1–5 fxn	9 months	84% of symptomatic patients	3
Sheehan [48]/ Retrospective	40/ 110/ 0	Mixed	17.3 in 1 fxn (range, 10–24)	12.7 months	85%	0
Wang [32]/ Phase I and II trial	149/166/ 79	Mixed	30 in 5 fxn of 27 in 3 fxn	15.9 months	No pain based on BPI: 26% increased to 54% at 6 months Opioid use: 28.9% decreased to 20.0% at 6 months	0
Amdur [49]/ Phase I and II trial	21/ 25/ 12	Mixed	15 in 1 fxn	N/A	43%	0

(Continued)

Table 28.2 (*Continued*)

Series/type	No. of patients/ Tumors/ No. of tumors with prior EBRT	Patient type	Dose (Gy)	Follow-up	Pain control or improvement of neurologic symptoms	Radiation myelopathy
Garg [33]/ Phase I and II trial	60/ 61/ 0	Mixed	16–24 Gy in 1 fxn	20 months (mean)	18 vs 13 patients pain free at 3 and 6 months vs baseline Reduced pain levels (based on BPI) at 3 and 6 months vs baseline	0
Mahadevan [50]/ Retrospective	60/ 81/ 81	Previously irradiated	24 in 3 fxn or 25–30 in 5 fxn (if tumor touched cord)	12 months	65%	4 patients developed neurologic deficits from tumor progression
Jin [35]/ Retrospective	24/ 31/ 0 (myeloma)	Spinal cord compression	16 in 1 fxn (range, 10–18)	11.2 months	71% with neurologic deficits improved	0
Ryu [36]/ Retrospective	62/ 85/ 0	Spinal cord compression	16 in 1 fxn (range, 12–20)	11.5 months	81% with neurologic deficits improved	0

EBRT, external beam radiation therapy; fxn, fraction/s; BPI, Brief Pain Inventory germ cell tumors, is surgical decompression followed by post-operative external beam radiation therapy in patients with good KPS. This approach has been proven to be superior to external beam radiation therapy alone in a randomized phase III trial [34].

Investigators from Henry Ford Hospital from Detroit, Michigan, have pioneered the use of SBRT for radiosurgical decompression of epidural spinal cord compression. In the first study, 24 patients with 31 myeloma lesions presenting with epidural spinal cord compression were treated with single fraction SBRT to a dose of 10–18 Gy with 5 of the 7 patients with baseline neurologic deficits achieving improvement or normalization of function after treatment [35]. No radiation-induced myelopathy was observed. In another study from the same group, 62 patients with 85 lesions causing metastatic epidural compression from non-radiosensitive tumors were treated with single fraction SBRT to a dose of 12–20 Gy, and neurologic improvement was observed in 81% of patients [36]. Similar to the previous study, no radiation myelopathy was observed. Table 28.2 summarizes the details of these studies.

Bone metastasis

The standard treatment for uncomplicated bone metastasis is external beam radiation therapy. Based on evidence from multiple randomized phase III trials, as documented in the ASTRO bone metastasis guideline, a single fraction of 8 Gy is preferred. In most circumstances, with the exception of spinal locations, OARs are typically remote from the treatment field. As a result, highly conformal techniques are not typically used. Occasionally, bone metastases from radioresistant histologies such as renal cell carcinoma and melanoma are treated with ablative radiation dose regimens using highly conformal techniques, in an aim to improve local tumor and pain control (Figure 28.2). However, data on the use of highly conformal radiation therapy for non-spinal bone metastasis are very limited in the literature. Recently, the group from The Methodist Hospital reported the treatment outcomes of 18 patients with 24 painful bone metastases treated with SBRT to a dose of 24–40 Gy in 3–5 fractions. A dose response was observed for pain control, and a dose of 40 Gy in 5 fractions was associated with a shorter time to achieve pain relief. There were no grade 2 or higher toxicities [37].

Adrenal metastasis

Most adrenal metastases are asymptomatic lesions that are discovered on diagnostic imaging studies during the staging work-up of the primary cancer. Some patients may have visceral or somatic type pain due to enlarging adrenal lesions, and palliative radiation therapy may be given for symptomatic control [38]. SBRT has been used to treat adrenal metastasis either as a local therapy for oligometastatic disease or for rapid symptomatic control. In most studies, most or all of the patients with baseline pain achieved pain relief. In the

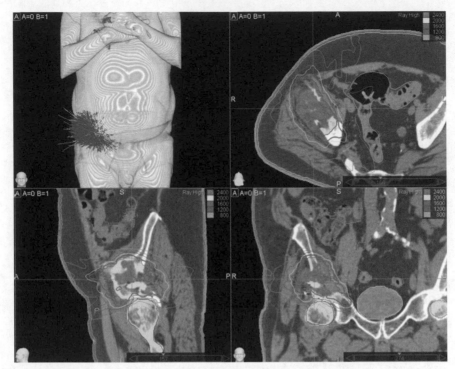

Figure 28.2 CyberKnife-based stereotactic body radiotherapy for the treatment of a single large painful right iliac bone metastasis from renal cell carcinoma; a dose of 24 Gy in 3 fractions was prescribed to 70%; OARs included the right femoral head and the small bowels (see Plate 28.2).

studies from University of Rochester and The Ohio State University, all the patients with baseline pain achieved pain control [38,39].

Toxicities associated with palliative radiotherapy using advanced technologies

The risk of complications associated with conventional radiation therapy is usually very low since most patients receive a relatively low dose of radiation and they may not survive long enough to develop complications. With the use of advanced technology, the radiation dose is typically escalated and hypofractionated regimens are frequently used. As a result, complications not observed in conventional palliative radiation therapy sometimes occur when advanced radiation therapy techniques are used.

Although SRS for brain metastases has resulted in an improved local tumor control and overall survival in some patients, complications such as radiation-induced seizures and necrosis have been observed [40,41]. When SBRT is delivered for spinal metastasis, complications such as radiation myelopathy

(RM), vertebral compression fracture (VCF), and pain flare have been observed [15,42–44]. RM is a catastrophic complication related to the maximum point dose delivered to the spinal cord [42–44]. In SBRT, a focal high dose of radiation is given to the whole or part of the vertebra and a very steep dose gradient is typically generated between the treated target volume and the spinal cord. As a result, even the slightest set-up and intrafractional variation may result in overdosing of the spinal cord. The risk of VCF is higher with SBRT compared to conventional external beam radiation therapy, and it is related to radiographic appearance and location of the vertebra [44,45]. Recent data from the University of Toronto have also shown that radiation dose per fraction is a predicting factor for VCF as well [46]. Pain flare is also a phenomenon observed rarely in conventional external beam radiation therapy but not uncommonly in SBRT [15].

Conclusion

With the availability of advanced technology, radiation oncologists are now able to deliver a higher dose of radiation to a target volume while still sparing normal tissues or OARs. Among all those treatments, SRS has been investigated in randomized phase III trials, and there is level I evidence to support its use in patients with 1–3 or 1–4 brain metastases alone or as a boost [16–19]. Other advanced radiation therapy technologies have shown promises in terms of symptomatic control in other settings, such as SBRT for painful spinal metastasis [15]. However, there are limited data comparing SBRT with standard external beam radiation therapy in a randomized fashion. For some oncologic emergency situations such as spinal cord compression, the use of highly advanced techniques such as SBRT may not be the most appropriate treatment outside of a clinical trial setting since additional time is needed for treatment preparation and neurologic symptoms may progress during that interval.

At this time, for most clinical situations, more data are needed to better define the role of those advanced radiation therapy techniques in the palliative setting. The RTOG has completed a phase II trial of single fraction SBRT for spinal metastasis and is enrolling patients for the phase III portion to compare single dose SBRT and single 8 Gy dose of external beam radiation therapy (www.rtog.org). The results of these and other trials will certainly better define the niches most appropriate for the use of these exciting technologies.

References

1. Lo SS, Fakiris AJ, Chang EL, et al. Stereotactic body radiation therapy: a novel treatment modality. Nat Rev Clin Oncol 2010; 7: 44–54.
2. Lindquist C, Paddick I. The Leksell Gamma Knife Perfexion and comparisons with its predecessors. Neurosurgery 2007; 61(3 Suppl): 130–140; discussion 140–141.

3. Allen AM, Pawlicki T, Dong L, *et al*. An evidence based review of proton beam therapy: the report of ASTRO's emerging technology committee. *Radiother Oncol* 2012; **103**: 8–11.

4. Das IJ, Downes MB, Corn BW, *et al*. Characteristics of a dedicated linear accelerator-based stereotactic radiosurgery-radiotherapy unit. *Radiother Oncol* 1996; **38**: 61–68.

5. Special report: stereotactic radiosurgery for intracranial lesions by gamma beam, linear accelerator, and proton beam methods. *Tecnologica MAP Suppl* 1999; **Jan**: 26–27.

6. Bucholz RD, Laycock KA, Cuff LE. CyberKnife stereotactic radiosurgery for intracranial neoplasms, with a focus on malignant tumors. *Technol Cancer Res Treat* 2010; **9**: 541–550.

7. Gibbs IC. Frameless image-guided intracranial and extracranial radiosurgery using the Cyberknife robotic system. *Cancer Radiother* 2006; **10**: 283–287.

8. Das S, Isiah R, Rajesh B, *et al*. Accuracy of relocation, evaluation of geometric uncertainties and clinical target volume (CTV) to planning target volume (PTV) margin in fractionated stereotactic radiotherapy for intracranial tumors using relocatable Gill-Thomas-Cosman (GTC) frame. *J Appl Clin Med Phys* 2011; **12**: 3260.

9. Lo SS, Fakiris AJ, Papiez L, *et al*. Stereotactic body radiation therapy for early-stage non-small-cell lung cancer. *Expert Rev Anticancer Ther* 2008; **8**: 87–98.

10. Jaffray D, Kupelian P, Djemil T, *et al*. Review of image-guided radiation therapy. *Expert Rev Anticancer Ther* 2007; **7**: 89–103.

11. Nutting C, Dearnaley DP, Webb S. Intensity modulated radiation therapy: a clinical review. *Br J Radiol* 2000; **73**: 459–469.

12. Lo SS, Chang EL, Suh JH. Stereotactic radiosurgery with and without whole-brain radiotherapy for newly diagnosed brain metastases. *Expert Rev Neurother* 2005; **5**: 487–495.

13. Lo SS, Chang EL, Yamada Y, *et al*. Stereotactic radiosurgery and radiation therapy for spinal tumors. *Expert Rev Neurother* 2007; **7**: 85–93.

14. Lo SS, Sahgal A, Wang JZ, *et al*. Stereotactic body radiation therapy for spinal metastases. *Discov Med* 2010; **9**: 289–296.

15. Sahgal A, Larson DA, Chang EL. Stereotactic body radiosurgery for spinal metastases: a critical review. *Int J Radiat Oncol Biol Phys* 2008; **71**: 652–665.

16. Andrews DW, Scott CB, Sperduto PW, *et al*. Whole brain radiation therapy with or without stereotactic radiosurgery boost for patients with one to three brain metastases: phase III results of the RTOG 9508 randomised trial. *Lancet* 2004; **363**: 1665–1672.

17. Chang EL, Wefel JS, Hess KR, *et al*. Neurocognition in patients with brain metastases treated with radiosurgery or radiosurgery plus whole-brain irradiation: a randomised controlled trial. *Lancet Oncol* 2009; **10**: 1037–1044.

18. Aoyama H, Shirato H, Tago M, *et al*. Stereotactic radiosurgery plus whole-brain radiation therapy vs stereotactic radiosurgery alone for treatment of brain metastases: a randomized controlled trial. *JAMA* 2006; **295**: 2483–2491.

19. Kocher M, Soffietti R, Abacioglu U, *et al*. Adjuvant whole-brain radiotherapy versus observation after radiosurgery or surgical resection of one to three cerebral metastases: results of the EORTC 22952-26001 study. *J Clin Oncol* 2011; **29**: 134–141.

20. Tsao MN, Rades D, Wirth A, *et al*. Radiotherapeutic and surgical management for newly diagnosed brain metastasis(es): an American Society for Radiation Oncology evidence-based guideline. *Pract Radiat Oncol* 2012; **2**: 210–225.

21. Mehta MP, Tsao MN, Whelan TJ, *et al*. The American Society for Therapeutic Radiology and Oncology (ASTRO) evidence-based review of the role of radiosurgery for brain metastases. *Int J Radiat Oncol Biol Phys* 2005; **63**: 37–46.

22. Roberge D, Parker W, Niazi TM, Olivares M. Treating the contents and not the container: dosimetric study of hair-sparing whole brain intensity modulated radiation therapy. *Technol Cancer Res Treat* 2005; **4**: 567–570.

23. Welsh JS, Mehta MP, Mackie TR, *et al*. Helical tomotherapy as a means of delivering scalp-sparing whole brain radiation therapy. *Technol Cancer Res Treat* 2005; **4**: 661–662.

24. Marsh JC, Gielda BT, Herskovic AM, *et al*. Sparing of the hippocampus and limbic circuit during whole brain radiation therapy: a dosimetric study using helical tomotherapy. *J Med Imaging Radiat Oncol* 2010; **54**: 375–382.

25. Marsh JC, Godbole RH, Herskovic AM, *et al*. Sparing of the neural stem cell compartment during whole-brain radiation therapy: a dosimetric study using helical tomotherapy. *Int J Radiat Oncol Biol Phys* 2010; **78**: 946–954.

26. Gondi V, Tolakanahalli R, Mehta MP, *et al*. Hippocampal-sparing whole-brain radiotherapy: a "how-to" technique using helical tomotherapy and linear accelerator-based intensity-modulated radiotherapy. *Int J Radiat Oncol Biol Phys* 2010; **78**: 1244–1252.

27. Gondi V, Tome WA, Marsh J, *et al*. Estimated risk of perihippocampal disease progression after hippocampal avoidance during whole-brain radiotherapy: safety profile for RTOG 0933. *Radiother Oncol* 2010; **95**: 327–331.

28. Aoki M, Abe Y, Hatayama Y, *et al*. Clinical outcome of hypofractionated conventional conformation radiotherapy for patients with single and no more than three metastatic brain tumors, with noninvasive fixation of the skull without whole brain irradiation. *Int J Radiat Oncol Biol Phys* 2006; **64**: 414–418.

29. Aoyama H, Shirato H, Onimaru R, *et al*. Hypofractionated stereotactic radiotherapy alone without whole-brain irradiation for patients with solitary and oligo brain metastasis using noninvasive fixation of the skull. *Int J Radiat Oncol Biol Phys* 2003; **56**: 793–800.

30. Gerszten PC, Burton SA, Ozhasoglu C, *et al*. Radiosurgery for spinal metastases: clinical experience in 500 cases from a single institution. *Spine* 2007; **32**: 193–199.

31. Sahgal A, Chou D, Ames C, *et al*. Image-guided robotic stereotactic body radiotherapy for benign spinal tumors: theUniversity of California San Francisco preliminary experience. *Technol Cancer Res Treat* 2007; **6**: 595–604.

32. Wang XS, Rhines LD, Shiu AS, *et al*. Stereotactic body radiation therapy for management of spinal metastases in patients without spinal cord compression: a phase 1-2 trial. *Lancet Oncol* 2012; **13**: 395–402.

33. Garg AK, Shiu AS, Yang J, *et al*. Phase 1/2 trial of single-session stereotactic body radiotherapy for previously unirradiated spinal metastases. *Cancer* 2012; **118**: 5069–5077.

34. Patchell RA, Tibbs PA, Regine WF, *et al*. Direct decompressive surgical resection in the treatment of spinal cord compression caused by metastatic cancer: a randomised trial. *Lancet* 2005; **366**: 643–648.

35. Jin R, Rock J, Jin JY, *et al*. Single fraction spine radiosurgery for myeloma epidural spinal cord compression. *J Exp Ther Oncol* 2009; **8**: 35–41.

36. Ryu S, Rock J, Jain R, *et al*. Radiosurgical decompression of metastatic epidural compression. *Cancer* 2010; **116**: 2250–2257.

37. Jhaveri PM, Teh BS, Paulino AC, *et al*. A dose-response relationship for time to bone pain resolution after stereotactic body radiotherapy (SBRT) for renal cell carcinoma (RCC) bony metastases. *Acta Oncol* 2012; **51**: 584–588.

38. Chawla S, Chen Y, Katz AW, *et al*. Stereotactic body radiotherapy for treatment of adrenal metastases. *Int J Radiat Oncol Biol Phys* 2009; **75**: 71–75.

39. Guiou M, Mayr NA, Kim EY, *et al*. Stereotactic body radiotherapy for adrenal metastases from lung cancer. *J Radiat Oncol* 2012; **1**: 155–163.

40. Liu Y, Xiao S, Liu M, *et al.* Analysis of related factors in complications of stereotactic radiosurgery in intracranial tumors. *Stereotact Funct Neurosurg* 2000; **75**: 129–132.

41. McKenzie MR, Souhami L, Caron JL, *et al.* Early and late complications following dynamic stereotactic radiosurgery and fractionated stereotactic radiotherapy. *Can J Neurol Sci* 1993; **20**: 279–285.

42. Sahgal A, Ma L, Gibbs I, *et al.* Spinal cord tolerance for stereotactic body radiotherapy. *Int J Radiat Oncol Biol Phys* 2010; **77**: 548–553.

43. Sahgal A, Ma L, Weinberg V, *et al.* Reirradiation human spinal cord tolerance for stereotactic body radiotherapy. *Int J Radiat Oncol Biol Phys* 2012; **82**: 107–116.

44. Rose PS, Laufer I, Boland PJ, *et al.* Risk of fracture after single fraction image-guided intensity-modulated radiation therapy to spinal metastases. *J Clin Oncol* 2009; **27**: 5075–5079.

45. Boehling NS, Grosshans DR, Allen PK, *et al.* Vertebral compression fracture risk after stereotactic body radiotherapy for spinal metastases. *J Neurosurg Spine* 2012; **16**: 379–386.

46. Cunha MV, Al-Omair A, Atenafu EG, *et al.* Vertebral compression fracture (VCF) after spine stereotactic body radiation therapy (SBRT): analysis of predictive factors. *Int J Radiat Oncol Biol Phys* 2012; **84**(3): e343–9.

47. Gibbs IC, Kamnerdsupaphon P, Ryu MR, *et al.* Image-guided robotic radiosurgery for spinal metastases. *Radiother Oncol* 2007; **82**: 185–190.

48. Sheehan JP, Shaffrey CI, Schlesinger D, *et al.* Radiosurgery in the treatment of spinal metastases: tumor control, survival, and quality of life after helical tomotherapy. *Neurosurgery* 2009; **65**: 1052–1062; discussion 1061–1062.

49. Amdur RJ, Bennett J, Olivier K, *et al.* A prospective, phase II study demonstrating the potential value and limitation of radiosurgery for spine metastases. *Am J Clin Oncol* 2009; **32**: 515–520.

50. Mahadevan A, Floyd S, Wong E, *et al.* Stereotactic body radiotherapy reirradiation for recurrent epidural spinal metastases. *Int J Radiat Oncol Biol Phys* 2011; **81**: 1500–1505.

Index